Film and the Chinese Medical Humanities

"This collection of film studies brings together the creative work of China's most talented filmmakers as they reflect on contemporary social problems, work out in narratives and images an original analysis of what's wrong with us (as individuals, as a society, and in cultural settings), and as they propose paths to redemption."
                                — **Judith Farquhar**, Max Palevsky Professor Emerita,
                                Department of Anthropology, University of Chicago

Film and the Chinese Medical Humanities is the first book to reflect on the power of film in representing medical and health discourse in China in both the past and the present, as well as in shaping its future.

Drawing on both feature and documentary films from mainland China, the chapters each engage with the field of medicine through the visual arts. They cover themes such as the history of doctors and their concepts of disease and therapies, understanding the patient experience of illness and death, and establishing empathy and compassion in medical practice, as well as the HIV/AIDs epidemic during the 1980s and 1990s and changing attitudes towards disability. Inherently interdisciplinary in nature, the contributors therefore provide different perspectives from the fields of history, psychiatry, film studies, anthropology, linguistics, public health and occupational therapy as they relate to China and people who identify as Chinese. Their combined approaches are united by a passion for improving the cross-cultural understanding of the body and ultimately healthcare itself.

A key resource for educators in the Medical Humanities, this book will be useful to students and scholars of Chinese Studies and Film Studies as well as global health, medical anthropology and medical history.

Vivienne Lo is Senior Lecturer and the convenor of the UCL China Centre for Health and Humanity, UK. Vivienne's core research concerns the social and cultural origins of acupuncture, therapeutic exercise, and food and medicine.

Chris Berry is Professor of Film Studies at King's College London, UK. He researches Chinese-language cinemas and other Chinese-language screen-based media.

Guo Liping is Professor of English and Vice Dean in the School of Health Humanities, Peking University, China. Her research interests include narrative medicine and medical humanities education.

Routledge Advances in Asia-Pacific Studies

Film and the Chinese Medical Humanities

Edited by
Vivienne Lo, Chris Berry
and Guo Liping

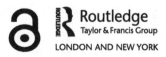
Routledge
Taylor & Francis Group
LONDON AND NEW YORK

First published 2020
by Routledge
2 Park Square, Milton Park, Abingdon, Oxon OX14 4RN

and by Routledge
52 Vanderbilt Avenue, New York, NY 10017

Routledge is an imprint of the Taylor & Francis Group, an informa business

First issued in paperback 2021

British Library Cataloguing-in-Publication Data
A catalogue record for this book is available from the British Library

Library of Congress Cataloging-in-Publication Data
Names: Lo, Vivienne, editor. | Berry, Chris, 1959 April 28– editor. | Guo, Liping, 1969– editor.
Title: Film and the Chinese medical humanities / edited by Vivienne Lo, Chris Berry and Guo Liping.
Identifiers: LCCN 2019028228 (print) | LCCN 2019028229 (ebook) | ISBN 9781138580299 (hardback) | ISBN 9780429507465 (ebook) | ISBN 9780429017407 (adobe pdf) | ISBN 9780429017384 (mobi) | ISBN 9780429017391 (epub)
Subjects: LCSH: Medicine in motion pictures. | Public health in motion pictures. | Public health—China.
Classification: LCC PN1995.9.M44 F55 2020 (print) | LCC PN1995.9.M44 (ebook) | DDC 791.43/653—dc23
LC record available at https://lccn.loc.gov/2019028228
LC ebook record available at https://lccn.loc.gov/2019028229

ISBN: 978-1-138-58029-9 (hbk)
ISBN: 978-1-03-208524-1 (pbk)
ISBN: 978-0-429-50746-5 (ebk)

Typeset in Times New Roman
by Apex CoVantage, LLC

Contents

**14 Food-related *Yangsheng* short videos among the retired
   population in Shanghai** 226
   XINYUAN WANG AND VIVIENNE LO

Figures

Contributors

Hongwei Bao is Associate Professor in Media Studies at the University of Nottingham, where he also codirects the Centre for Contemporary East Asian Cultural Studies. He holds a PhD in Gender and Cultural Studies from the University of Sydney. His research primarily focuses on queer theory and activism in China, with an emphasis on queer films and community media. His works have been published in *Cultural Studies, Culture Unbound, Global Media and China, Health, Culture and Society, Interventions, Queer Paradigms* and *The JOMEC Journal*. He is the author of *Queer Comrades: Gay Identity and Tongzhi Activism in Postsocialist China* (2018).

Chris Berry is Professor of Film Studies at King's College London. In the 1980s, he worked for China Film Import and Export Corporation in Beijing, and his academic research is grounded in work on Chinese cinema and other Chinese screen-based media, as well as neighbouring countries. He is especially interested in queer screen cultures in East Asia; mediatized public space in East Asian cities; and national and transnational screen cultures in East Asia. Together with John Erni, Peter Jackson, and Helen Leung, he edits the Queer Asia book series for Hong Kong University Press. Prior to his current appointment, he taught at La Trobe University in Melbourne, The University of California, Berkeley, and Goldsmiths, University of London.

Michael J. Clark is an Honorary Lecturer and Tutor for UCL's China Centre for Health and Humanity and the Centre for Multidisciplinary and Intercultural Inquiries, and he was formerly a Visiting Lecturer and Tutor at the Centre for the Humanities and Health, King's College London. He has published on the representation in film and television of various aspects of medicine and biology, especially pain, cloning, and genetics, on the role of 'wounded healer' figures in medical film and television dramas and the place of film studies in Chinese medical humanities as well as on aspects of the history of psychiatry. Together with Dr Catherine Crawford (University of Essex) he co-edited the collection *Legal Medicine in History* (1994).

Erminia Colucci is Senior Lecturer in the Department of Psychology at Middlesex University. She uses arts-based and visual methods, particularly photography and ethnographic film-documentary, in her research, teaching, and advocacy work in Cultural and Global mental health. Her key interests are human rights violations in mental health, suicide prevention, violence against women, and first-hand stories of people with lived experience of mental illness and suicide. She is also affiliated to the Global and Cultural Mental Health Unit, Centre for Mental Health, University of Melbourne.

Guo Liping has an MA in English and a PhD in the history of science and technology. She is currently Professor of English and Vice Dean at the School for Health Humanities, Peking University (formerly the Institute for Medical Humanities, PKU). Her research interests include narrative medicine and medical humanities education, as well as literature and medicine. Her passion is helping physicians use the tools of narrative medicine to enhance doctorpatient communication in China.

Marta Hanson is Associate Professor of the history of East Asian medicine in the Department of the History of Medicine, Johns Hopkins University (2004–present). Her book is titled *Speaking of Epidemics in Chinese Medicine: Disease and the Geographic Imagination in Late Imperial China* (London: Routledge, 2011). She was senior co-editor of *Asian Medicine: Tradition & Modernity* for five years (2011–2016). Her publications engage with a wide range of issues within the history of Chinese medicine, disease, and the body, cross-cultural medical history, and the history of public health in East Asia.

Therese Hesketh is Professor of Global Health at the Institute of Global Health, UCL. She is also Director of the Centre for Global Health and holds a Professorship at Zhejiang University. She has a background in pediatrics and public health and has worked in China for over 30 years as a clinician, a manager and a researcher. Her research is concerned with many aspects of population health and epidemiology in China with a focus on interventions.

Derek Hird is Senior Lecturer in Chinese Studies at Lancaster University and Deputy Director of the Confucius Institute there. His research interests include Chinese migrant men's experiences in London and Chinese white-collar masculinities. Recent publications include *Men and Masculinities in Contemporary China* (with Geng Song) (2014), 'Making class and gender: White-collar men in postsocialist China', in *Changing Chinese Masculinities: from Imperial Pillars of State to Global Real Men*, ed. Kam Louie, 137–56 (Hong Kong: 2016), and 'Moral Masculinities: Ethical Self-fashionings of Professional Chinese Men in London', *Nan Nü 18.1* (2016): 115–147.

Lili Lai is Associate Professor of Anthropology at the School of Health Humanities, Peking University. Lai's research interests focus on the body, everyday life, and medicine. Her book, *Hygiene, Sociality, and Culture in Contemporary China: The Uncanny New Village*, was published in 2016 by Amsterdam University Press. Her current research mainly concerns the modern production of traditional knowledge and the social historical conditions of public health in rural China.

Vivienne Lo is Senior Lecturer and Director of the China Centre for Health and Humanity at UCL. She is well published in the history of medicine in China with a particular interest in visual culture and the cross-cultural transmission of technical knowledge. She initiated the first-ever postgraduate module on Chinese Film and the Body, and the China and the Medical Humanities website YiMovi (www.yimovi.com).

Susan McDonough is an occupational therapist and education and service development consultant working to promote cultural safety, engage diverse communities and improve the cultural responsiveness of mental health providers and practitioners. She has taught anthropology and sociology and worked in community and correctional mental health settings as well as internationally in community-based rehabilitation. Her current postgraduate research at Latrobe University examines the way bilingual and bicultural practitioners contribute to the well-being of immigrant and refugee communities. Victorian Transcultural Mental Health, St Vincent's Hospital, Melbourne College of Science, Health and Engineering, La Trobe University, Melbourne.

Leon Antonio Rocha is Senior Lecturer in Chinese History and Society at the University of Lincoln. He is currently working on two book-length projects, *Harnessing Pleasure: Imagining Chinese Sexuality in the Twentieth Century* and *Needham Questions*. The former is a global history of the conceptualisations of 'Chinese sexuality' in medico-scientific and popular discourses in the twentieth century, while the latter considers the work of British Sinologist and biochemist Joseph Needham (1900–1995) and places the monumental *Science and Civilisation in China* project in historical and philosophical context.

Daniel Vuillermin is Lecturer at the School of Health Humanities at Peking University and a section editor of the *Palgrave Encyclopaedia of the Health Humanities*. Vuillermin is an editor of the *Chinese Medical Humanities Review* and formerly the biographical dictionary *Who's Who in Australia* (2008) and has published in journals including *a/b: Auto/Biography Studies*, *Life Writing*, and the *Journal for Modern Life Writing Studies*, among others. His current research focuses on narrative medicine and rare disease in China.

Nashuyuan Serenity Wang is a PhD candidate in History at UCL. Her research project concerns psycho-geography and the travels of the suffering female body in the twenty-first century-Chinese cinema of dislocation. She graduated from the University of Warwick (2017 BA: Film and Television Studies) and UCL (2018 MA: Film Studies). She is currently the judge and film reviewer for the Beloit International Film Festival and a journalist for *Chinese Weekly*.

Wang Xiaomin is a post-doctoral researcher in the School of Public Health at Zhejiang University. She received her doctorate from Zhejiang University and her main research interest is the prevention of anti-microbial resistance.

Xinyuan Wang is a post-doc researcher in Anthropology at UCL, where she received her PhD and MSc degrees. She was a researcher in the 'Why We Post – Global social media impact study'. Wang was co-author and translator of the Chinese version of *Digital Anthropology* (Horst and Miller eds, 2013). Her most recent books are *How the World Changed Social Media* (co-author, 2016) and *Social Media in Industrial China* (2016).

Zhou Xudong is Associate Professor in the School of Public Health at Zhejiang University. He studied for his doctorate at Zhejiang University and his main research interest is health systems and reform in the Chinese context.

Introduction

Vivienne Lo, Chris Berry and Guo Liping

Film and the Chinese Medical Humanities is the first book to reflect on the power that the moving image has to represent medical and health discourse in China in the past and present, and to shape its future. Its chapters all represent the Medical Humanities' long-term interest in engaging with the field of medicine through the visual arts. They include, but are not limited to, analyses of those Chinese films that speak to the traditional themes of the field: the history of doctors and their concepts of disease and therapies, understanding the patient experience of illness and death, and establishing empathy and compassion in medical practice, as well as medical ethics.

Medical Humanities is inherently interdisciplinary and commonly uses literature, theatre, and the visual arts in participatory ways to actively address these themes. The authors in this volume themselves variously represent a broad interdisciplinary mix of medical history, medicine and psychiatry, film studies and filmmakers, anthropology, linguistics, global health, public health, traditional medicines, and occupational therapy as they relate to China and people who identify as Chinese. Their combined approaches are united by a passion for improving the cross-cultural understanding of the body, its identities and practices, and improvement of healthcare.

In recent years the term Health Humanities has been used alongside or in place of Medical Humanities, since it embraces all the ways in which healthcare involves those other than professional medical communities, including the self in self-care regimen. The Chinese context has unique perspectives and contexts to offer in this respect. Both fields are, however, largely dominated by Eurocentric practices in teaching. While there have been many historical and anthropological studies of 'other' non-European peoples' medical and healing practices, both fields have been slow to embrace non-European approaches and have therefore been criticised for their fundamentally 'Western' agenda, and their reliance on the classical European and American canons of medicine, literature, and art to think with (Hooker and Noonan 2011).

There is no doubt that, as China moves rapidly into public-private partnerships in healthcare, after the American model, that many of the traditional approaches of Medical Humanities, as listed earlier, are essential for maintaining and developing a humane and effective medical system. Yet, there are other ways in which the use of Chinese films can help the reader understand the conditions of health and the body. Fundamental to a number of the chapters are observations about the body aesthetics of a uniquely Chinese humanistic discourse.

The compassionate Chinese society, according to contemporary national-ist debates, should be grounded in Confucian concepts (Feng 2018). These would include *ren* 仁, the quality that makes individuals and society 'human' or 'humane' (Graham 1989: 18–22). This Neo-Confucianism of the last decade has been placed at the centre of a post-socialist Chinese humanistic ethics, uncriti-cally ignoring the social and gender inequalities embedded in Confucian tradition and re-casting ancient Chinese philosophies for the twenty-first century (Dear 2012). Among Chinese filmmakers, especially the pioneers of documentary and docu-drama, there is critical work which challenges the state to live up to its Neo-Confucian claims and to make adequate provisions for the most vulnerable communities in society.

With the popular and pervasive rise of religion in late twentieth and twenty-first century China, particularly Buddhism and Daoism, there has also been a grass-roots revival of the plural ways in which people in China have understood and dealt with illness, spiritual and psychological crises, old age and death, people with differently-abled bodies and minds, of diverse sexuality and gender identi-ties. As will be evident from the following chapters, film and filmmakers inter-weave China's plural traditions as they reflect and constitute all these embodied states.

The study of medicine and the body in China through film can therefore offer new insights into the state of the nation through an intimate engagement with China's mainstream and popular health traditions. It also illustrates radically dif-ferent conceptions of state, community, and individual. We will see in these pages how the body as a site of personal cultivation, social conformity or political con-testation is all made visible in film.

The work here has grown out of a Wellcome Trust-sponsored collaboration between UCL, PKU, and King's College London. It has emerged in particular through our teaching of Medical and Health Humanities to Chinese students, which focuses on the use of film. In this context the volume is related to the development of YiMovi (www.yimovi.com), a website which draws attention to documentary and feature films of Medical Humanities interest. On YiMovi you will find further analysis by many of the authors in this volume and others together with relevant film clips, many of which were generously provided by the film directors themselves. We are particularly indebted to the contributions of key team members Patrizia Liberati and Michael J. Clark and those who have also contributed to editing the texts, Dolly Yang and Penelope Barrett. The develop-ment of the website, and of this volume, has brought up critical points of cultural difference and has highlighted the unique challenges that the Chinese-speaking worlds face.

In the 2013 edition of the online journal of the *Social and Behavioural Sci-ences*, John Harley Warner pointed out that Medical Humanities has inherited the 'discourse of deficiency' from History of Medicine (Warner 2013: 322). That is, both fields serve as a kind of guilty conscience for the sciences and for the medical profession, which are increasingly forgetting the human side of sickness and dying, yet neither has had much direct utility in transforming medical practice. Inspired by our collective decades worth of research and teaching of China's Medical Humanities and Film Studies we would argue for a more positive and inclusive vision of the value of this particular combination of disciplines and hope that both this volume and YiMovi make a small contribution to articulating effective new directions.

Medical humanities pedagogy

Medical Humanities in China was inspired by the Medical Humanities movement in the United States. Like their American counterparts, the humanities scholars in medical schools have been the champions of the field. The Chinese Medical Humanities began in the 1980s, developed in the 1990s and prospered after 2000. Peking University Health Science Center leads the development of Medical Humanities in China. It began to teach the history of medicine to medical students in 1946, medical psychology in 1979, bioethics in 1988, and health law in 1991. Later, medical anthropology, medical sociology, and literature and medicine were offered as elective courses. Medical educators all agree that the humanities play a very important role in the training of healthcare professionals (Zhang and Chen 2006: 31); the Medical Humanities are a 'boon companion or supportive friend' (Brody 2011: 6) to medical practice and biomedical science. On the one hand, there is an urgent need to enhance the 'Medical Humanities competence' (*yixue renwen suzhi* 医学人文素质) of medical students and healthcare professionals. On the other hand, the discipline-oriented didactics of these courses in large lecture halls has not lived up to the high expectations of it – such teaching seems to aim at producing 'lesser' historians of medicine, bioethicists, and health law experts among medical students rather than making them humane carers with the ability to reflect on their own practice and profession more broadly. Therefore, efforts to achieve the 'integration' of Medical Humanities are beginning to focus on themes such as birth, aging, and death, rather than on disciplines such as the history of medicine or bioethics.

It seems to be the consensus of Medical Humanities educators worldwide that 'medical students can be a tough audience for the Medical Humanities' since they have 'an uncanny ability to parse the curriculum and divine what parts of their coursework will be more or less . . . (useful in their) assessments, regardless of what their professors say' (Jones *et al.* 2015: 637). When looking 'west' for inspiration to improve the efficacy of Medical Humanities education, Chinese Medical Humanities educators find that various livelier alternative means have been employed to achieve this end through film, literature, music, visual arts, and theatre.

In China, medical colleges usually do not employ people trained in music, and the visual and performing arts – they tend to hire from the more 'academic' disciplines for Medical Humanities education. Furthermore, unlike in those countries where Medical Humanities as a field is more advanced, a mechanism of incorporating visual and performing artists into extramural Medical Humanities education is yet to be developed in China. Therefore, literature and film rather than the visual and performing arts are most often chosen as alternative means for Medical Humanities education, because 'films not only can be used to help healthcare providers develop skills in the human dimension of medical practice. They can also promote enthusiasm for learning, highlight themes, enhance discussion and reflection' (Colt *et al.* 2011: v).

In medical schools, there are two main approaches to education in the field. The utilitarian approach of teaching literature (and film studies) constitutes the 'ethical route' (Coles 1979) where literary works and films are presented as more fully developed ethical cases or examples for students. This approach is deeply rooted in the medical school psyche. The other approach is advocated by literary scholars and is called the 'aesthetic route' (Trautmann 1978) where readers read literature closely, trying to find out how analysis of the formal elements like visual structure, metaphor, and narrator help to create the theme. However, the two approaches are not necessarily exclusive. Cinemeducation helps the two merge. Colt, Quadrelli, and Friedman argue that, by using films to teach medical ethics, viewers can 'voice opinions, argue contradictory positions, display their emotions, and justify their perspectives based on external evidence, their personal experiences and what actually happens in the fictional narrative of the cinematographic experience' (2011: v).

However, true to the insights of Claire Hooker and Estelle Noonan, the bulk of films used in the Chinese Medical Humanities classrooms are 'Western' films (especially films in the English language), such as *Frankenstein* (1931), *Patch Adams* (1998), and *Wit* (2001) to name just a few. Medical educators in both China and abroad have started to ask whether there is a need to develop a specifically Chinese Medical Humanities, and whether the use of Chinese films will be more instrumental in improving empathy, enhancing compassion, sensitivity, and gaining surrogate experiences of patients' suffering (Clark 2016; Guo *et al.* 2016).

Humanities and film studies

The publication of the essays in this volume is evidence not only of increased awareness of different medical cultures, but also of the growing role of audio-visual cultures in the transmission of those cultures. In these circumstances, film studies can bring a range of valuable methodologies to Medical Humanities for the analysis of films, television programmes, video clips, GIFs, and all the other audio-visual forms proliferating across our screens today. These methodologies include the systematic analysis of how viewers combine narrative, camerawork, editing, lighting, sound, music, and all the other components of the cinema to produce meaning, or the semiotics of the cinema (Metz 1974). This approach to understanding meaning through systematic analysis provided the foundation for the initial mapping of cinematic genres, auteur styles, national cinemas, and so forth in the early days of the discipline of film studies.

Since then, work on 'body genres' such as horror or weepies (Williams 1991) has led to a new focus that combines analysis of meaning with analysis of affect. This approach has developed so that affect is understood to include both emotions and feelings and also pre-cognitive bodily apprehensions, such as a thriller making you jump even before your mind can process what is happening. It has grown to encompass all the ways in which the cinematic text is haptic (Marks 2000), or felt in the body. All of this is also useful for analysing newer communication technologies, such as the addictive qualities of the touch screen (Alter 2017).

For Medical Humanities, these approaches not only enable an understanding of cinema that goes beyond meaning. They also open up to possibilities for a better understanding of how audio-visual media can engage not only medical practitioners as part of their education, but also patients. This engagement includes not only communicating health messages, as in Hesketh's essay here on campaigns to promote awareness of antibiotic resistance. It also includes the potential therapeutic effects of engagement with the audio-visual, as in the production of video self-narratives in Colucci and McDonough's chapter on mental health and minority communities in Melbourne, Australia. For film studies, as it moves to an expanded understanding of the cinematic as extending across all manner of platforms from the movie theatre out to the mobile phone, Medical Humanities offers a new partner for research into the cinematic, not only as reflecting or representing what is going on in the world but also as shaping the world.

Introducing the chapters

The book is divided into four sections: 'Cross-cultural histories of the body and its care'; 'Film and the public sphere'; 'Improving the education and training of health professionals'; and 'Transforming self-health care in the digital age'.

The essays in Part 1, 'Cross-cultural histories of the body and its care', mobilise film as a vernacular discourse that can generate alternative medical histories and unsettle received wisdom about health and care. Chapter 1, Vivienne Lo's 'Dead or alive? martial arts and the forensic gaze' examines the depiction of early twentieth-century-detective work in Peter Chan's film *Wuxia* as staging just such a tension. On the one hand, there are modern understandings of the body as an object with an anatomy, newly introduced in the era when the film is set. On the other, there is the Buddhist and martial arts approach to the body as an ever-changing living product of its relationships with other beings and the world around it. The other chapters come closer to the present. Chapter 2, Leon Antonio Rocha's 'How to be a good Maoist doctor: *An Ode to the Silver Needle under a Shadowless Lamp* (1974)' examines this lesser known Cultural Revolution-era film by the great director Sang Hu. It demonstrates how the film's argument in favour of the Red masses versus expert doctors because the masses dare to develop acupuncture anaesthesia is also an empowerment of vernacular knowledge. Chapter 3, Michael J. Clark's 'Self-care, *Yangsheng*, and mutual aid in Zhang Yang's *Shower* (1999)' shows how the film stages a contrast between vernacular and long-established understandings of well-being and self-care in the bath-house culture of old Beijing and the notions of progress driving the demolition of the bath-house in which the film is set. Derek Hird's Chapter 4, 'Sentiments like water: unsettling pathologies of homosexual and sadomasochistic desire' examines the struggle between a policeman and the gay man he arrests in another 1990s film, Zhang Yuan's *East Palace, West Palace*. It argues that the film narrates this contest as undermining both the modern era and highly conservative ideas about homosexuality and masculinity by invoking older Chinese ideas about multiple and alternative masculinities that continue to circulate through, for example, opera culture.

Part 2, 'Film and the public sphere', focuses on films that attempt to change public thinking about health. Chapter 5, 'The fever with no name: genre-bending responses to the HIV-tainted blood scandal in 1990s China' looks at *Love for Life*, the film adaptation of Yan Lianke's novel, *Dream of Ding Village*, about the HIV-AIDS crisis produced by hygiene failures in blood-buying campaigns. Marta Hanson considers these works as cultural responses that go beyond a purely medical analysis of the problem to point to failures of power and larger patterns of culpability. Lili Lai's Chapter 6, '*Fortune Teller*: the visible and the invisible' analyses Xu Tong's remarkable documentary as an effort to make the lives of disabled people and their everyday struggles in China more visible. Chapter 7, '*Longing for the Rain*: journeys into the dislocated female body of urban China', by Vivienne Lo and Nashuyuan Serenity Wang, incorporating the responses of students, is also concerned with an attempt to make the invisibility of middle-class mental health issues visible. The chapter considers Yang Lina's feature film about the descent into psychosis of a Beijing housewife and her efforts to find a cure, from visiting a shaman to communal chanting at a Buddhist monastery. The article sees the film not only as a portrait of self-care and mental health in contemporary Beijing, but also as a study in female collective solidarity and support.

Part 3 turns to what film can contribute to a long-held mission of the 'Medical humanities: improving the education and training of health care professionals'. Chapter 8, 'The gigantic black citadel: *Design of Death* and medical humanities pedagogy in China' by Guo Liping, analyses classroom experience. It explores how a film can open up self-reflexive discussion about taboo topics like unreasonable prolongation of life and abuse of power in the healthcare field. Chris Berry's Chapter 9, '*Blind Massage*: sense and sensuality' considers how a film about blind *tuina* masseurs communicates what it believes is the experience of blindness, providing an educational opportunity for inducing empathy. However, Berry argues that the film achieves empathy less by visual techniques that mimic blindness and sight loss than by highlighting the sense of touch that the cinema audience lacks as surely as the blind lack sight. In Chapter 10, 'Cinemeducation and disability: an undergraduate special study module for medical students in China', Daniel Vuillermin analyses student responses to films about disability to see how their understandings of and empathy towards disabled people changed as a result of the module. A particular emphasis is placed on different responses to Western and Chinese films and their usefulness in the Chinese context.

The final section of the book is Part 4, 'Transforming self-health care in the digital age'. All the essays in this part are crucially shaped in one way or another by the opportunities that digital media provide. Chapter 11 is Therese Hesketh's 'Raising awareness about anti-microbial resistance: a nationwide video and arts competition for Chinese university students using social media'. As well as online voting for works that try to communicate the dangers of overprescribing antibiotics, the project examined in the chapter used the web to disseminate the successful entries from the competition. In Chapter 12, 'Queer Comrades: digital video documentary and LGBTQ health activism in China', Hongwei Bao focuses on a health activist website that functions as a platform for short web documentaries aimed at the LGBTQ communities. He argues that as well as communicating practical messages about self-care, the documentaries on the site demonstrate how good health is also dependent on changing social and political perception. Chapter 13 is 'Recovering from mental illness and suicidal behaviour in a culturally diverse context: the use of digital storytelling in cross-cultural medical humanities and mental health' by Erminia Colluci and Susan McDonough. It reports on an Australian mental health project to reach ethnic communities, including the Chinese, by working with patients to produce digital videos about their experiences. Originally intended to reach out to the wider community, this process of video-making also had unexpected therapeutic benefits. Finally, Wang Xinyuan and Vivienne Lo in 'Food-related *Yangsheng* short videos among the retired population in Shanghai' look at the enthusiastic viewing and sharing of short online videos about healthcare by the elderly in Shanghai, using their smartphones. Drawing on Traditional Chinese Medicine, they eagerly disseminate recipes for seasonally appropriate food and other recommendations. Contemporary technology has integrated ancient knowledge into the everyday, using the lively, engaging, and concise qualities of audio-visual media.

Bibliography

Alter, A. (2017) *Irresistible: The Rise of Addictive Technology and the Business of Keeping Us Hooked*, Harmondsworth: Penguin.

Brody, H. (2011) Defining the Medical Humanities, *Journal of Medical Humanities*, 32: 1–7.

Clark, M.J. (2016) With China in Mind: Reflections on Film, Medicine, the Body and Teaching Chinese Medical Humanities, in C. Vullermin and L.P. Guo (eds.) *Chinese Medical Humanities Review*, Beijing: Peking University Medical Press, pp. 9–28.

Coles, R. (1979) Medical Ethics and Living a Life, *The New England Journal of Medicine*, 301 (8): 444–6.

Colt, H., Quadrelli, S. and Friedman, L.D. (2011) *The Picture of Health: Medical Ethics and the Movies*, New York: Oxford University Press.

Dear, D. (2012) Chinese Yangsheng: Self-help and Self-image, *Asian Medicine: Tradition and Modernity*, 7 (1): 1–33.

Feng, E. (2018) China Nationalism Unleashes Boom in Confucian Schooling, *Financial Times*, 4 December 2018, www.ft.com/content/a5bd3212-d75a-11e8-a854-33d6f82e62f8, accessed 9 April 2019.

Graham, G. (1989) *Disputers of the Dao: Philosophical Argument in Ancient China*, La Salle, IL: Open Court.

Guo, L., Wei, J., Li, Y. and Li, H. (2016) Medical Humanities and Empathy: An Experimental Study, in C. Vuillermin and L.P. Guo (eds.) *Chinese Medical Humanities Review*, Beijing: Peking University Medical Press, pp. 29–35.

Hooker, C. and Noonan, E. (2011) Medical Humanities as Expressive of Western Culture, *Medical Humanities*, 37: 79–84.

Jones, D., Greene, J., Duffin, J. and Warner, J.H. (2015) Making the Case for the History of Medicine in Medical Education, *Journal of the History of Medicine and Allied Sciences*, 70 (4): 623–52.

Marks, L. (2000) *The Skin of the Film: Intercultural Film, Embodiment, and the Senses*, Durham: Duke University Press.

Metz, C. (1974) *Film Language: A Semiotics of the Cinema*, trans. M. Taylor, New York: Oxford University Press.

Tong, K. (2017) Confucianism, Compassion (Ren) and Higher Education: A Perspective from the Analects of Confucius, in P. Gibbs (ed.) *The Pedagogy of Compassion at the Heart of Higher Education*, Netherlands: Springer, pp. 113–26.

Trautmann, J. (1978) The Wonders of Literature in Medical Education, in D. Self (ed.) *The Role of the Humanities in Medical Education*, Norfolk, VA: East Virginia Medical School, pp. 32–44.

Warner, J.H. (2013) The Humanizing Power of Medical History: Responses to Biomedicine in the 20th-Century United States, *Procedia Social and Behavioral Sciences*, 77: 322–9.

Williams, L. (1991) Film Bodies: Gender, Genre, and Excess, *Film Quarterly*, 44 (4): 2–13.

Zhang, D. and Chen, Q. (eds.) (2006) *Zhongguo yixue renwen jiaoyu: lishi, xianzhuang yu qianjing* (Medical Humanities Education in China: Past, Present and Future) 中国医学人文教育：历史、现状与前景, Beijing: Peking University Medical Press.

Part 1

Cross-cultural histories of the body and its care

1 Dead or alive?

Martial arts and the forensic gaze

Vivienne Lo

The contemporary worldwide addiction to the forensic-medical gaze, the power to see both the patterns of brutality inscribed on a body and the moral truths about *whodunit*, how and why they did it, and sometimes with whom, took a fascinating turn in Peter Chan's (Chen Kexin 陳可辛) Chinese martial arts film *Dragon* (2011), hereafter referred to by its Chinese title *Wuxia* 武俠, 'Martial Chivalry'. In a brilliant twenty-first century appropriation of both ancient Chinese medical traditions and the much-loved forensic detective genre, *Wuxia* pushes the martial arts epic in a new direction with a minute visual analysis of the anatomy and physiology of the martial arts body. Throughout the film a series of slow-motion replays and fast-paced montages juxtapose martial arts action with stills that draw on images from China's medical past, and footage generated by modern medical imaging technologies. With this collage of perspectives, Chan participates in a twenty-first-century zeitgeist which disrupts the binary conventions that pit West against East; modernity against tradition; reductionism against holism; science against religion; objective anatomy against the subjective subtle body; and mind against body. In today's world, the global balance of power is changing and new forms of cross-cultural scientific knowledge and natural philosophy are required to keep up.

The critical value of this film for the Medical Humanities lies in the way it both reflects and delivers these larger cultural 'truths' about the nature of science and medicine for a general audience. Recent transcultural histories of anatomy and forensic science also undermine the pervasive politics of conventional medical histories. It is no longer tenable to situate the rise of anatomical science entirely in a modern Europe with all its attendant assumptions about Western progress and processions of great white men of superior learning and insight. As Peter Chan's film delivers its cinematic riposte to an unreconstructed Western narrative of scientific modernity, and instead outlines for us a unified and transcendent body of Chinese cultural genius, we are drawn in to a multi-faceted and compelling political vision, at once transnational in its production and intended audiences, and national in its powerful representation of an ethnically diverse one-China (Berry and Farquhar 2006: 195).

Chan's film draws on elements of both of the two main sub-genres of the martial arts film genre, the fast-action choreographed bare-fist fight of the *kungfu* film, and the romance, chivalry, and running-up-walls, flying-through-the-air fantasy tales of martial errantry characteristic of the genre from which the film takes its Chinese name, *wuxia*. While the film draws on the aesthetics of both these cinematic traditions, the themes of honour and chivalry characteristic of the *wuxia* sub-genre are uniquely developed into an analysis of how martial arts moral philosophy is encoded in the living body itself (Teo 2009: 17–37).

The relationship that develops between the two main protagonists of this film, Xu Baijiu徐百九and Liu Jinxi 劉金喜 (formerly known as Tang Long), highlights a persistent modern Chinese dilemma about the nature of truth and individual responsibility, here revealed in anatomical expertise about living and dead bodies. On the one hand Xu Baijiu, the forensic detective, played by Taiwanese-Japanese superstar Takeshi Kaneshiro金城武, subtly references the largely unacknowledged Japanese contribution to Chinese modernity, and particularly medicine, during the early twentieth century (Elman 2005: 396–8; Andrews 2014: 69–88). In his dogged determination to get to the bottom of the crimes Xu suspects Liu Jinxi (Donnie Yen) to have committed in an earlier phase of his life and under a different identity, we find in Xu's character the Chinese awakening to theories and practices of universal law, modern science and rationality, and concomitant notions of citizenship. For Xu, evidence is dispassionate and objective and there is only one, scientific version of the truth: 'only physiology and the law don't lie' (c.f. Elman 2005: 372–432).

On the other hand, we have Donnie Yen (Yan Zidan 甄子丹), famous for his portrayal of *Ip Man* (*Ye Men* 葉問 2008; sequels 2010, 2016), the gentle-mannered, educated originator of Wing Chun style *kungfu*. Xu Baijiu's forensic examination of Liu Jinxi's living body exalts and almost eroticises the martial arts body, its combination of suppleness and muscularity, calm acuity of the senses and glowing skin, but also clandestinely celebrates the way in which it embraces the lawless honour and justice code of the *jianghu* 江湖 (literally, 'rivers and lakes'), a Chinese equivalent of the Wild West (Teo 2009: 18–19). Liu Jinxi represents a traditional Buddhist understanding of the martial arts. For him, individual actions have multiple external causes (Wright 1959: 108–27). Personal redemption lies in transcending the karma of one's birth, in this case as heir to the chief of an exceptionally violent Xixia 西夏 (Tangut) clan known as the 72 Demons. But ultimately this can only be achieved through tremendous personal sacrifice in order to counter 'the fabric of existence [which] is controlled by a myriad of karmic threads, [in which] everything is connected, no one truly has free will, we are all accomplices'. In juxtaposing these various natural-philosophical and religious perspectives visually, as contrasting body cultures, the film challenges the singular Western anatomical 'gaze' and its claim to universal truth with a fascinating and uniquely Chinese relativism.

Two nationalistic impulses are held in dynamic tension throughout the film. The first is the drive to regenerate China as a modern, scientific nation that gained pace among nineteenth- and early twentieth-century Chinese reformers and revolutionaries, for whom the image and objective investigation of the anatomical and forensic body were emblematic, just as they were in Europe and North America at the time (Asen 2009; Elman 2005: 388–96, 400–3). The second is the persistent claim of Chinese particularity regarding the superhuman potential of the living body, epitomized by a subjective, traditional understanding of the body in movement: a kind of cultural genius that is embodied in the spectacular visual culture of martial arts performances and Chinese opera alike.

Wuxia offers a further opportunity to interrogate a new style of patriotic masculinity as expressed through the martial arts body. In the 1980s the iconic martial arts hero Bruce Lee embodied the transnational tensions of his time, 'Lee as Hong Kong; Lee as cultural and/or diasporic China; Lee as Third World anti-imperialist; Lee as Asian American Champion' (Berry and Farquhar 2006: 197–204). Thirty years on, China is in a much stronger and less equivocal position. After the economic miracle, the 1997 return of Hong Kong, and the inexorable growth of China's power and international standing, *Wuxia* looks back to China's earlier internal struggles and extols the power and beneficence of political unity for a multi-ethnic state. This political message is intertwined with notions of Chinese cultural superiority and is conveyed in the narrative of Liu Jinxi's renunciation of his minority roots. Redeeming himself from a violent past among the Xixia people, he rejects the lawless autonomy of the nomads. Separatism, we are given to understand, is best transcended through peaceful elective membership of the majority by enlightened individuals (Berry and Farquhar 2006: 197–204).

Xixia was a medieval term for the kingdom or empire of the Buddhist Tangut people, who are not now included among China's officially recognised ethnic minorities. The negative representation of this pre-modern group in the film does not, therefore, run the risk of offending any living community, but obliquely illustrates contemporary China's ideal relationship with its 55 recognised ethnic minorities (the concept of the Han Chinese as a 56th category, self-identifying as a majority ethnicity). The historic Buddhism of the Xixia people (Gaowa 2007) is in fact a vehicle for one of the film's dénouements, as the main character Liu Jinxi undergoes a radical lifestyle transformation in order to achieve a separation from his brutal father, foregoing a violent inheritance and professing a new, more enlightened form of Buddhism among the submissive 'ethnic minority' of the villagers (the men and boys of the village still wear their hair in the pigtails that signify submission to the old Manchu dynasty, and also by implication to the new Chinese Republic represented in the film by Xu Baijiu and his police superior, and, by inference for the viewer, to Communist China itself).

There is also broader cultural significance to be found in the film through the multiple transnational processes at work at all levels of production. Peter Chan Ho-sun is himself a truly transnational director: born in Hong Kong and raised in Bangkok, he studied cinema in the United States at the UCLA film school before returning to Asia in the early 1980s. He began work in the Hong Kong film industry as second assistant director to John Woo in *Heroes Shed No Tears* (*Yingxiong wulei* 英雄無淚, 1986), and as a location manager to Jackie Chan in *Project A II* (*A jihua xuji* A 計劃續集, 1987) and *Armour of God* (*Longxiong hudi* 龍兄虎弟, 1986), before moving on to producing and directing his own films in the late 1980s. Twenty movies later, he eventually joined Steven Spielberg at

Dreamworks. *Wuxia* marks the first film appearance in seventeen years of veteran *wuxia* film idol Jimmy Wang Yu (*One Armed Swordsman – Dubi dao* 獨臂刀, 1967, and *The Chinese Boxer* (*Longhu dou* 龍虎斗, 1970), who is widely regarded as the first authentic *kungfu* star. As we will see, in its final scenes, *Wuxia* pays direct homage to the *One Armed Swordsman*, whose loss of one arm has been linked not only to male castration anxieties and the homoerotic nature of the martial arts, but also to the theme of severing links with patriarchal obligation, a choice which is highlighted in the final scenes of this film (Zhang 2004: 178).

The interlinking transnationalities of the director and of the various genres of martial arts and forensic detective films that play out in *Wuxia* have produced a remarkable visual demonstration of cross-cultural body consciousness, which challenges many long-standing orientalist assumptions. The film calls into question Eurocentric biases about the history of the body and its care, and embodies a distinctively Chinese ethic of modernity and citizenship. For these reasons it is an excellent subject for the Medical and Health Humanities. It is important for its expression of Asian body and health-related beliefs and practices that have gone global in recent times. But it is even more significant in the context of this volume as a contemporary commentary on an old set of prejudices in the practice of medical history which for centuries have shaped perspectives on global power dynamics according to the now outdated binary opposition of East and West (Figure 1.1).

Set six years after the Xinhai revolution (1911), when imperial China has already come to a violent end, the action of the film takes place in the context of the troubled beginnings of the modern Chinese state. The authority of the new Republican government and the peace of communities in the hinterland of China are challenged by roaming bandits and local warlords on horseback. In a rural village in the far south-west of China (Yunnan), the plot of *Wuxia* unfolds as we discover that Liu Jinxi, a seemingly meek and law-abiding paper-maker, is actually Tang Long 唐龍, a notorious killer and beloved son of a much-feared chief of a Xixia clan known as the *qisher disha* 七十二地煞 (72 Demons). In an attempt to cast off his violent

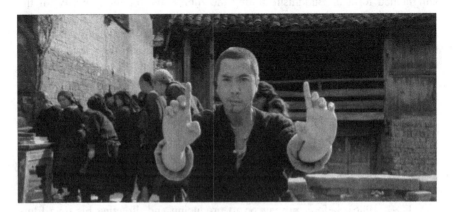

Figure 1.1 Donnie Yen as Liu Jinxi in *Wuxia* (2011)

and vengeful past, Tang has absconded from his clan and married a local woman, Yu 玉 (Tang Wei 湯唯), from the Yunnan village where the film is set. Settled there, he takes the village clan's surname. Yu has been deserted by the father of her oldest son, and Tang, now Liu Jinxi, a model villager, has integrated himself into the idyllic life of the village as the saviour of the spurned woman. Together, by the start of the film, they have given birth to another son. Life is beautiful: cows graze on the roofs of the wooden huts, and the day moves to the gentle rhythm of the paper presses; while the warm browns, reds, and rich greens of the countryside lull the viewer into a false sense of security. Yu is a modest and beautiful adornment to the narrative, a natural product of her native lands, but after a promising start she largely fades into the background and her character is never well developed. The couple seem to be open and gentle with each other, and there are unmistakable suggestions of a strong physical bond between them, but no romance or passion is allowed to distract from the strange relationship that develops between the two male leads, since in traditional male-dominated *wuxia* films celibacy and male camaraderie are the homosocial norms (Figures 1.2a and b).

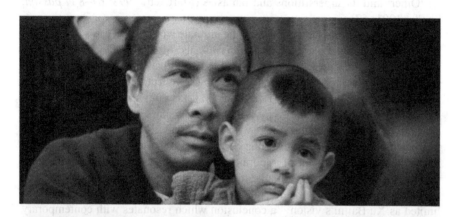

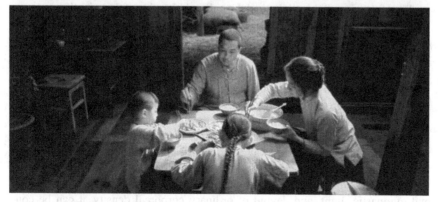

Figure 1.2 (a) and (b) Tang Long's new identity

On an otherwise normal day in this rural paradise, Liu gets into a fight with two notorious bandits and kills them both, in an apparently accidental sequence of events, while attempting to protect the elderly couple who run the village shop and inn. The rest of the film focuses on the investigation and eventual exposure of Liu Jinxi's false identity by Xu Baijiu, the detective, by means of an analysis of both the forensic evidence provided by the corpses of the villains themselves, and the unique qualities of the martial arts body. As Xu examines the battered cadavers of the bandits, peering through his 1920s-style spectacles and covering his nose delicately with a white handkerchief, all the political hierarchies embodied in the superior gaze of modern science and its claim to definitive knowledge are challenged by the camera as it follows the feeble, asthmatic, and neurotic figure of the detective. His furtive observation casts a veil of doubt, trespassing from all angles into the lives and bodies of Liu's family, disturbing and undermining the balance of the community, even intruding into their marital bed and day-to-day religious ceremonies. With this uncomfortable visual construction of the practices of science and modernity, the film begins to question the legitimacy of the concomitant eroticisation of a vanquished oriental 'Other' and its superstitions and fantasies (Marchetti 1993: 67–8 *et passim*; Shohat 1991: 57).

Xu Baijiu's nocturnal intrusions into the intimate workings of Liu's living body, his nausea-inducing examination of the criminals' lifeless bodies, the grotesque visions of decaying flesh crawling with flies, all impart a perverse eroticism to the processes involved in the discovery of objective truth and implicitly cast the viewer as voyeur. Xu's neurotic reflections on Liu's guilt are punctuated by brief but ghastly flashbacks of the Xixia clan's previous mass murders, disrupting the slow peaceful imagery of the village with fast intercut glimpses of bodies hung up like butchers' carcasses, and dangling corpses. With these nightmarish visions of Xu's single-minded pursuit of a morally superior universal justice, and his fixation with discovering an immutable truth, the film further suggests that the late nineteenth- and early twentieth-century cultures of science and empiricism are as limited as Xu Baijiu's vision – a conclusion which resonates with contemporary studies of the rise of objectivity and the cultural histories of the scientific communities of the mid-nineteenth century that created modern notions of truth (Daston and Galison 2007).

In contrast to the cadavers, the living and comparatively robust and healthy qualities of the superhuman martial arts body are revealed cumulatively as the story unfolds and as Xu Baijiu slowly gathers evidence to indict Liu. These unique qualities are particularly vividly displayed in a replay of the initial fight scene where, in a fiction within the fiction, the figure of the bespectacled detective himself is introduced into the frames in order to direct the viewer's gaze to the minutiae of the action. In this way Xu deconstructs the double homicide scene, proving that Liu was not an innocent victim of the thugs, but a highly skilled fighter, and that his body is a well-trained and disciplined killing machine. Supple and gymnastic, light, and devoid of ordinary corporeal density, it can be controlled at will through *qinggong* 輕功 (body lightening *kungfu*).

As Liu's true identity is revealed, he suddenly undergoes a cinematographic metamorphosis. Gone is the modest village papermaker, whose self-effacing loyalty to the village community and his family has previously been built up first in long shots of the luscious landscape; then in medium shots from the side, as he engages with his family, from above, as he cowers beneath the shop counter agonising about whether to reveal his secret martial strength; and finally, pinned down beneath the villain's body, apparently the victim of a vicious attack. Instead, for the first time, he stares directly into the camera, striking a powerful and alert 'horse stance', arms and hands squarely ready for combat, his eyes ablaze and intent upon his opponents. With that iconic Donnie Yen image, and others which follow later depicting his father's and the Xixia clan's physical prowess, Xu demonstrates a unique and persistent Chinese belief that the true martial artist:

- has extraordinary control of the breath: he 'breathes once every ten counts to collect *qi* at the core';
- 'can control the flow of his *qi* and his mental state';
- is protected by a field of power and 'radiates *qi* that repels even flies';
- has enhanced body *qi*, which promotes superhuman healing of wounds;
- has a body hardened like diamond that blades bounce off, as in the Vajrapāni (*Jingang shen* 金剛神) martial traditions (Shahar 2012).

More than anything else, the martial artist has a sophisticated knowledge of the anatomy of death. By juxtaposing modern hi-tech and classical Chinese anatomical and physiological images, the film encourages the viewer to imagine that Chinese people have always visualised the internal bodily organs, the musculature, and the skeleton, as being in a natural relationship with the subtle body of *qi*, the non-material power behind life and generation. The opening titles are framed by images of the blood circulation seen from inside the body that were in fact unknown anywhere in the pre-modern world, with floating platelets and shots from inside the arteries and capillaries. Startling visions of the corporeal then punctuate the film throughout. From the introductory sequence, which involves a painful if comic scene of Liu's son having a tooth extracted by his older stepbrother, through much of the subsequent action, the loss of a tooth becomes a recurring motif. The location of one of the villain's displaced teeth, which has torpedoed into a medicinal wine jar, leaving a neat circular hole, demonstrates the speed and accuracy of Liu's blows (Figure 1.3).

Central to the visual narrative are modern interpretations and maps of Chinese subtle and corporeal anatomy represented in black outline on sepia background, which rather unsubtly reference pre-modern medical manuscripts. They interrupt the flow of the story as the detective relates how the main protagonist has killed the thugs in the village shop professionally and made it look accidental to those standing by: Liu Jinxi, he demonstrates, has superior knowledge of the circulation of *qi*, the acupuncture point system, and the death points of the martial

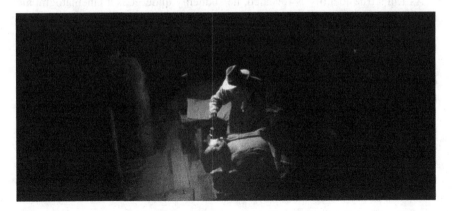

Figure 1.3 Xu Baijiu examining the corpse of one of the villains

arts. Throughout, the language of twentieth-century anatomy is inserted into traditional explanations. Here are just a few of Xu Baijiu's explanations of what lies beneath the surface:

- The death of Villain 1: It is major trauma to the vagus nerve that actually caused his death; Liu Jinxi had punched the *Taiyang* 太陽 acupoint on the villain's temple.
- The death of Villain 2: Liu Jinxi delivered a blow to the *Yunmen* 雲門 point which 'caused a blood clot blocking the blood flow, resulting in congestion of the arteries and cardiac arrest'.
- The constitution of Villain 2: The propensity to cardiac arrest was caused by a level of gluttony that impaired his *qi*. This gluttony was the result of 'an overdeveloped *Renying* 人迎 point, because normally the *Renying* point controls hunger'.
- Antidote to poison: One must treat bodily and personality flaws together using acupuncture. In Xu Baijiu's case this meant treating his own inappropriate 'empathy' for a child who, it transpires, was a pathological serial poisoner, who had killed his own parents and poisoned Xu himself. Xu used the acupoint *Danzhong* 膻中, to 'cure' his own misplaced empathy and treated the poisoning itself with the acupoint *Tiantu* 天突.
- As the two protagonists ultimately join forces against the chief of the 72 Demons, Xu induces the apparent death of Liu Jinxi/Tang Long, and then brings him back to life before it is too late – unfortunately, in the middle of the wake, as his *jianghu* warrior brothers circle his not-quite-dead-corpse on horseback. In the process of Liu's living death, Xu describes the stages he passes through: the brink, degeneration, and the final death; all can be induced by acupuncture, and acupressure to the vagus nerve.

Xu's explanations are accompanied by images of the beating heart, nerves, blood splattering, and scans of the skeletal structure, interspersed with modern charts of acupuncture. The images disrupt the narrative with a sense of urgency, and contrast with the portrayal of the weak and troubled detective using images shot in darkness and from oblique downward angles that emphasise his psychologically traumatised condition. In contrast, Liu Jinxi's concealed mastery of the anatomy of death is subtle and subjective; his control of his own robust and living body is deployed only to protect the vulnerable villagers. The camera gazes upwards at him, as if at an invulnerable hero. Captivated by Donnie Yen's physical beauty and prowess, his ability to fly through the air, and pivot his body effortlessly against walls, the audience chooses to forget the violence of Liu Jinxi's past and believes in the possibility of redemption – not only the redemption of Liu's past, but also of a Chinese past full of superstition and magic as negatively perceived and portrayed by early twentieth-century reformers, a view further reinforced by the banning of martial arts films in China in 1931 and then again in the People's Republic for being 'superstitious' and 'feudal' (Berry and Farquhar 2006: 225).

Our self-divided heroes, it transpires, share a past full of guilt. Liu's violent past is matched by Xu Baijiu's obsession with rationality and the unwavering rule of law which stems from his mistaken trust for the poisoner-child and its consequences. We discover that in recompense for his youthful mistake, he accused his own father-in-law of selling fake drugs, a family betrayal which led to the old man's suicide. The subsequent estrangement from his wife is filmed in a dark, cold light, and when contrasted to the warmth and colour of the Liu family's rural life, it feels as bleak and joyless as the corpses of the dead villains themselves. In the course of the film, the corruption of local government and the dire consequences of Xu's obsession with bringing Liu to justice, which ultimately triggers the near destruction of the village by the Xixia clan, call seriously into question the idea of a fair, universal, and benevolent rule of law. But to understand how all these modern and ancient currents blend so easily together requires an introduction to the history and historiography of anatomy and forensic medicine in China, and also to the transnational history of the detective novel and film.

Chinese anatomy and surgery

Dissection and anatomy as medical practices have frequently been associated with the divergence of Greek and Asian medicine (Kuriyama 1999). A European visual style beginning with Renaissance illustrations of the internal organs and the skeletal body is commonly cited as marking the birth of modern medical science, and dissection and anatomy have become emblematic of a Western civilisation with unique claims to fostering modernity and progress (Kemp and Wallace 2001: 158). In contrast to the Western anatomical gaze, medical historians writing about China have tended to suggest that the supposed body view of Chinese tradition focuses on a physiology of yin and yang in dynamic transformation, unified by *qi*, a view that emphasises the subjective and imaginary realm where the human body is subordinate both to the state and to the larger forces of the cosmos.

This historical divergence, I will argue, has been seriously overstated in a misrepresentation of history which downplays the transnational development of anatomical ideas, and devalues the astro-medical tradition in both European and Arabic medicine (Goody 2006; Akasoy *et al.* (eds.) 2008). A new wave of scholarship has begun to challenge the orthodox view prevalent in both Euro-American *and* modern Chinese history of medicine that historically, the Chinese did not 'do anatomy' (Despeux 2005; Wang 2018; Hu 2018; Chen 2007; Wang and Fuentes 2018; Berlekamp *et al.* 2015; Li Jianmin, *forthcoming*). We can see in these studies an increasing amount of evidence that medicine in imperial China, like medicine in Greece and Rome, was concerned with the musculature and sinews, both healthy and diseased, damaged, and dead – and that skin-deep surgery and sometimes even deep surgical procedures are scattered throughout historical medical records (Harper 1998: 97–8).

Increasingly, the anatomised body and the truths it reveals are a research topic for contemporary historians of Chinese medicine. The earliest recorded dissections occurred as early as 16 CE, in the Han dynasty, when we have details of how the executed bodies of criminals were disembowelled and their organs weighed, measured, and reflected upon (Despeux 2005: 57; *Huangdi neijing Lingshu* 12). However, ancient Chinese physicians could no more carry out deep abdominal surgery based on this information than could physicians in ancient Greece and Rome. In 1041 CE, there was another famous dissection, this time of the abdomen of the executed rebel Ou Xifan 歐希範. Artists published drawings of his internal organs. A similar set of drawings called after their artist, Yanluozi 煙蘿子 (fl. 936–941 CE), are a direct source for two illustrations contained in Li Jiong's 李駉 commentary on *The Canon of Eighty-One Problems (Bashi yi nan jing 八十一難經)* of 1269 (Despeux 2005; Berlekamp *et al.* 2015; Lo and Barrett 2018) (Figure 1.4).

The Yanluozi images are explicitly concerned with the forms of the internal organs upon which adepts would meditate in inner alchemy in the pursuit of transcendence and enlightenment. In this illustrated medical genre, we can see how anatomical images sit side-by-side with descriptions of a body made up of many spirits and body gods from medieval Chinese medical and Daoist traditions. But by including the Yanluozi images in his sequence, Li Jiong also related them to the pulse and to *qi* circulation, and suggested the permeable boundaries between medicine and religion, the anatomical and the subtle body, in the tradition of inner alchemy. Most of the Yanluozi images were copied in a 1313 Persian study of Chinese Medicine called *The Treasure Book of the Ilkhans on the Branches of the Chinese Sciences (Tansūqnāma-i Īlkhān dar funūn-i ʿulūm-i Khatāʾī)*. Under the direction of the scholar-physician Rashīd al-Dīn (d. 1318), images of the internal organs were included, but without anything to identify their original connection to Daoist inner alchemy or cosmology (Berlekamp *et al.* 2015) (Figure 1.5).

Most likely, these images of the internal organs found a place in the *Tānsūqnāma* not because of what they signified about Chinese medicine or alchemy, but because

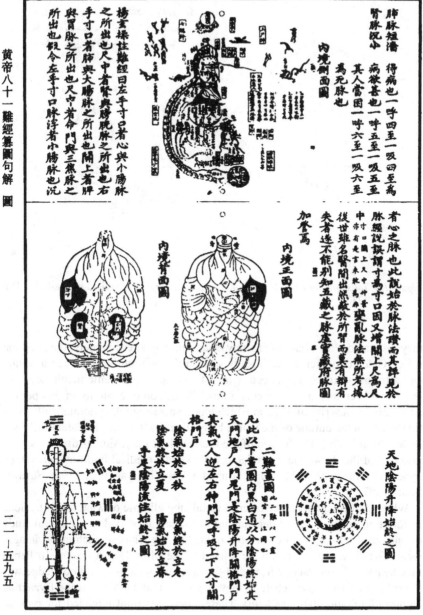

Figure 1.4 *The Canon of Eighty-One Problems* – originally edited by Li Jiong 1269

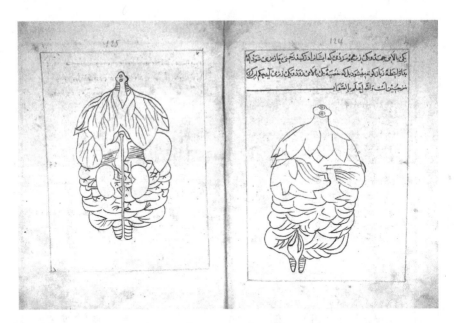

Figure 1.5 Tansūqnāma-i Īlkhān dar funūn-i 'ulūm-i Khatā'ī compiled by Rashid al Din
1313

they resonated with what Persian physicians already knew, namely, the attention
which Galenic medicine had already paid to the relationship between anatomy
and astrology-astronomy. Indeed, within the history of Galenic medicine, there
may have been a resurgent interest in the illustration of anatomy in this period,
as a Latin manuscript of 1292 in which blood vessels are diagrammatically positioned within the outline of the whole body suggests (Oxford, Bodleian MS Ashmole 399, fol. 19r.). By the end of the fourteenth century, similar diagrams were
also part of the Perso-Islamic trajectory of Galenic medical tradition, when they
appeared in the work of Mansur b. Ahmad b. Yusuf b. Ilyas (fl. c. 1390) (Savage-
Smith 1997).

   While the Persian evidence offers a tantalising glimpse of what might be done
in future to enhance our understanding of the late medieval transcultural study
of anatomy, it is far from clear how influential the Chinese anatomical images
were. The alchemical charts were printed in the Ming Daoist Canon. In Persia
they again took manuscript form and the accompanying textual knowledge was
the subject of academic debate by physicians from as far West as the Byzantine
empire (Terzioğlu 1974: 288–96). These works were not intended for popular
consumption, and to this day this transnational history of anatomy is not well
known. I do not, therefore, offer this abbreviated history of anatomy in China in
order to suggest that the writers and directors of *Wuxia* were consciously engaging
in propaganda about the priority of Chinese scientific knowledge. Rather, I hope

that it will help to redress the bias of influential histories of medicine in the last centuries and highlight the political issues at stake in the illustration of anatomy. However, in *Wuxia*, the representation of the anatomy of dead bodies emerges through different transnational processes that have shaped literary and film versions of the forensic detective story.

The forensic detective in Chinese literature and film

Historical evidence for a genre of forensic case histories demonstrates that a lively tradition of Chinese forensic medicine dates back over two thousand years to pre-imperial times. Two cases recorded in a manuscript from the Shuihudi 睡虎地 burial site (closed c. 217 BCE), the *Fengzhen shi* 封診式 (Models for Sealing and Physical Examinations), are of particular interest in this regard. Protocols labelled *xun yu* 訊獄 (interrogating in legal trials) and *zhi yu* 治獄 (the conduct of legal trials) in the text set out the requirements of officials in trying legal cases, and reflect the practical administration of one aspect of early Chinese law.

Among cases of livestock theft, robbery, and avoiding conscription, there are descriptions of the official inspection of injured and dead bodies, very similar to those depicted in *Wuxia*. Details of one 'death by injury' were recorded as being investigated by the *lingshi* 令史 (Magistrates' Clerk) and tell of the direction and manner in which the body of a man was lying, the tears in the victim's clothing, the blade wounds on the left temple and on his back, measurements of the wounds, and the nature of the blood seepage, as well as the approximate time of death and circumstances in the neighbourhood at the time of the death (Hulsewé 1985: 00):

> *Death by injury: Statement of a Criminal Investigation:*
>
> X's head had a blade wound in one place on the left temple and in two places on the back running lengthways/perpendicular, each (wound) measuring four *cun* 寸 (Chinese inches, an adaptable measurement geared to individual body sizes), in each case one *cun* wide like clefts made with an axe; the corners of the brain at the temple were both seeping blood, and the head, back and ground were all soiled and the size [of what?] cannot be determined. The remaining (body) was all intact.

Another record is of 'death by hanging', and describes the position of the hanged man and the thickness and placement of the rope in order to ascertain whether the hanging was the result of suicide or murder. Establishing motives for suicide was also an essential part of the investigation. It records:

> *Death by hanging: Statement of a criminal investigation:*
>
> A and B were ordered to take Bing's corpse to the court of (forensic) examination. On examination it was necessary to first look carefully at the marks and personally visit the place of death; to look immediately at the rope and

bindings, whether there were still marks where the ties were; to look at whether the tongue protruded or not, what was the drop from the head and feet to the ground; was there loss of urine?

(*Shuihudi Qinmu zhujian* 睡虎地秦墓漢簡 1990: 147–63)

In this case murder was suspected because the tongue did not protrude, the mouth and nose did not sigh, the marks from the rope did not bruise, and the rope was tight and could not be removed. This is the earliest extant record of forensic-medical investigation in China and perhaps anywhere in the world.

Better known than these ancient-world case histories, which have only been discovered in tombs in the twentieth century, are the many commented editions of Song Ci's 宋慈 (1186–1249) instructions to coroners, *Xiyuan jilu* 洗冤集錄 (A Collection of Records on the Washing Away of Wrongs) (McKnight 1982). Here is one of a set of images from the *Xiyuan jilu* as they were printed in the 1856 edition, *Xiyuan lu xiangyi* 洗冤錄詳義 (A Collection of Records on the Washing Away of Wrongs with Detailed Explanations), with a detailed commentary by Xu Lian 許槤 (1787–1862) (Figure 1.6).

These early studies reveal over a millennium of consistent activity in recording the observations of civil servants working with the judiciary in the investigation of dead bodies. They deal with a set of problems at the heart of forensic-medical examinations that differentiate the accidental from the deliberate or self-inflicted

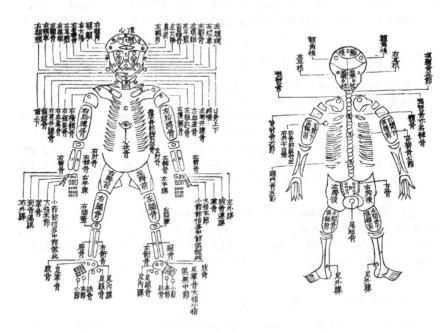

Figure 1.6 Xiyuan lu xiangyi, commentary by Xu Lian (1787–1862)

wound, suicide from murder, pre- from post-mortem wounds, and natural or accidental from unnatural death, exposing those like Liu Jinxi who try to make cul-
pable homicide appear accidental, and those who try to make suicide look like
murder in order to incriminate their enemies. These texts reveal a Chinese body
that is very far from the classical Chinese medical body essentialised by historians
and anthropologists, a physical body that even in death can tell revealing stories
about the true circumstances of life.

More germane to historical influences on the production of *Wuxia*, we can find
antecedents to the figure of Xu Baijiu and his gaze on the bandits' bodies in the
forensic detectives of popular literature. Charting the changing cultural manifes-
tations of the forensic detective story, which has taken one form or another in
China since the sixteenth century, would be a major undertaking, so I will just
sketch the bare bones of this transnational history as they relate to the themes of
this chapter.

The most popular of the characters we will meet is Di Renjie 狄仁杰, in English, Judge Dee, loosely based on a magistrate and official of the Tang court of
that name.

Di Renjie the historical figure (c. 630–c. 700) was born to a lineage of prefects
and rose to prominence in the Tang court under Emperor Gaozong 唐高宗. He
was much favoured by the extraordinary Wu Zetian 武則天, Gaozong's empress
and the only woman to have ruled in her own right as emperor, whom he served
as a close confidante and adviser. An influential military general (Fifth Commander against the Turks) and Secretary General to the Supreme Court, Di was
a member of the Imperial Censorate, with a well-known tendency to challenge
authority. There is, however, scant evidence that he ever carried out the kind of
forensic investigation that he was celebrated for in the eighteenth-century detective novel written in his name, *Di Gong'an* 狄公案 (Cases of Judge Dee). While
he is recorded as having remonstrated at court on behalf of people who had been
unfairly convicted, the only court case which he presided over for which we have
any precise details involved him bringing a ghost to trial and sentencing it to be
burnt (*Taiping guangji* 298/3; MacMullen 1993).

The more credible real-life detective hero who has captured the imaginations of
four centuries of Chinese readers is the Song dynasty Judge Bao 包公, Bao Zheng
包拯 (999–1062). Two examples of *gong'an* 公案 (crime case fiction) written in
the form of novels about him date from an earlier time than those attributed to Di
Renjie, having been published in the Ming dynasty (1368–1644):

- *Cases of A Hundred Families Judged by Dragon-Design Bao* (*Bao longtu
  baijia gong'an* 包龍圖百家公案) written by An Yushi (安遇时) in 1594.
- *Cases Judged by the Dragon-Design* (*Longtu gong'an* 龍圖公案), an anonymous account including several chapters from the previous book.

Both of these historical figures, Bao Zheng and Di Renjie, have been periodically
reinvented, in order to cater for a popular Chinese appetite for murder mysteries

laced with gruesome details. During the late nineteenth and twentieth centuries, this appetite has been further stimulated by diverse transnational influences such as the professionalisation of forensic medicine and science, Victorian gothic horror stories, and Hollywood's hugely successful *Crime Scene Investigation* series (2000–2015). Dr Edmond Locard (1877–1966), the 'Sherlock Holmes of France', set up the first police scientific laboratory for investigating crime and criminals in Lyon in 1910, and codified the principles of modern forensic-scientific practice in his *Traité de Criminalistique* (7 Vols., 1931–35). For Locard, modern forensic science was the silent witness which could be interrogated to reveal the truth about past crimes, based on his so-called 'Exchange Principle' that 'every contact leaves a trace' (Kirk 1953). These scientific developments did not go unnoticed in China, where interest in forensic science fitted neatly into the twentieth-century negotiation between traditional Chinese forensic methods, largely legal in context, and the emergence of new medico-legal and forensic-scientific specialisms in Europe and America (Freidson 1970; Svarverud 2011; Asen 2012).

In 1896, less than ten years after their first publication, Sir Arthur Conan Doyle's (1859–1930) first detective stories were translated into classical Chinese to great acclaim, followed in 1916 by *The Complete Stories of Sherlock Holmes* in 44 stories. The success of the translation was further assured by the favourable reaction of such giants of the Chinese literary world as Cheng Xiaoqing 程小青 (1893–1976), who went on to mimic Holmes and Watson's rational scepticism and penetration of the deeper truths of life in his own Shanghai-style short stories (Wong 2007).

In the same years that Sherlock Holmes was taking root in China, the popular depiction of the Chinese detective in American B movies was, at first sight, not so complimentary, particularly since both Bela Lugosi (*Count Dracula*, 1931) and Boris Karloff (*Frankenstein* 1931) were sometime *yellowfaces* in the *Mysterious Detective*, innumerable *Mr Wong* (1935) movies, and *Charlie Chan at the Opera* (1936). Karloff had also played the evil Dr Fu Manchu (*The Mask of Fu Manchu*, 1932), and there are certain formal elements, such as the laboratory setting, that are common to both the depiction of the evil oriental genius and the Hawaii-based detective. But the character of the Chinese detective was both conventional and unique and broke the famously negative depiction of the threatening and often sickly oriental in US movies (Fuller 1996: 56). No doubt the more sinister aspects of the oriental villain bled across genres, but the archetypal Chinese screen detective was a generally good-natured character endowed with 'enigmatic traits such as psychic abilities, highly developed powers of observation and razor-sharp deductions that dazzle and amaze other characters' (Fuller 1997: 151). Their shared laboratory settings associate these characters with the science of detection, and while still partaking of the oriental 'other', the Chinese detective in America was an agent of the state, a patriotic and heroic oriental who was 'without exception, depicted as a loyal servant of any number of chosen institutions of Western authority' (*ibid.*: 86). 'Strangely conversant with the criminal mind, yet equally at home among the cultivated, rich and powerful' (*ibid.*: 151), the oriental detective's 'subtle discrediting of the West, this constant insistence on the superior finesse of the yellow races in the presence of homicide, is something which every red-blooded American should resent' (Review of *Mr Wong in Chinatown, New York Times* 31 July 1939.9). The Euro-American characterisation of the Chinese detective therefore remained ambivalent until the arrival in English literature of Di Renjie.

Di Renjie took some time to re-emerge in the twentieth century, coming to Europe by a circuitous route via Japan, but by the 1960s he had achieved global renown. The apparently insatiable appetite of the British for the exotic and salacious mysteries of the Orient took a new and murderous turn with Robert van Gulik's (1910–67) hugely successful 24 mystery detective stories. Van Gulik based his original fiction on his own translation of the eighteenth-century cases of Di Renjie, which were published as *The Celebrated Cases of Judge Dee* in 1949. The series was completed (between 1957 and 1968) while van Gulik was working in the Dutch Foreign service in Asia. Van Gulik's potent mixture of sex (during the same years he published an influential book of erotic coloured prints of uncertain provenance) (van Gulik 1951) and murder is exemplified in the *Chinese Bell Murders* (van Gulik 1958). In this story, a young butcher's daughter, the lover of a hapless candidate for the imperial examiners, is raped and murdered by an irredeemable thug who poses as a mendicant monk.

All these productions have formed the basis for what I suggest is a massive late-twentieth- to twenty-first-century revival of interest in forensic medicine and science, stimulated by the international success of van Gulik's Judge Dee stories, the arrival of American and British TV series and films in China in the last 15 years, together with a pride and familiarity in the antiquity of the forensic science detective novel in China. In Hong Kong, the hugely popular 22-part *Xiyuan lu* 洗冤錄 series, which began in 1999, draws on Song Ci's 宋慈 twelfth-century instructions to coroners, mixed in with the cases of Judge Bao.

There have been five Central China TV television seasons featuring Judge Dee (Fu *et al.* 2004–18) and recent films include Tsui Hark's award-winning *Detective Dee and the Mystery of the Phantom Flame* (*Di Renjie zhi tongtian diguo* 狄仁傑之通天帝國 2010) and *Young Detective Dee: Rise of the Sea Dragon* (*Di Renjie zhi shen zhi shendou long wang* 狄仁傑之神都龍王 2013).

There is no doubt that *Wuxia* owes much to this twentieth-century crossfertilisation of the forensic detective genre between London, Shanghai, Hollywood, and Hong Kong. It would therefore be wrong to conclude that the forensic detective in *Wuxia* is unattractive to a Chinese audience. Read against the backdrop of the racial stereotyping of American and UK genres of the inter-war period, the figure of the Chinese detective had many positive qualities of intelligence, commitment, and flexibility. Xu Baijiu's craving for a *truth* that reveals itself through forensic examination lies precisely within this negotiation between the depiction of traditional and modern professional forensic frameworks. For him, culpability and responsibility are definitively located in bare facts, the more naked and stripped of cultural meaning the better. But according to our film, this is a worldview that requires a contemporary moderation that scientises Chinese tradition.

In many respects, both main protagonists are troubled heroes who embody old Chinese stereotypes of masculinity, the *wen* 文 (literary scholar) and the *wu* 武 (martial warrior), and yin-yang polar opposites (and represent the kinds of sons and heirs that all traditional Chinese mothers have apparently aspired to produce). But in Chinese tradition both are essential to the health of each other, as two sides of the same phenomenon. The Chinese scholar, pale from his mental exertions in the study, and delicate in constitution from lack of exercise, is reinvented here as a representative of rationality, science, and modernity, and the transcending of emotion. In recent years Chinese passion for similar fictional characters in modern adaptations of the Holmes (*Fuermosi* 福尔摩斯) story has intensified with a craze for forensic science novels, TV documentaries, and movies. *Crime Scene Investigation* is a nationwide hit, and so is Benedict Cumberbatch, the most determinedly asexual actor to be voted 'Sexiest Man Alive' (*Daily Mail* 2 October, 2013). His interpretation of Sherlock Holmes makes him the latest clean-shaven effete scholarly figure to have taken young Chinese girls by storm, just like their UK counterparts (BBC China blog 2 January, 2014).

The other clean-shaven, delicate forensic scientist with hairless creamy skin who has stirred the passions of many young Chinese girls in cyberspace is the inimitable Johnny Depp, now known for his rather more hirsute role as Captain Jack Sparrow in the *Pirates of the Caribbean* series (dir. Verbinski, Marshall, Ronning and Sandberg 2003, 2006, 2007, 2011, 2017). Compare his vulnerable forensic gaze in Tim Burton's *Sleepy Hollow* (1999) with the nervous, intense gaze of Xu Baijiu. Like Xu Baijiu, the *Sleepy Hollow* detective Ichabod Crane has trouble with a father figure, who has killed his mother for her practice of witchcraft and superstition. Both characters are therefore victims of paternal traumas that have disfigured their lives, and both have to battle with and overcome what is represented as a pathological patriarchal principle in the course of their respective films (Figure 1.7a and b).

We can vouch for this fascination with the forensic detective genre and its cross-cultural genius among our students, for as one recent UCL graduate tells me about the latest in the Judge Bao genre:

> Apart from *Zhong'an liuzu* 重案六组 (Special Detective Squad) my favourite one is *Shaonian bao qingtian* 少年包青天, especially the first series. I was fascinated by this TV series as a little girl largely because I was drawn to its mysterious enchantment in relation to traditional Chinese culture. It has made detective narratives a way of informing me about Chinese ethnicity, myth, folklore, ghost stories, as well as traditional medicine practices (and a lot more). Yet it also seeks a fairly good balance between so-called supernatural beliefs and apparently scientific and logical explanations at the end of each case. In a word, it made me feel an urge to belong to a culture that is both mysterious and cool.
>
> (personal communication with Lulu Wang,
> UCL 2015)

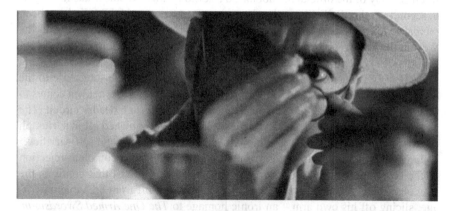

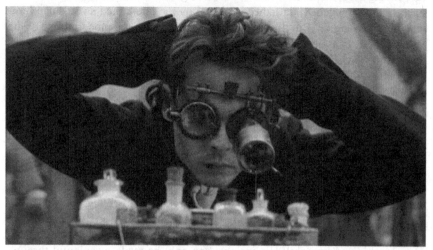

Figure 1.7 (a) and (b) Medicine bottles and the forensic gaze. Depp and Takeshi get to the bottom of things . . .

Conclusion

I will leave further reflections on the apparent fascination of young Chinese women with homoerotic male relationships to another occasion. But Lulu's fascination with the 'cool' and ethnically seductive Chinese detective genre and the way it strikes a 'balance between so-called supernatural beliefs and seeming scientific and logical explanations' neatly brings this chapter to a conclusion. We have come a long way from the kind of analysis that contrasts the cosmologised Chinese body with the anatomised Greek body. Historians like Li Jianmin (*forthcoming*) and Catherine Despeux (2005) have given us new histories of anatomy, dissection, and surgery for China, and Asen and Wu of the modern Chinese forensic body of the official handbooks, a tradition which we know has its origins in second-century BCE China. The legendary Bao Gong and Di Renjie have been recreated for a modern China that claims at least an equivalent expertise to the West in the discovery of moral truths through reading the inanimate body. As Xu Baijiu sides with Liu Jinxi and comes to his aid in the counter-attack on Tang Long (Liu)'s father with an acupuncture needle jabbed into the foot close to the acupoint *Yongquan* 湧泉, and some more at the back of his neck, heaven comes to their aid as a bolt of lightning connects the needles to form a deadly circuit. The Xixia chief is electrocuted, and a violent separatist past is finished off in a triumph of cross-cultural cooperation, traditional medicine, electricity, and self-sacrifice.

Tang Long's journey to become Liu Jinxi has involved a complete rejection of the separatist violence of his forefathers. In a bizarre twist that confirms the new order that is contemporary China, he cuts himself off from his violent heritage, slicing off his own arm – an ironic homage to *The One Armed Swordsman*, since Liu's estranged Xixia father is played by the one-armed swordsman himself, Jimmy Wang Yu. But this final act also subverts the pre-modern trope of the severing of flesh as an act of Confucian altruism to feed the ailing body of one's parents. In *Wuxia*, Liu Jinxi severs his lineage and sacrifices his blood tie to his father in a filial act to the more forward-looking, multicultural China that he has chosen to join.

In the negotiation of truth between these two men it becomes clear that they are in fact two complementary and interdependent aspects of the same struggle for survival. Together, they represent a uniquely Chinese brilliance, one able to resolve the tensions between anatomical science and cultural heritage that had embodied the longstanding nineteenth- and twentieth-century national spiritual crisis. In contrast to Liu Jinxi's seamless ability to deal with complex and fluid social and moral situations, and the flexibility of his living body, Xu Baijiu's voyeuristic anatomical gaze and his obsession with objectifying both living and dead bodies does not engage with real people, but rather appears quasi-pornographic and immoral. His insights can only be made meaningful through a collage of modern and traditional knowledge wherein the boundaries between life and death can ultimately be negotiated through Traditional Chinese Medicine. Liu's flexibility is physiologised: a mastery, at once scientific and anatomical yet simultaneously supernatural, of the martial arts body, a body that, phoenix-like, revives from the dead as Liu and Xu come together for a single common purpose. Together, the two protagonists embody a new national pride, keen to represent multicultural genius, a strong body of the people, with a long synthetic history. This ideal is one that embraces the past with a fluid, relative science and morality that is more than fit for the challenges of the future – both dead and alive, empathetic, emotional, but simultaneously rational and ready for whatever the future may bring. Despite the failure of the bodies of the Boxers to ward off European bullets with their bare hands in 1901, and countless less than totally convincing attempts to prove the Chinese martial arts in physical contests, despite the failure to identify corporeal counterparts to *qi* or the channels of acupuncture, the magic of *Wuxia* lives on. In the spirit of China's nineteenth- and early-twentieth-century reception of European science, more than a hundred years later the martial artists are still 'doing it on their own terms' (Elman 2005), flying through the air, running up walls, and leaping over rooftops to re-balance global dynamics for the twenty-first century.

Filmography

American Dreams in China (Zhongguo hehuo ren 中國合伙人*)*, dir. Peter Chan (Chen Kexin 陳可辛),2013.

Armour of God (Longxiong hudi 龍兄虎弟*)*, dir. Jackie Chan (Cheng Long 成龍), 1986.

Charlie Chan at the Opera, dir.H. Bruce Humberstone, 1936.

The Chinese Boxer (Longhu dou 龍虎斗*)*, dir. Jimmy Wong Yu (Wang Yu 王羽), 1970.

Detective Dee and the Mystery of the Phantom Flame (Di Renjie zhi tongtian diguo 狄仁傑之通天帝國*)*, dir. Tsui Hark (Xu Ke 徐克), 2010.

Dracula, dir. Tod Browning, 1931.

Dragon (Wuxia 武俠*)*, dir. Peter Chan (Chen Kexin 陳可辛), 2011.

Frankenstein, dir. James Whale, 1931.

Heroes Shed No Tears (Yingxiong wulei 英雄無淚*)*, dir. John Woo (Wu Yusen 吳宇森), 1986.

Ip Man (Ye Men 葉問*)*, dir. Wilson Yip (Ye Weixin 葉偉信), 2008, and sequels 2010, 2016.

The Mask of Fu Manchu, dir. Charles Brabin, 1932.

The Mysterious Detective, Mr Wang, dir. William Nigh, 1935.

One Armed Swordsman (Dubi dao 獨臂刀*)*, dir. Jimmy Wang Yu, 1967.

Pirates of the Caribbean, dir. Verbinski, G., Marshall, R., Ronning J. and Sandberg E. 2003; sequels 2006, 2007, 2011, 2017.

Project A II (A jihua xuji A 計劃續集*)*, dir. Jackie Chan, 1987.

Sleepy Hollow, dir. Tim Burton, 1999.

Young Detective Dee: Rise of the Sea Dragon (Di Renjie zhi shen dou longwang 狄仁傑之神都龍王*)*, dir. Tsui Hark, 2013.

TV series

Crime Scene Investigation, Zuicker, A.E. *et al.* 15 Seasons, 2000–15.

Detective Di Renjie (Shentan Di Renjie 神探狄仁杰*)* Series 1–6, dir. Qiang Yanqiu 钱雁秋, 2004.

Bibliography

Primary sources

Bao *Longtu baijia gong'an* 包龍圖百家公案 (Cases of A Hundred Families Judged by Dragon-Design Bao), An Yushi 安遇时 (1594) modern edn: Guben xiaoshuo jicheng bianji weiyuanhui 古本小説集成編輯委員會 (eds.) (1991) *Bao Longtu baijia gong'an* 包龍圖百家公案, Shanghai: Shanghai guji chubanshe.

Bao *Longtu gong'an* 龍圖公案 (Cases Judged by the Dragon-Design), Anon. Bodleian MS Ashmole 399, fol. 19r., Oxford (1292).

Fengzhen shi 封診式 (Models for Sealing and Physical Examinations), Shuihudi tomb, Yunmeng County, Hubei, closed 217–16 BCE., modern edn: Shuihudi Qin mu zhujian zhengli xiaozu 睡虎地秦墓整理小組 (1990) *Shuihudi Qinmu zhujian* 睡虎地秦墓竹簡, Beijing: Wenwu chubanshe.

Huangdi *bashiyi nanjing* 黃帝八十一難經 (The Canon of Eighty-One Problems), Li Jiong 李駉 (ed.) (1269) printed in *Huangdi bashiyi nanjing zuan tu jujie* 黃帝八十一難經纂圖句解 in *Zhengtong Daozang* 正統道藏 (1436–49), Shanghai: Hanfen lou.

Huangdi *neijing* 黃帝內經 (The Inner Canon of the Yellow Emperor), Anon. c. Han dynasty (202 BCE – 220 CE); *Suwen* 素問 (Plain Questions), edn Wang Bing 王冰 (c. 710–805); *Lingshu* 靈樞 (The Numinous Pivot), modern edn: Guo Aichun 郭靄春 (ed.) (1992) *Huangdi neijing suwen jiaozhu* 黃帝內經素問校注, Beijing: Renming weisheng chubanshe and Guo Aichun 郭靄春 (ed.) (2010) *Huangdi neijing lingshu jiaozhu yuyi* 黃帝内经灵枢校注语译, Guiyang: Guizhou jiaoyu chubanshe.

Taiping *guangji* 太平廣記 (Extensive Records of the Taiping Era, Li Fang 李昉 (925–966), completed 978, modern edn: Yan Yiping 嚴一萍 (ed.) (1970) *Taiping guangji fu jiaokan ji* 太平廣記附校勘記, Taibei: Yiwen yinshu guan.

Tansūqnāma-i *Īlkhān dar funūn-i 'ulūm-i Khatā 'ī* (The Treasure Book of the Ilkhan on Chinese Science and Techniques) (1313) Rashīd al-Dīn Faẓl Allāh (d. 1314), Süleymaniye Library, Aya Sofya, Istanbul.

Xiyuan *lu* 洗冤錄 (Treatise for Washing Away Injustice), Song Ci 宋慈, 18th century, modern edn: Wang Youhuai *et al.* (eds.) (1916) *Chongkan buzhu xiyuan lu jizheng: 5 juan* 重刊補註洗冤錄集證 :5 卷, [Shanghai]: Guangyi shuju.

Secondary sources

Andrews, B. (2014) *The Making of Modern Chinese Medicine, 1850–1960*, Honolulu: University of Hawai'i Press.

Akasoy, A., Burnett, C. and Yoeli-Tlalim, R. (eds.) (2008) *Astro-Medicine: Astrology and Medicine, East and West*, Florence: Sismel.

Asen, D. (2009) Vital Spots, Mortal Wounds, and Forensic Practice: Finding Cause of Death in Nineteenth-century China, *East Asian Science, Technology, and Medicine*, 3 (4): 453–74.

———. (2012) Dead Bodies and Forensic Science: Cultures of Expertise in China, 1800–1940, PhD thesis, Columbia University.

Berlekamp, P., Lo, V. and Wang, Y. (2015) Administering Art, History, and Science in the Mongol Empire, in A. Landau (ed.) *Pearls on a String: Art in the Age of Great Islamic Empires*, Baltimore and Seattle: Walters Art Museum and Washington University Press, pp. 53–85.

Berry, C. and Farquhar, M. (2006) *China on Screen: Cinema and Nation,* New York: Columbia University Press.

Chen Baogong 陳實功 (2007) *Waike Zhengzong* 外科正宗 (Orthodox Manual of External Medicines), Beijing: Renmin Weisheng Chubanshe.

Daston, L. and Galison, P. (2007) *Objectivity*, New York: Zone Books.

Despeux, C. (2005) Visual Representations of the Body in Chinese Medical and Daoist Texts from the Song to the Qing Period (tenth to nineteenth century), trans. P. Barrett, *Asian Medicine: Tradition and Modernity*, 1 (1): 10–52.

Elman, B. (2005) *On Their Own Terms*, Cambridge, MA and London: Harvard University Press.

Freidson, E. (1970) *Profession of Medicine*, New York: Dodd, Mead & Co.

Fuller, K.F. (1996) Masters of the Macabre: The Oriental Detective, *The Spectator*, 17 (1): 55–69.

———. (1997) Hollywood Goes Oriental: CaucAsian Performance in American Cinema, PhD thesis, Northwestern University.

Gaowa, S. (2007) A Review of Tangut Buddhism, Art and Textual Studies, *International Dunhuang Project, British Library*, http://idp.bl.uk/downloads/Tangut.pdf, accessed 1 June 2018.

Goody, J. (2006) *The Theft of History*, New York: Cambridge University Press.

Harper, D. (1998) *Early Chinese Medical Literature: The Mawangdui Medical Manuscripts*, London and New York: Kegan Paul International.

Hu Xiaofeng 胡曉峰 (2018) A Brief Introduction to Illustration in the Literature of Surgery and Traumatology in Chinese Medicine, in V. Lo and P. Barrett (eds.) *Imagining Chinese Medicine*, Leiden: Brill, pp. 183–96.

Hulsewé, A.F.P. (1985) *Remnants of Ch'in Law: An Annotated Translation of the Ch'in Legal and Administrative Rules of the 3rd Century B.C. Discovered in Yun-meng Prefecture, Hu-pei Province, in 1975*, Leiden: Brill.

Kemp, M. and Wallace, M. (2001) *Spectacular Bodies: The Art and Science of the Human Body from Leonardo Till Now*, Berkeley: University of California Press and Hayward Gallery.

Kirk, P. (1953) *Crime Investigation: Physical Evidence and the Police Laboratory*, New York: Interscience Publishers, Inc.

Kuriyama, S. (1999) *The Expressiveness of the Body and the Divergence of Greek and Chinese Medicine*, New York: Zone.

Li Jianmin 李建民 (*forthcoming*) Anatomy and Surgery, in V. Lo and M. Stanley-Baker (eds.) *Routledge Handbook of Chinese Medicine*, London and New York: Routledge.

Lo, V. and Barrett, P. (eds.) (2018) *Imagining Chinese Medicine*, Leiden: Brill.

Lu Gwei-djen and Needham, J. ([1980] 2002) *Celestial Lancets: A History and Rationale of Acupuncture and Moxa*, London: RoutledgeCurzon.

MacMullen, D. (1993) The Real Judge Dee: Ti Jen-chieh and the T'ang Restoration of 705, *Asia Major*, Third Series, 6 (1): 1–81.

Marchetti, G. (1993) Romance and the Yellow Peril, Berkeley, Los Angeles and London: University of California Press.

McKnight, B. (1982) *The Washing Away of Wrongs: Forensic Medicine in Thirteenth-Century China*, Ann Arbor: University of Michigan Center for Chinese Studies.

Savage-Smith, E. (1997) The Depiction of Human Anatomy in the Islamic World, in F. Maddison and E. Savage-Smith (eds.) *Science Tools and Magic: Part One: Body and Spirit, Mapping the Universe*, vol. 12 of Nasser D. Khalili Collection of Islamic Art, London: The Nour Foundation in association with Azimuth Editions and Oxford University Press, pp. 14–24.

Shahar, M. (2011) The Diamond Body, in V. Lo (ed.) *Perfect Bodies*, London: British Museum Research Publications, pp. 121–30.

Shohat, E. (1991) Gender and the Culture of Empire: Toward a Feminist Ethnography of the Cinema, *Quarterly Review of Film and Video*, 13 (1/3): 45–84.

Svarverud, R. (2011) Re‐constructing East Asia: International Law as Inter‐cultural Process in Late Qing China, *Inter-Asia Cultural Studies*, 12 (2): 306–18.

Taylor, K. (2005) *Chinese Medicine in Early Communist China, 1945–1963: A Medicine of Revolution*, London and New York: RoutledgeCurzon.

Teo, S. (2009) *Chinese Martial Arts Cinema: The Wuxia tradition*, Edinburgh: Edinburgh University Press.

Terzioğlu, A. (1974) 'Ilkhanischen Krankenhäuser'. Die Ilkhanischen Krankenhäuser und die Einflüsse der islamischen Medizin auf Byzanz zu dieser Zeit, in *Proceedings of the*

XXIII International Congress of the History of Medicine, London, 2–9 September 1972, London: Wellcome Institute for the History of Medicine.

Van Gulik, R. ([1949] 1976) *Celebrated Cases of Judge Dee: An Authentic Eighteenth-century Chinese Detective Novel, Translated and with an Introduction and Notes*, New York: Dover Publications Inc. First published as *Dee Goong an: Three Murder Cases Solved by Judge Dee*, Tokyo.

———. (1951) *Erotic Colour Prints of the Ming Period*, Tokyo: Privately Printed.

———. (1958) *The Chinese Bell Murders*, London: Michael Joseph.

Wang Shumin 王淑民 and Fuentes, G. (2018) A Survey of Images from the Chinese Medical Classics, in V. Lo and P. Barrett (eds.) *Imagining Chinese Medicine*, Leiden: Brill, pp. 29–50.

Wong, T.C. (2007) *Sherlock in Shanghai*, Honolulu: University of Hawaii Press.

Wright, A.F. (1959) *Buddhism in Chinese History,* Stanford, CA: Stanford University Press.

Wu, Y-L. (2015) Between the Living and the Dead: Trauma Medicine and Forensic Medicine in the Mid-Qing, *Frontiers of History in China*, 10 (1): 38–73.

Zhang Yingjin (2004) *Chinese National Cinema*, New York and London: Routledge.

2 How to be a good Maoist doctor

An Ode to the Silver Needle under a Shadowless Lamp (1974)

Leon Antonio Rocha

Adapted from a short play written by the Shanghai Chest Hospital Amateur Art Group (*Shanghai shi xiongke yiyuan yeyu wenyi chuangzuozu* 上海市胸科医院 业余文艺创作组), *An Ode to the Silver Needle under a Shadowless Lamp* (*Wuyingdeng xia song yinzhen* 无影灯下颂银针, 1974, also known as *Song of Acupuncture Treatment*, but hereinafter *Silver Needle*)[1] was one of a small handful of films about medicine released during the latter part of the Cultural Revolution (1966–1976). What makes *Silver Needle* remarkable as a primary source is its subject matter: it is the only Chinese film from the period that portrays the practice of 'acupuncture anaesthesia' (*zhenci mazui* 针刺麻醉 or *zhenma* 针麻) in an urban hospital setting. Other Cultural Revolution films on medicine and healthcare focussed exclusively on the 'barefoot doctors' (*chijiao yisheng* 赤脚医生) – rural residents who received some medical training and delivered basic healthcare to China's vast countryside and frontier regions (Fang 2012; Scheid 2013: 261–2; Lan 2015; Pang 2017: 101–34).[2] *Silver Needle* celebrates acupuncture anaesthesia as one of the crowning achievements of Traditional Chinese Medicine in combination with Maoist ideology (Hsu 1996; Taylor 2005: 138–9; Hayot 2009: 207–45). The film also presents a model of the revolutionary doctor dedicated to serving the Chinese masses. *Silver Needle* dramatises a protracted debate on the political status of expertise and experts which began after the establishment of the People's Republic of China (PRC) in 1949, further intensified in 1957–1958, and reached a climax during the late 1960s and early 1970s (Lynteris 2013: 58–89; Andreas 2009).

Silver Needle is a 40-minute film, directed by the veteran 'Second Generation' filmmaker Sang Hu 桑弧 (1916–2004), who first became well-known in the late 1940s for his collaborations with Eileen Chang (Zhang Ailing) 张爱玲 (1920–1995) (Xiao Zhiwei 1988; Zhongguo dianyingjia xiehui dianying shi yanjiubu 1982). After the Communists came to power in 1949, Sang continued to have a distinguished career. Even though a 'lifelong non-communist', Sang somehow survived the Anti-Rightist Movement of 1957 and the Cultural Revolution (Pickowicz 2013: 116). However, Sang did not make any films between 1966 and 1973; *Silver Needle*, released in 1974, was Sang Hu's first film since *Shanghai Spring* (*Shanghai zhi chun* 上海之春, 1965). As Paul Clark (2008: 111) explains, 'feature film production effectively stopped for the first four years of the Cultural

Revolution . . . film required a proper "cleansing of the ranks" before being given the task of taking the new culture to China's audiences'. By around 1970, the first film adaptations of the so-called eight 'model performances' (*yangbanxi* 样板戏) were released; new films such as *Silver Needle* which were not based on the eight model performances emerged only after 1972 'when Mao Zedong, Zhou Enlai and other state leaders pointed out the paucity of cultural works available to their audiences' (Clark 2008: 75).[3] The lead character of Sang Hu's *Silver Needle*, Dr Li Zhihua 李志华, is an anaesthesiologist. She is from a proletarian background and is devoted equally to serving her patients and to advancing Mao Zedong Thought. Dr Li is played by Zhu Xijuan 祝希娟 (1938–), one of the most recognisable faces from mid-twentieth-century Chinese cinema, celebrated for her debut role as Wu Qionghua 吴琼花 in *Red Detachment of Women* (*Hongse niangzi jun* 红色娘子军, dir. Xie Jin 谢晋, 1961) for which Zhu won the first Hundred Flowers Award for Best Actress (Lu Wei 2006; Donald 2000: 1).

The action of *Silver Needle* takes place in 1972, in the wards of the Shanghai People's Hospital (*Shanghai renmin yiyuan* 上海人民医院). Old Yang (Lao Yang 老杨), played by Lou Jicheng 娄际成 (1934–), is a steel worker who has fallen seriously ill.[4] Dr Li Zhihua suggests that Old Yang must have an immediate heart operation – probably to repair valves damaged by rheumatic fever – with acupuncture anaesthesia as opposed to chemical anaesthesia. However, Dr Luo 罗医生 (played by veteran character actor Qiu Shisui 邱世穗), the head of the Department of Surgery, rejects Dr Li's proposal. Dr Luo is worried that Old Yang's heart procedure will end in failure and will therefore irreparably tarnish the hospital's brilliant track record in administering acupuncture anaesthesia. A battle of wills unfolds between the young, idealistic, and passionate Dr Li, versus the older, risk-averse, and politically suspect Dr Luo.

In this chapter I will discuss how Sang Hu's *Silver Needle* projects specifically Maoist ethics, embodied by Dr Li Zhihua, a 'red expert' (*hongzhuan* 红专) who channels the spirit of the famous Canadian surgeon and Communist martyr Norman Bethune (1890–1939, in Chinese Bai Qiu'en 白求恩). First, I shall explore the debate on scientific and medical expertise during the early Communist era, drawing on insights from Christos Lynteris' work on the genealogy of 'selflessness' in Maoist China (Lynteris 2011, 2013), before turning to *Silver Needle* and analysing its representation of the good, Maoist, Bethunian doctor.

The good doctor: from Norman Bethune to Dr Li

As Christos Lynteris has discussed, immediately after the establishment of the PRC in 1949, a number of urgent questions arose in the field of medicine:

> Is medicine inherently bourgeois, or [are] its theory and practice originally progressive and only politically distorted by its enclosure into bourgeois educational, clinical and governmental institutions? Are medical doctors class enemies of the insurgent proletariat, or should they be treated like other intellectuals . . . If medical doctors are indeed malleable, what measures and

criteria should be applied to affect reform? How should revolutionaries guard against the potential medical 'fifth-column', in terms of both bourgeois doctors and bourgeois theory and work-style, corrupting the revolution? Will bourgeois medical science eventually give way to some sort of proletarian medicine, or is a rupture necessary for its overcoming?

(Lynteris 2013: 6)

This set of questions could be – and had been – raised with respect to just about *any* field of expertise as the Chinese Communist Party (CCP) seized long-term power (Schmalzer 2008; Fan 2012; Mullaney 2012; Hudecek 2014). But it was particularly pressing for China to deal with its medical structures (Lampton 1977; Taylor 2005). Simply put, the capacity to monitor and regulate the health of its population – by containing diseases and epidemics, intervening in fertility and childbirth, keeping built environments hygienic, and so on – was vital to any modern nation-state, regardless of its political ideology, in maintaining the productivity of its labour force for economic development and ensuring the security of its territory and the legitimacy of its rule. When the CCP took power in 1949, they inherited a country that was ravaged after decades of war. With severely limited resources, Mao's government had to co-opt the public health infrastructure left behind by the Kuomintang and put together a Ministry of Health by employing the biomedical personnel and 'turncoat' officials who had previously served under Chiang Kai-shek. China also had to rely on scientific advisors 'on loan' from the Soviet Union. This became a serious problem for Mao as this bourgeois and often Western-trained biomedical elite was 'terrified by the perceived vulgarity of the battle-worn guerrillas', and was threatening to form a new bloc of technocrats and experts who were far removed socially and politically from both the urban proletariat and the rural peasants (Lynteris 2011: 31). They passively shunned or even actively obstructed Mao's project to revolutionise all social relations in China. The Patriotic Health Campaign of 1952, launched in connection with allegations that the United States had used biological weapons in the Korean War, consisted of nationwide mobilisation of civilians to eliminate disease vectors (Rogaski 2002, 2004: 285–99). Mao simultaneously pushed back against the medical elite by challenging their ability to manage the epidemiological crisis (Lynteris 2011: 26).

It was in this political setting that the life and legacy of Norman Bethune emerged as a *point de capiton* for the debates on the status of medical expertise, and the politically correct mentality and conduct of practitioners. Bethune was a Canadian doctor and communist who served as a frontline surgeon for the Anti-Fascists during the Spanish Civil War. He then travelled to China and volunteered for the Communist Eighth Route Army. At the Yan'an Revolutionary Base during the Second Sino-Japanese War, Bethune cut his finger while operating on a wounded Chinese soldier, contracted septicaemia and died in November 1939 (Hannant 1998; Allan and Gordon 2009; Stewart and Stewart 2011). A month later, Mao penned a eulogy entitled 'In Memory of Norman Bethune', which hailed Bethune as a 'martyr' and instructed all communists to 'learn [Bethune's] spirit of absolute selflessness' (Mao Zedong 1939). In *Silver Needle*, the heroine Dr Li Zhihua quotes directly from Mao's memorial while gazing at a propaganda poster of Bethune, whom she regarded as her role model (11:48–12:16). When 'In Memory of Norman Bethune' (*Jinian Bai Qiu'en* 纪念白求恩) was first published in 1939, it was 'little more than a typical acknowledgement of the bravery and self-sacrifice of a man who had devoted his medical skill in the fight against social injustice' (Lynteris 2011: 22). But the Bethunian 'spirit of absolute selflessness' was subsequently resurrected twice – in the early years of the PRC, and then again during the Cultural Revolution – to make two very different arguments (Lynteris 2013: 58–89).

The first resurrection of Bethune was carried out by Fu Lianzhang 傅连璋 (also known as Nelson Fu, 1894–1968). Fu was a doctor in western medicine who participated in the Long March (1934–1936), treated top CCP leaders in the 1940s, and after 1949 was appointed Vice-Minister of Health and President of the Chinese Medical Association (CMA). According to Lynteris, in December 1952 Fu delivered a commemorative lecture entitled 'What We Should Learn from Dr Bethune's Revolutionary Humanitarianism', which was printed in the *Chinese Medical Journal* in May 1953 (Lynteris 2011: 24). Fu's interpretation of Mao's memorial was simple: Bethune's achievement was that he was able to sublimate his personal interest into the collective interest. But in order to sublimate, one first had to 'cultivate'. Bethune was able to serve the Chinese soldiers and sacrifice himself in the way that he did precisely because he had been able to develop those exceptional surgical skills beforehand – without the interference of non-experts. In other words, one had to become a 'professional expert' first and then become 'politically red' (Lynteris 2011: 31). This was Fu and the CMA's attempt to mitigate the effects of Mao's mass mobilisation: the masses could be mobilised in (for example) public health campaigns but they had to be led by experts, and these experts had to be given the safe space to acquire knowledge so that they could make profound contributions to revolutions.

Bethune then largely disappeared from medical discourse, resurfaced in November 1965, near the start of the Cultural Revolution (Lynteris 2011: 32). After the failure of the Great Leap Forward (1958–1962), Mao resigned as Chairman of the PRC. Liu Shaoqi 刘少奇 (1898–1969) and Deng Xiaoping 邓小平 (1904–1997) stepped in to bring order and stability back to the country. The result was the restoration and then dramatic expansion of a privileged, centralised class of technocratic specialists and professional experts who were tasked with economic development, agricultural management, and administrative regularity. Mao's egalitarian and revolutionary vision was abandoned. The inequality between urban and rural China resurfaced, if not worsened, as scarce resources were ring-fenced for cities and strategic industries. In the famous 1965 'Directive on Public Health', Mao voiced his displeasure at the disparity between urban and rural healthcare provision, and accused the Ministry of Health of catering to '[only] 15% of the total population of the country . . . this 15% is mainly composed of gentlemen, while the broad masses of the peasants do not get any medical treatment'. Mao sarcastically suggested renaming the

Ministry of Health the 'Ministry of Urban Health, the Ministry of Gentlemen's Health, or even . . . [the] Ministry of Urban Gentlemen's Health' (Mao 1965). Under attack, the CMA published an article entitled 'Norman Bethune, the Great Champion of Internationalism' (1965) and recycled Fu Lianzhang's interpretation of Bethune from 1952, emphasising that Bethune's 'spirit of ever seeking fresh knowledge and improving his professional skill' enabled him to perform his selfless acts (Lynteris 2011: 32).

In 1966, the second resurrection of Bethune took place in the pages of the *People's Liberation Army Daily* (*Jiefang junbao* 解放军报), at that point the mouthpiece of Mao loyalist Marshall Lin Biao 林彪 (1907–1971). As Lynteris explains, the 21 December 1966 *People's Liberation Army Daily* editorial recast Mao's 'In Memory of Norman Bethune' as a 'powerful weapon to eradicate self-interest and foster public interest' (Lynteris 2011: 34). Doctors had to change their 'world outlook' (*shijieguan* 世界观) to a proletarian one, embodied by Bethune, which entailed 'complete devotion to the public interest [and] the concept of saving people wholeheartedly, the communist spirit of utter devotion to others without any thought of the self' (*ibid.*). By contrast, the bourgeois world outlook – 'self-interest, selfishness, advancing one's own interests at the expense of others, and extreme individualism' – had to be purged (*ibid.*). The *People's Liberation Army Daily* editorial was then followed by a string of articles in the *China Medical Journal*, which relentlessly criticised counter-revolutionary doctors who believed in the supremacy of individual skill, who accumulated expertise for the sake of fame and fortune, and who blindly worshipped foreign ideas and Western science (*ibid.*: 35–6). All this amounted to a radical reversal of Fu Lianzhang's 1952 vision of the Bethunian ideal doctor. Fu had argued that it was meticulous self-cultivation that allowed medical professionals to contribute to the Communist cause, whereas the Cultural Revolution iteration exalted the 'spirit of absolute selflessness' as the foundation of medical practice and treated expertise with suspicion if not outright hostility. Towards the end of 1966, as Barbara Mittler points out, Mao's Bethune memorial, 'Serve the People' (*Wei renmin fuwu* 为人民服务; Mao 1944), and 'The Foolish Old Man Who Removed the Mountains' (*Yugong yishan* 愚公移山; Mao 1945) were 'considered the best vehicle[s] for transmitting the core of Mao's thought to the masses'. The teaching of these 'Three Constantly Read Articles' (*lao san pian* 老三篇) was assured, 'starting in kindergartens when it was based on pictures and continuing to the higher levels' (Mittler 2012: 203). With this larger historical background in mind, we can now return to *Silver Needle*.

Saving lives (*Jiuming* 救命) and revolutionising lives (*Geming* 革命)

The first scene of *Silver Needle* occurs at the Shanghai Steel Factory (*Shanghai gangtie chang* 上海钢铁厂). The film quickly introduces Dr Li Zhihua as the camera rapidly zooms into a brightly lit medium close-up (Figure 2.1). Dr Li's political purity is immediately established: she is a young doctor who regularly

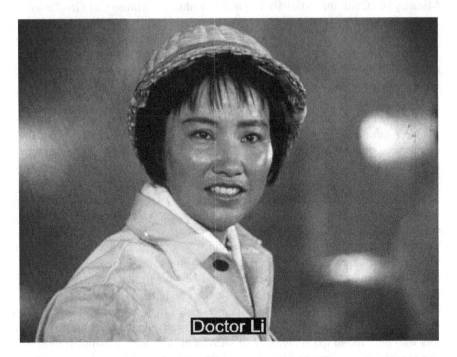

Figure 2.1 A medium close-up that establishes the heroine of *Silver Needle*, Dr Li Zhihua

volunteers at the steel mill when she is off-duty, and cheerfully carries out physical labour (*laodong* 劳动) alongside the male steelworkers. Old Yang, an elderly worker, has a heart attack and Dr Li escorts him to the hospital.

In the second scene Dr Luo, the antagonist of *Silver Needle*, makes his appearance, delivering a closing speech at a conference with other senior colleagues and Communist Party officials. He boasts of the hospital's record in administering acupuncture anaesthesia in 92 successful operations. Conflict between Dr Li and Dr Luo is foreshadowed during the diagnosis of Old Yang. Dr Li argues that an operation carried out by Dr Luo's deputy Dr Ding 丁医生, aided by acupuncture anaesthesia, is the only cure for Old Yang's rheumatic heart disease. However, Dr Luo simply places the patient under 'further observation'. Dr Li's colleague Dr Feng (Xiaofeng 小冯) comments, 'Dr Luo's reluctant to take responsibilities. He's keen on introducing acupuncture anaesthesia experiments, but has become a lot more conservative about operations now'.

Dr Ding asks Dr Luo to reconsider Dr Li's proposal. Dr Luo says that Dr Li's ideas are 'very good and bold', but 'we need to slow things down'. He explains that '[the] 92 operation experiences are highly appreciated' by CCP officials, and orders Dr Ding to handpick a bunch of 'safer' patients who can be easily operated on and cured, so that the hospital can 'accomplish 100 [successful] operations in the shortest amount of time'. Dr Luo then secretly pulls out a discharge notice from his drawer and fills in Old Yang's details, and thus reveals his deceitful and manipulative nature.

The next scene in the film is crucial as Dr Li and Dr Luo are pitted against each other for the first time. Dr Li discovers that Dr Luo has signed a discharge notice for Old Yang; she asks Old Yang to stay put and angrily confronts Dr Luo. Dr Luo uses Old Yang's medical history to point out that his liver is functioning badly and he cannot take conventional anaesthetics. When Dr Li reiterates that they could try acupuncture anaesthesia, Dr Luo retorts that he has 'never seen such a severely ill patient operated on in that way', and he does not wish to jeopardise the hospital's brilliant track record. Dr Li argues that acupuncture anaesthesia is a 'newborn thing' (*xinsheng shiwu* 新生事物), and reminds Dr Luo that doctors must first and foremost serve the 'workers, peasants and soldiers' (*gongnongbing* 工农兵) and should not 'serve ourselves with their illnesses'.[5] When Dr Luo suggests that 'even in advanced foreign countries' a patient like Old Yang would be impossible to treat, Dr Li proudly declares that, as long as they 'embrace profound proletariat feelings' and 'explore [China's] medical treasure', they will be able to accomplish what Western bourgeois capitalist nations cannot. Here Dr Li is referring to Mao's 1958 slogan, 'Chinese medicine is a great treasure-house and should be diligently explored and improved upon' (Scheid 2002: 70; Taylor 2005: 120). When the debate ends in stalemate, Dr Li decides that they should 'listen to the leaders' and the masses' opinions' and appeals to the Shanghai People's Hospital's CCP branch.

The film then cuts to the end of the CCP branch committee meeting, and another key character is introduced – Master Chen (Chen shifu 陈师傅), the CCP branch secretary (*dang zhibu shuji* 党支部书记). Chen is not a physician but appears to work as a janitor at the hospital. He lends his support to Dr Li's treatment proposal, because it shows 'the great affection that the medical personnel holds for workers, peasants and soldiers'. Chen impresses on Dr Li that this case is not 'just about curing Old Yang's illness', but really 'a battle to protect Chairman Mao's revolutionary medical care and public health line (*geming yiliao weisheng luxian* 革命医疗卫生路线), and solidify the achievements of the Cultural Revolution'. Old Yang's case constitutes a 'leap' of Mao's philosophy into the domain of everyday medical practice.

The next sequence is the most important in *Silver Needle*. Dr Li stares at a propaganda poster of Norman Bethune operating on a wounded Chinese soldier in an abandoned temple, which the camera zooms into (Figure 2.2 and 2.3).[6] We hear Dr Li's thoughts,

> Comrade Bethune's spirit, his utter devotion to others without any thought of self, was shown in his great sense of responsibility in his work and his great warm-heartedness towards all comrades and the people. Every communist must learn from him.

This is a verbatim quotation from Mao's famous 'In Memory of Norman Bethune' (1939). Dr Li looks out of the window and sees two enormous billboards which

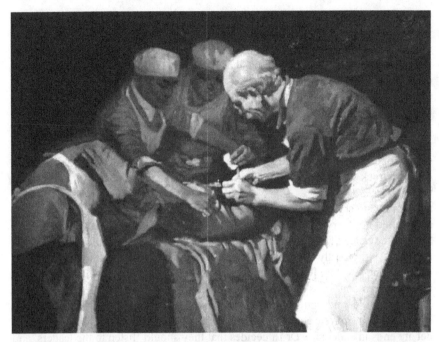

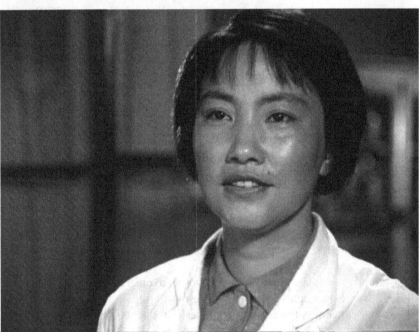

Figure 2.2 and 2.3 Dr Li gazes at a propaganda poster of Norman Bethune. We hear Dr Li's thoughts in a voice-over; she quotes directly from Mao

read 'Long Live the Great Proletarian Cultural Revolution' (*wuchan jieji wenhua da geming wansui* 无产阶级文化大革命万岁) and 'Long Live Chairman Mao' (*Mao zhuxi wansui* 毛主席万岁), and feels energised and empowered.

At this point of the film, it becomes abundantly clear that Dr Li and Dr Luo represent diametrically opposite 'world outlooks' (*shijieguan* 世界观) – proletarian/Bethunian (in the second, Cultural Revolution version of how his legacy was understood) versus bourgeois/reactionary. Dr Li is a 'descendant of the working class'; she is much younger than Dr Luo, and belongs to a generation that holds the future of medicine in China. It is hinted that Dr Li has received her medical training after the PRC has been established, and would thus be less tainted by any hangover of bourgeois ideology and institutions. In that regard, Dr Li is even 'purer' than Norman Bethune who, after all, came from capitalist Canada. On the other side is Dr Luo, the supervisor of surgery. Dr Luo belongs to an older generation of elite physicians who had already been practising medicine in the pre-PRC period. He wears polished leather shoes and spectacles, which are cinematic signifiers of 'class incorrectness' (Clark 2008: 141). Dr Li's character exemplifies Mao's 'revolutionary medical care and public health line', whereby the primary function of medicine and healthcare is to facilitate socialist construction – serving the workers, peasants, and soldiers wholeheartedly. Dr Li is well-versed in the Maoist classics, and readily consults the CCP branch leadership to ensure that she is following the correct path. For Dr Li the intrusion of the 'masses' (in the form of Master Chen) into therapeutic decision-making, and even into the operating theatre later on in the film, is entirely natural. Dr Luo's major interaction with the CCP, on the other hand, is to gloat over the hospital's track record with acupuncture anaesthesia; he is presumably trying to curry favour with officials in order to advance his own career. His careerism is also reflected in his foot-dragging which, as we will see, escalates into attempts to sabotage both Dr Li and Dr Ding.

With the CCP branch leadership's affirmation, Dr Li visits other hospitals and clinics to research Old Yang's medical history. It emerges that a decade ago, Yang was the recipient of a botched procedure at a different hospital, which actually worsened his heart condition. Back in the Shanghai People's Hospital, Old Yang is upbeat and talks to his fellow patients about the amazing power of acupuncture anaesthesia. When Dr Li does her rounds in the wards – mopping the floor herself in another selfless act of kindness and care – Old Yang recalls the steps in his operation that Dr Li has asked him to memorise. Dr Li interjects, 'During the operation, tell me when you feel thirsty so I can feed you oranges!' and Old Yang bursts into song, 'Besides eating oranges, I will sing revolutionary model operas: "Nothing will defeat the Communists!"'

Old Yang spells out what is at stake:

You treat the workers, peasants and soldiers like a family. I was operated on in Hujiang 沪江 Hospital and those aristocrats didn't care for workers at all. The revisionist medical care and public health line (*xiuzheng zhuyi yiliao weisheng luxian* 修正主义医疗卫生路线) must be criticised. For now, I'm not just your patient but also your comrade protecting Chairman Mao's revolutionary medical care line!

Dr Li clutches Old Yang's hands and exclaims, 'Let's win this battle together!'

In the corridor, Dr Ding expresses his doubts about the operation. Dr Luo appears to have been undermining his junior colleague's confidence by feeding Dr Ding 'a lot of materials', putting forward 'too many difficult issues' regarding Old Yang's procedure, and repeatedly reminding Dr Ding of the hospital's achievement thus far in acupuncture anaesthesia. Dr Li replies emphatically, looking directly into the camera and addressing the viewer thus:

> When the Party and the People need us to step forward, how can we flinch from difficulties and danger? Treating Master Yang's illness isn't just a matter of saving lives (*jiuming* 救命); it's for revolutionising life (or simply 'revolution', *geming* 革命)! We've the duty to help him recover as soon as possible, so that he can contribute to socialist construction for years and decades to come. Master Yang's operation isn't just about technical issues. It's a battle between two lines. Don't be a blind believer in this foreign mumbo-jumbo (*yangbenben* 洋本本). Let's go among the masses!

This speech is followed by an extended montage of Dr Li and Dr Ding consulting their colleagues. Dr Ding enthusiastically shows the fruit of their research to Du Luo. Once again Dr Luo's attitude is contemptuous; he claims that 'even the most experienced doctor dare not try the operation'. This time Dr Luo threatens Dr Ding explicitly, telling him not to throw away his career over a pointless case. Dr Ding furiously walks away and says that he will continue studying acupuncture anaesthesia with Dr Li. When he arrives at Dr Li's office, the door is left ajar and Dr Ding makes a shocking discovery. Dr Li has been experimenting on herself with dangerous acupuncture points and procedures. She asks her colleague Dr Feng to 'stick [the needle] further in to enhance stimulation', even though the needle's depth is 'already beyond the prescribed range' and Dr Li risks having her pleura punctured (Figure 2.4). Dr Li heroically says, 'to ensure the safety of Old Yang's operation, we've got to take some risks! . . . Be brave!' Dr Feng resumes in tears, while Dr Ding leaves without alerting his two colleagues.

Old Yang has another heart attack, and Dr Li argues that the operation must be performed without further delay. However, at an all-staff meeting, Dr Luo continues to be obstructive and wants to transfer Old Yang to the Department of Internal Medicine. This sparks a climactic showdown between Dr Li and Dr Luo. Dr Luo again reiterates that the hard work in accumulating 92 successful acupuncture anaesthesia cases will go to waste if Old Yang's operation fails. Dr Li accuses Dr Luo of using acupuncture anaesthesia 'to pursue personal fame and fortune (*mingli* 名利)'; Dr Luo in turn attacks Dr Li for treating patients like laboratory animals. Dr Feng reveals that Dr Li has been selflessly experimenting with acupoints on her own body. Dr Ding discloses the earlier conversation in which Dr Luo orders him to select a bunch of 'easy' patients to operate on

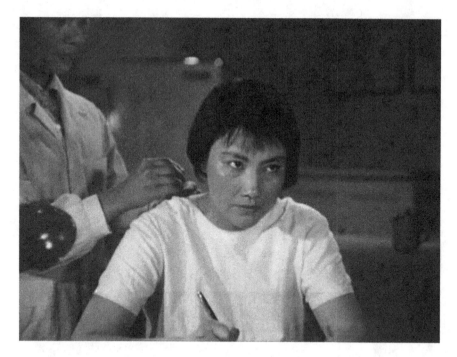

Figure 2.4 Dr Li sacrifices herself through self-experimentation

with acupuncture anaesthesia, to reach the target of 100 cases. Dr Ding chastises Dr Luo, 'After the Great Proletarian Cultural Revolution, why do you still behave like this?' Stunned by Dr Ding's insubordination, and sensing the anger among his colleagues, Dr Luo feebly complains, 'Is this not going too far?'

Dr Li replies that there is no such thing as 'going too far' (*tai guofen* 太过分), echoing the rhetoric in Mao Zedong's 'Report on an Investigation into the Peasant Movement in Hunan' (1927). She delivers a long speech (Figure 2.5):

> Don't think that after revisionism has been criticised during the Great Proletarian Cultural Revolution, that there'll be no more struggles (*douzheng* 斗争). No! Things never stay calm under the shadowless lamp. The bourgeoisie are competing with us at any moment for the scalpel. If we aren't vigilant, and deviate from Chairman Mao's revolutionary line, then revisionism will be restored! Take Master Yang for example. More than a decade ago, he was hospitalised for his heart condition. That hospital was called Hujiang Hospital. At that time, Master Yang actually improved with medication. But a surgeon, in his pursuit of personal fame and fortune, hastily operated on Master Yang. Because of the doctor's sloppy surgery, Master Yang's heart was permanently damaged. His heart disease got worse after he was discharged. That's why he's such a severely ill patient now. Today, can we forget the

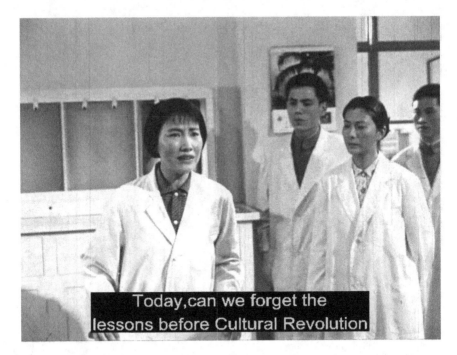

Figure 2.5 Dr Li, supported by other junior doctors, delivers a long speech against Dr Luo, in the climactic conflict between the two that resembles a 'struggle session'

lessons from the Cultural Revolution? Can we forget the workers', peasants' and soldiers' criticisms of the bourgeois Ministry of Gentlemen's Health, and drive Master Yang out of our hospital?

Humiliated, Dr Luo storms out of the meeting. Dr Li takes over and calls on her colleagues to 'let Mao Zedong Thought guide our silver needles and our scalpels'. In the next scene Master Chen, the CCP branch secretary, tells Dr Li that the CCP is paying a great deal of attention to Old Yang's case. Master Chen will summon help to 'keep on criticising [Dr Luo's] ideology of seeking fame and fortune' and 'to straighten him out in practice'. Dr Li finds Dr Luo sitting alone in the hospital gardens. Dr Luo confesses that he was the one who operated on Old Yang a decade ago – a fact that Dr Li already knows from her research into Old Yang's medical history. She tells Dr Luo:

Throughout the Cultural Revolution, the Party has saved many medical practitioners from an erroneous line, hoping that they'll progress with Chairman Mao's revolutionary line. However, not everybody can follow through. . . . Things that have happened today are very serious. In the past you rushed to operate, but today you dare not approve the operation. Your behaviour is different but the essence is the same. It's the bourgeois thought of pursuing personal fame and fortune.

As Dr Li checks on Old Yang in the middle of the night, she discovers that Old Yang has written a 'Statement of Determination' (*juexin shu* 决心书), in which he thanks Chairman Mao and the doctors. Old Yang hopes that the doctors can gain knowledge for the betterment of humankind, regardless of his operation's outcome. The following day, Dr Li and Dr Luo walk in front of 'Big Character Posters' (*dazibao* 大字报) plastered all over the hospital's bulletin boards – in a long lateral tracking shot – which all vehemently criticise Dr Luo's bourgeois and revisionist mentality (Figure 2.6). After being shown Old Yang's Statement, Dr Luo admits that he has 'lost his way again' and that it is 'very difficult to reform one's world outlook' (*shijieguan gaizhao* 世界观改造).

Old Yang's operation finally takes place, with Dr Ding acting as chief surgeon and Dr Li maintaining anaesthesia through acupuncture and an electrical amplifier, as well as Master Chen observing. Old Yang is conscious throughout. Dr Luo loiters in the corridor, fearing judgment from his junior colleagues. Master Chen urges Dr Luo to stop being 'trapped in [his] own circle', and he joins the surgical team. The operation hits a snag and there appears to be a 'misplaced artery' and heavy bleeding, and Old Yang's blood pressure plummets. This is fixed when

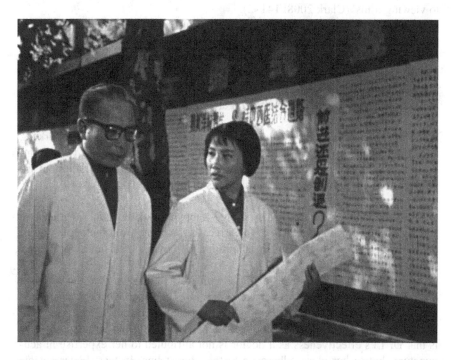

Figure 2.6 A long lateral tracking shot as Dr Li and Dr Luo walk in front of 'Big Character Posters'

Dr Li stimulates an additional set of acupoints. A fully conscious Old Yang takes a sip of orange juice. The operation is a resounding success and the team accompanies Old Yang back to the ward. A patient asks if Dr Luo has taken part in the operation, and he replies, 'No, our comrades have carried out a great operation on me!'

Tellingly, *Silver Needle* does suggest the possibility of reform and conversion for a reactionary like Dr Luo. When Dr Luo protests that accusations of him 'pursuing fame and fortune' have gone 'too far', in fact Dr Li has not gone far enough. She never mentions to her colleagues or reports to the CCP that Dr Luo was the culprit behind the botched surgery carried out on Old Yang at Hujiang Hospital. Dr Li, as the perfect Maoist doctor, must be politically steadfast and vigilant, and is able to struggle against co-workers – including people in positions of authority – who have deviated from the Maoist line and whose selfishness, if left unrectified, is infectious and corrupting. Nevertheless, the perfect Maoist doctor must also allow 'deviants' to see the errors of their ways, with the assistance of the Party. At the end of the film, Dr Luo admits that his junior colleagues have 'changed his heart' (*huanxin* 换心) and he joins the progressive side. As Paul Clark points out, characters who are permitted to reform their political outlook are a major innovation in late-Cultural Revolution cinema; they are called 'change characters' (*zhuanbian renwu* 转变人物) and the emergence of these characters is 'best explained with reference to the naturalistic expectations audiences brought to viewing films' (Clark 2008: 141–2).

In the penultimate scene, Master Chen speaks into the camera: 'Acupuncture anaesthesia is a newborn socialist thing. Only through the Great Proletarian Cultural Revolution could medicine make such remarkable progress'. Old Yang thanks Chairman Mao for giving him a 'second life' and holds aloft an acupuncture needle with gratitude and pride (Figure 2.7). Dr Li takes the needle, looks at the audience, and has the final word (Figure 2.8):

> This silver needle represents Chairman Mao's great care towards workers, peasants and soldiers. We must firmly carry out Chairman Mao's revolutionary line, and serve workers, peasants and soldiers better! This traditional silver needle will make great contributions to humankind!

The film finally ends with Dr Li visiting a happy and healthy Old Yang, back in action at the Shanghai Steel Mill, which recalls the scene from the beginning of the film when Dr Li volunteers her labour and thereby maintains close proximity with the proletariat.

Acupuncture anaesthesia was extremely unlikely to have worked the way that *Silver Needle* portrays – if it ever worked at all. The scene where a 'misplaced artery' is found in Old Yang's heart and is miraculously fixed by Dr Li is particular jarring because it seems scientifically impossible. But the larger point here is that Dr Li's effectiveness as a doctor is not attributed to her expertise in acupuncture, but to her close adherence to the Maoist line. In fact, *Silver Needle* promotes a political epistemology that highlights self-sacrifice and de-emphasises

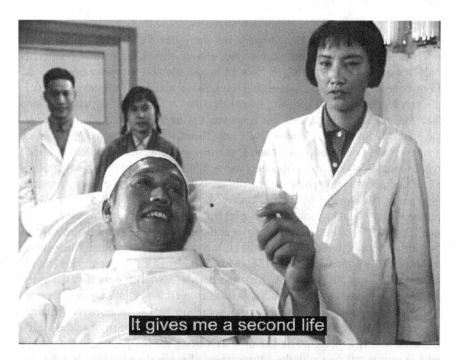

It gives me a second life

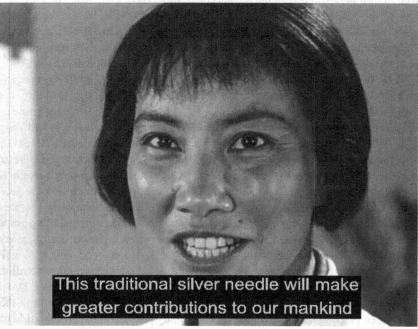

This traditional silver needle will make greater contributions to our mankind

Figure 2.7 and 2.8 Old Yang holds the eponymous 'silver needle' and thanks Chairman Mao; Dr Li looks into the camera

expertise – the Cultural Revolution interpretation of the Bethune story. Dr Li does investigate Old Yang's medical history, but she is never shown to consult scientific manuals or acupuncture scholarship, and dismisses the research materials that Dr Luo feeds to Dr Ding as 'foreign mumbo-jumbo' (*yangbenben* 洋本本) from bourgeois nations. Instead, selfless, self-sacrificial self-experimentation is the privileged means to generate knowledge that is empirical, experiential, and therefore reliable. Dr Li tests the acupoints on herself and records the analgesic effects before using them on Old Yang. There is nothing particular 'Chinese' about self-experimentation, of course; the history of western medicine is filled with examples of doctors deliberately exposing themselves to pathogenic materials or toxins that yielded new cures (Altman 1998). But self-experimentation also aligns with Mao's influential philosophical essay 'On Practice' (1937), in which he argues that 'human knowledge arise[s] from practice and in turn serve[s] practice' (Mao 1937). This epistemology is anti-'book-worship', and is designed to 'negate the predictive or guiding role of theory, and the consequent hegemony of "experts"' (Schmalzer 2008: 126). Moreover, Dr Li's self-experimentation is hazardous; she could potentially puncture her chest wall leading to a collapsed lung (pneumothorax). The operation is itself dangerous – Old Yang is a severely ill patient undergoing heart surgery – but somehow Dr Li's manoeuvres with her needles avert disaster. The film highlights, once again, the 'spirit of selflessness': a doctor who is willing to risk her own well-being for her patient, and a patient who in turn is satisfied with the advancement of medical knowledge and the victory of the Maoist line even if he dies from the procedure. *Silver Needle* suggests that risk-taking behaviours can reap fantastic, truly transformative rewards. A risky medical operation is analogous – or even identical – to risky revolutionary politics, hence Dr Li's proclamation about 'saving and revolutionising lives'.

There are clear ambivalences and contradictions in *Silver Needle*'s propagandist messages. Even setting aside the issue of efficacy and (im)plausibility, the film shows that acupuncture anaesthesia can really only play a supporting role to open-heart surgery. Ultimately, it is the chief surgeon Dr Ding who saves Old Yang using a Western medical treatment and Western surgical techniques. Moreover, Old Yang's surgery has to be carried out with the aid of acupuncture anaesthesia because, clinically speaking, he is too severely ill to take conventional anaesthetics. In other words, acupuncture anaesthesia is something of which Chinese people should feel immensely proud – it works when western medicine fails – but it is simultaneously a *last resort*. Finally, to a modern viewer, there is something gratifying about a workplace drama in which an earnest junior female doctor stands up against a scheming senior male manager for a greater good. *Silver Needle* is unencumbered with any subplots regarding romantic relationships or familial attachments. But it is not a straightforward tale of feminist empowerment. Dr Li relies on a male mentor in Master Chen, who appears at key points in the film – the committee meeting that reaffirms Dr Li's treatment protocol, the organisation of 'big character posters' that attack Dr Luo – to uphold the CCP line. Nevertheless, given that the archetype of the 'selfless doctor' remains tremendously powerful in popular imagination and in the self-fashioning of the medical profession around the world, a Cultural Revolution propaganda film like *Silver Needle* opens up fascinating historical, comparative questions on medical politics and ethics.

Notes

1 The English name of the film is sometimes given as *Song of Acupuncture Treatment*, for example in the 2003 Guangzhou Beauty Media DVD edition. As far as I can tell the film has no official English name, and I do not use *Song of Acupuncture Treatment* because it does not adequately translate the Chinese original.
2 Notable films about medicine from the 'Cultural Revolution decade' include: *Spring Shoots* (*Chunmiao* 春苗, 1975, dir. Xie Jin 谢晋); *Red Rain* (*Hongyu* 红雨, 1975, dir. Cui Wei 崔嵬); *By the Yanming Lake* (*Yanming hu pan* 雁鸣湖畔, 1976, dir. Gao Tianhong 高天红); *Youth* (*Qingchun* 青春, 1977, dir. Xie Jin 谢晋). All these films are specifically about Chinese farmers who become 'barefoot doctors'.
3 In addition, Paul Clark has produced statistics on feature film production between 1949 and 1986 (Clark 1987: 185). In 1974, 17 films (including *Silver Needle*) were made.
4 Lou Jicheng is, incidentally, the father of 'Sixth Generation' director Lou Ye 娄烨 (1965–), whose film *Blind Massage* (*Tuina* 推拿) is discussed by Chris Berry in this volume.
5 The term *xinsheng shiwu* 新生事物 ('newborn thing' or 'new socialist thing') was developed by the Gang of Four, often employed during the Cultural Revolution. It 'functioned as a kind of open bank account, in which the radical faction could deposit everything it considered as an achievement' (Landsberger 2016).
6 The propaganda painting used in the film (see Figure 2.2) is based on a photograph of Norman Bethune, taken by Wu Yinxian 吴印咸 (1900–1994) at Sunjiazhuang 孙家庄 village in Laiyuan 涞源 County, Hebei Province in 1939. (Zhiyuan Chen 2013; Zhen Ni 2002: 69–72; Pratt n.d.)

Filmography

An Ode to the Silver Needle Under a Shadowless Lamp (*Wuyingdeng xia song yinzhen* 无影灯下颂银针), dir. Sang Hu 桑弧, 1974.

By the Yanming Lake (*Yanming hu pan* 雁鸣湖畔), dir. Gao Tianhong 高天红, 1976.

Red Detachment of Women (*Hongse niangzi jun* 红色娘子军), dir. Xie Jin 谢晋, 1961.

Red Rain (*Hongyu* 红雨), dir. Cui Wei 崔嵬, 1975.

Shanghai Spring (*Shanghai zhi chun* 上海之春), dir. Sang Hu 桑弧, 1965.

Spring Shoots (*Chunmiao* 春苗), dir. Xie Jin 谢晋, 1975.

Youth (*Qingchun* 青春), dir. Xie Jin 谢晋, 1977.

Bibliography

Allan, T. and Gordon, S. (2009) *The Scalpel, The Sword: The Story of Doctor Norman Bethune*, Originally published in 1952, Toronto: Dundurn.

Altman, L.K. (1998) *Who Goes First? The Story of Self-Experimentation in Medicine*, Berkeley: University of California Press.

Andreas, J. (2009) *Rise of the Red Engineers: The Cultural Revolution and the Origins of China's New Class*, Stanford: Stanford University Press.

Chen Zhiyuan (2013) Wu Yinxian (1900–1994), in Yuwu Song (ed.) *Biographical Dictionary of the People's Republic of China*, Jefferson, NC: McFarland & Co., p. 329.

Clark, P. (1987) *Chinese Cinema: Culture and Politics Since 1949*, Cambridge: Cambridge University Press.

———. (2008) *The Chinese Cultural Revolution: A History*, Cambridge: Cambridge University Press.

Donald, S.H. (2000) *Public Secrets, Public Spaces: Cinema and Civility in China*, Lanham, MD: Rowman & Littlefield.

Fan, Fa-ti (2012) "Collective Monitoring, Collective Defense": Science, Earthquake, and Politics in Communist China, *Science in Context*, 25: 127–54.

Fang Xiaoping (2012) *Barefoot Doctors and Western Medicine in China*, Rochester: University of Rochester Press.

Hannant, L. (ed.) (1998) *The Politics of Passion: Norman Bethune's Writing and Art*, Toronto: University of Toronto Press.

Hayot, E. (2009) *The Hypothetical Mandarin: Sympathy, Modernity, and Chinese Pain*, Oxford: Oxford University Press.

Hsu, E. (1996) Innovations in Acumoxa: Acupuncture Analgesia, Scalp and Ear Acupuncture in the People's Republic of China, *Social Science and Medicine*, 42: 421–30.

Hudecek, J. (2014) *Reviving Ancient Chinese Mathematics: Mathematics, History and Politics in the Work of Wu Wen-Tsun*, London: Routledge.

Lampton, D.M. (1977) *The Politics of Medicine in China: The Policy Process, 1949–1977*, Boulder, CO: Westview Press.

Landsberger, S. (2016) New Socialist Things, *Chineseposters.net*, https://chineseposters.net/themes/new-socialist-things.php, accessed 1 January 2018.

Li, Lan Angela (2015) The Edge of Expertise: Representing Barefoot Doctors in Cultural Revolution China, *Endeavour*, 39: 160–7.

Lu Wei 卢威 (2006) Hongse niangzi jun lianzhang Zhu Xijuan 红色娘子军连长祝希娟 (Zhu Xijuan the Company Commander in *Red Detachment of Women*), *Renmin ribao haiwai ban* 人民日报海外版 (People's Daily Overseas Edition), 13 January, www.people.com.cn/GB/paper39/16636/1464811.html, accessed 1 January 2018.

Lynteris, C. (2011) "In Memory of Norman Bethune": Two Resurrections of the "Spirit of Selflessness" in Maoist China, *Journal of the British Association for Chinese Studies*, 1: 21–48.

———. (2013) *The Spirit of Selflessness in Maoist China: Socialist Medicine and the New Man*, Basingstoke: Palgrave Macmillan.

Mao Zedong 毛泽东 (1927) Hunan nongmin yundong kaocha baogao 湖南农民运动考察报告(Report on an Investigation into the Peasant Movement in Hunan), 28 March 1927, www.marxists.org/reference/archive/mao/selected-works/volume-1/mswv1_2.htm, accessed 1 January 2018.

——— (1937) Shijian lun 实践论 (On Practice), www.marxists.org/reference/archive/mao/selected-works/volume-1/mswv1_16.htm, accessed 1 January 2018.

——— (1939) Jinian Bai Qiu'en 纪念白求恩 (In Memory of Norman Bethune), www.marxists.org/reference/archive/mao/selected-works/volume-2/mswv2_25.htm, accessed 1 January 2018.

——— (1944) Wei renmin fuwu 为人民服务 (Serve the People), www.marxists.org/reference/archive/mao/selected-works/volume-3/mswv3_19.htm, accessed 1 August 2019.

——— (1945) Yugong yishan 愚公移山 (The Foolish Old Man Who Removed the Mountains), www.marxists.org/reference/archive/mao/selected-works/volume-3/mswv3_26.htm, accessed 1 August 2019.

——— (1965) Zhongyang guanyu weisheng gongzuo de zhishi 中央关于卫生工作的指示 (Directive on Public Health), www.marxists.org/reference/archive/mao/selected-works/volume-9/mswv9_41.htm, accessed 1 January 2018.

Mittler, B. (2012) *A Continuous Revolution: Making Sense of Cultural Revolution Culture*, Cambridge, MA: Harvard University Asia Center.

Mullaney, T.S. (2012) The Moveable Typewriter: How Chinese Typists Developed Predictive Text during the Height of Maoism, *Technology and Culture*, 53: 777–814.

Ni Zhen (2002) *Memoirs from the Beijing Film Academy: The Genesis of China's Fifth Generation*, Durham, NC: Duke University Press.

Pang Laikwan (2017) *The Art of Cloning: Creative Production During China's Cultural Revolution*, London: Verso.

Pickowicz, P.G. (2013) *China on Film: A Century of Exploration, Confrontation and Controversy*, Lanham, MD: Rowman & Littlefield.

Pratt, L. (n.d.) Wu Yinxian, International Center of Photography, www.icp.org/browse/archive/constituents/wu-yinxian?all/all/all/all/0, accessed 1 January 2018.

Rogaski, R. (2002) Nature, Annihilation, and Modernity: China's Korean War Germ-Warfare Experience Reconsidered, *Journal of Asian Studies*, 61: 381–415.

———. (2004) *Hygienic Modernity: Meanings of Health and Disease in Treaty-Port China*, Berkeley: University of California Press.

Scheid, V. (2002) *Chinese Medicine in Contemporary China: Plurality and Synthesis*, Durham, NC: Duke University Press.

———. (2013) The People's Republic of China, in T.J. Hinrichs and L. Barnes (eds.) *Chinese Medicine and Healing: An Illustrated History*, Cambridge, MA: The Belknap Press of Harvard University Press, pp. 239–83.

Schmalzer, S. (2008) *The People's Peking Man: Popular Science and Human Identity in Twentieth-Century China*, Chicago: University of Chicago Press.

Stewart, R. and Stewart, S. (2011) *Phoenix: The Life of Norman Bethune*, Montreal: McGill-Queen's University Press.

Taylor, K. (2005) *Chinese Medicine in Early Communist China, 1945–63: A Medicine of Revolution*, London: Routledge.

Xiao Zhiwei (1988) Sang Hu (Li Peilin), in Yingjin Zhang and Zhiwei Xiao (eds.) *Encyclopaedia of Chinese Film*, London: Routledge, p. 296.

Zhongguo dianyingjia xiehui dianying shi yanjiubu 中国电影家协会电影史研究部 (ed.) (1982) *Zhongguo dianyingjia liezhuan* 中国电影家列传 (Biographies of Chinese Filmmakers), Beijing: Zhongguo dianying chubanshe, Vol. 6, pp. 391–403.

3 Self-care, *Yangsheng*, and mutual aid in Zhang Yang's *Shower* (1999)[1]

Michael J. Clark

Introduction

The concept of self-care in healthcare and medicine has become one of the most widespread and pervasive themes in contemporary debates and commentaries about health education, health maintenance, and health policy.[2] However, while there is broad agreement as to its importance, there is no one generally accepted definition of self-care. Self-care has been variously defined as 'care of the self without medical or other professional consultation' (Random House Dictionary 2017), 'the actions that individuals take for themselves, on behalf of and with others in order to develop, protect, maintain and improve their health [and] wellbeing' (Self-Care Forum U.K.) and

> The actions people take for themselves, their children and their families to stay fit and maintain good physical and mental health; meet social and psychological needs; prevent illness or accidents; care for minor ailments and long-term conditions; and maintain health and wellbeing after an acute illness [or injury].
>
> (U.K. Department of Health 2005)

According to Wikipedia, 'Self-care includes all health decisions [which] people, [either] as individuals or as consumers, make for themselves and their families to ensure they are physically and mentally fit' (Wikipedia: Self-Care). These and other definitions in common usage vary widely, notably with regard to the assumed scope of self-care (whether it is confined to physical and mental health, or extends more broadly to 'well-being' and psychosocial functioning); the extent to which self-help is seen either as a largely autonomous sphere of lay health choices or as an activity normally carried on in close collaboration with health professionals, and the extent to which self-care is seen as mainly a self-regarding activity or as a shared responsibility not only for the health of one individual but of his or her family, friends, neighbours, and co-workers (Easton 1993: 384–87; Webbe *et al.* 2013: 101–6).

But while such definitions undoubtedly help us to understand the importance of lay conceptions of health and the centrality of lay decision-making in healthcare choices, they scarcely do justice to the richness, complexity, and long histories of many of the ideas and practices included under the heading of 'self-care' both in Chinese and 'Western' medicine. In China, 'self-care' is closely associated, though not synonymous with, the concept and practice of *yangsheng* 養生, the traditional Chinese 'art of nurturing life' in all its various forms, whose origins may be traced back at least to the Han Dynasty, if not earlier (Lo 2001; Hinrichs and Barnes 2013: 11, 14, 69–70, 153–5, 166–7). Since the end of the Cultural Revolution and the partial relaxation of political controls over individual life-style and leisure choices which followed, *yangsheng* has undergone a consider-able revival in popularity, especially among older age groups in the cities, while in recent years there has also been a significant growth of hybrid commercialised forms of self-care which combine traditional Chinese health-related practices like *taiji, qigong,* and Buddhist meditation with new ideas and practices drawn from both modern Chinese and Western self-help movements and popular psychologies (Dear 2012; Farquhar and Zhang 2012; Farquhar 2013: 272–4).

In the discourse of western medicine and healthcare, the concept of self-care has a similarly long history and a variety of complex meanings. As Michel Foucault has emphasised, the idea and practice of self-care – or rather, of the 'Cultivation of the Self' – was already well established in Antiquity, and figures prominently in the works of philosophers and moralists such as Plato, Epictetus, Plutarch, Seneca, and Marcus Aurelius (Foucault 1990: 37–68), while for the Epi-cureans, philosophy itself was 'a permanent exercise in the care of oneself' (*ibid.*: 46). Subsequently, the classical tradition of self-care through self-cultivation went through many vicissitudes, partial revivals, and re-workings, but by the end of the twentieth century, for many people in the West, the 'care of the self' or 'self-cultivation' had become little more than a largely decontextualized, ad hoc com-bination of trendy health fads, including healthy dieting, jogging and exercise regimes, therapeutic dance routines, meditation, and self-help psychology.

In recent years, the classical Western discourse of self-cultivation, originally addressed to a gentlemanly and scholarly elite, has largely been replaced by a new, more impersonal and bureaucratic discourse concerning the strategic impor-tance attributed to self-care in the development of modern healthcare systems. In this view, self-care, which has been defined as 'the [intentional] care of one-self without medical, professional or other assistance or oversight' (Stedman's Medical Dictionary 2002, entry 'Self-Care'), is seen as accounting for most of the so-called 'continuum' or 'sliding scale of health care', up to around 80% of all healthcare in the U.K., according to one recent estimate by the U.K. Self-Care Forum (Self-Care Forum U.K.; Self-Care Continuum). British-based health educators and health economists believe that raising people's awareness of the benefits of self-care in the forms of healthy diets, regular moderate exercise, healthy and temperate life-style choices (giving up smoking, reducing alcohol consumption, etc.), and self-reliance in the treatment and management of minor common ailments and symptoms like winter coughs and sneezes can not only enhance people's health and well-being and prolong life but could also save the National Health Service up to £2 billion a year, according to the U.K. Self-Care

Forum (Self-Care Forum U.K.). Self-care is seen as a crucial form of primary care for patients with chronic conditions such as diabetes and heart disease, as well as some psychiatric conditions such as Obsessive-Compulsive Disorder, and self-care or self-management education, often seen as an essential first step towards 'patient activation' (Hibbard and Gilburt 2014),[3] is seen as complementing more traditional forms of patient education in such a way as to help people living with chronic conditions to enjoy a better quality of life. In the U.K., one week in every mid-November is officially designated 'NHS Self-Care Week', an event which has taken place every year since 2009, at first under the auspices of the Department of Health and subsequently of the national Self-Care Forum formed in May 2011 as a joint venture by the NHS Alliance, the Royal College of Nursing, the Royal College of General Practitioners, Public Health England, and the U.K. consumer health industry. The most recent such N.H.S. Self-Care Week was held on 12–18 November 2018, with the slogan 'Choosing Self-Care for Life' (N.H.S. Self-Care Week 2018). In October 2016, the English Local Government Association, which since 2013 has taken on important responsibilities for public health and health education in England and Wales, published *Helping People to Look After Themselves: A Guide on Self-Care*, to help local authorities devise and implement local strategies to promote self-care (Local Government Association for England and Wales 2016). At the launch of the new guide, the L.G.A. stated that 'Millions of visits to the doctor for coughs and colds are unnecessary' and advised people instead to visit their local pharmacies or the NHS Web site, claiming that greater self-reliance on the part of the public could help save general medical practitioners up to an hour's consulting time every day (Local Government Association Press Release 2016). Self-care, or 'Improving and maintaining your mental well-being', also features prominently on the Web site of Mind, the principal UK mental health charity backed by both psychiatrists and mental health service users (Mind 2018), and in much contemporary debate about how best to advise people living with mental health conditions to help themselves.

At the same time, self-care has taken on a variety of more specialised meanings in certain sub-sectors of the healthcare system. Thus self-care figures largely in modern nursing theory, where the 'self-care deficit theory' of the American nursing educator Dorothea Orem (1914–2007) has been highly influential as a way of defining the sphere of nursing as occupying the space between self-care, on the one hand, and specialised professional medical or surgical intervention on the other. Viewed in this light, the restoration or attainment of the maximum level of self-care appropriate to the condition and to the patient is seen as the ultimate goal of nursing (Orem 2001; Hartweg 1991; Nursing Theory; Theoretical Foundations of Nursing 2011). In the work of Donald Kalsched and other Jungian psychotherapists, self-care or, more precisely, 'the psyche's archetypal self-care system' (Kalsched 1996: 4), is understood as a deep psychological defence mechanism developed to protect young and growing personalities from the effects of overwhelming physical, emotional or psychological trauma through intra-psychical processes of dissociation, blocking, and 'splitting off' (*ibid.*: Chs. 1–6). This is a highly specialised usage which hardly enjoys widespread currency outside the rather select circles of Jungian analysis. But whether as a potential cure for the chronic deficits of healthcare systems in both developed and developing countries, as a means of successfully managing chronic physical or mental health conditions without the need for constant medical supervision, or as a key element of nursing theory and practice, raising the level of effective self-care through 'patient activation' is a pervasive theme in modern healthcare discourse and a key strategic goal of contemporary healthcare policy-making.

Self-care in Zhang Yang's *Shower*

All this may seem a far cry from the very concrete, small-scale, localized, and person-centred forms of self-care portrayed in the Chinese director Zhang Yang's 1999 tragi-comic film *Shower* 洗澡 (*Xi Zao*), a 'family drama' of father-son relationships set in an old-style privately owned Beijing communal bath-house.[4] But despite the distinctive setting of Zhang Yang's film and the great cultural distance between the very traditional, unmedicalised forms of healthcare and aids to well-being portrayed in *Shower* and the modern Western medical discourse around self-care and patient activation, the stark contrast between Chinese tradition and modernity within the film itself permits certain indirect but instructive comparisons to be made between Chinese and Western understandings of the role of self-care and mutual aid in the maintenance of health and well-being. *Shower* presents a vision of self-care among the mainly elderly and entirely male clientele of a somewhat dilapidated, unpretentious bath-house in an old *hutong* neighbourhood of Beijing which is in sharp contrast to the hurried, mechanical, and totally impersonal hygienic services provided in the fast-paced, money- and technology-dominated world of contemporary China, as shown in the unforgettable opening scene at the totally mechanised urban 'Shower Station'. In Old Liu's bath-house, the all-male and mostly elderly clientele enjoy the benefits of a person-centred culture of care based on the traditional creature comforts of the bath-house (massage, cupping, hairdressing, and pedicure, as well as bathing) and the values of personal service, face-to-face contact, mutual respect, and a broad measure of tolerance for the eccentricities and failings of others, all mediated through the physical and spiritual healing powers of water and massage. The bath-house serves as a refuge from the modern world where those clients fortunate enough to be able to spend several hours a day bathing can sip tea or rice wine, obtain relief from their various aches and pains, read the newspapers, play Chinese chess, gamble on fighting crickets, seek advice and guidance – or at any rate sympathy – for their marital and domestic woes, imagine themselves as operatic tenors, exchange gossip and insults, and generally pass the time in relaxing and mostly harmless pursuits. In the process, they learn to understand and appreciate each other's qualities, limitations, and foibles and in doing so, reaffirm and strengthen their common humanity. For the devoted proprietor Mr Liu, his two sons Da Ming and Er Ming, and their regular clientele, the bath-house serves as a kind of school in the art of living well which does as much to enhance their psychological and spiritual well-being, and ultimately their common humanity, as it does their bodily health and physical comfort.

Self-care, *Yangsheng* and mutual aid in *Shower*

In another context, all these various creature comforts and forms of healthy recreation would probably be regarded as aspects of *yangsheng*, the traditional Chinese art and practice of 'nurturing life' (Farquhar and Zhang 2012: 14–18, 21–2, 26–8). However, the relationship between the forms of physical therapy and pleasant pastimes depicted in *Shower* and the wider culture of *yangsheng* is not quite as straightforward as this might suggest. Indeed, if we take Judith Farquhar and Zhang Qicheng's book *Ten Thousand Things: Nurturing Life in Contemporary Beijing* (2012) as a guide, we find that while this book is all about *yangsheng*, the authors do not speak of 'Self-Care' as such. There is no entry 'Self-care' in the Index, although there are numerous references to 'Self-cultivation' (*zixiu* 自 修) and 'Self-health' (*ziwo baojian* 自我保健). Nor are there any references to bath-houses, bathing or water in the Index, although there are a few references to massage, particularly self-massage, and *qigong* and many to *taiji* and other aspects of Chinese medicine and healthcare which do not feature in the film (*ibid*.: 345–7). Several pages of Farquhar and Zhang's book are devoted to an appreciation of Ning Ying's 1993 film *For Fun* 找乐 (*Zhao Le*), which centres around the amateur outdoor performance of Chinese opera as a form of recreation, and there is also a brief discussion of Ning Ying's later film *Perpetual Motion* 无穷动 (*Wu qiong dong*) (2005), but curiously there are no references to Zhang Yang's *Shower* (*ibid*.: 90, 102–6). However, the film itself contains a number of scenes and visual clues which are clearly intended to place the physical comforts and amenities provided by the bath-house within a wider context of activities which are recognisably 'life-nurturing'. Thus we twice see a troupe of female fan-dancers rehearsing in the park very near to the bath-house entrance, along with a man in a shell-suit apparently practising *qigong*, while Old Liu and his younger son Er Ming's evening jogs through the park and the quarter take them past the local outdoor theatre in which Miao Zhuang, a shy fat boy who is one of the bath-house's regular clients and who fancies himself as a budding operatic tenor, attempts to give a rendition of 'O Sole Mio'. There are also a number of key scenes which clearly show that the three surviving members of the Liu family, father and sons, and at least some of their regular clients are fully aware of the deep psychological and symbolic resonance and even spiritual significance of water and of the bath-house as a kind of aquatic healing sanctuary. In addition to the dreamlike scenes harking back to the extraordinary sacrifices made by her peasant family to allow Er Ming's mother to take the traditional bath prescribed for the eve of a young girl's marriage in rural Shaanxi and to an epic Buddhist pilgrimage by an aged Tibetan grandmother and her granddaughter to bathe in a sacred, snowbound lake, there are a number of unmistakeable visual connections during the second half of the film to the idea of water as the source of all life, and as a gateway to the next world, to the maternal waters of the womb, and to immersion in water as a sign of both physical and spiritual rebirth and renewal. This is apparent not only in the scenes just described, but also in several others in which Er Ming slides beneath the waters of the bathhouse and holds his breath for a minute or more, at first in friendly competition with his father, but then latterly as a means of escape and possibly even suicide when faced with the abrupt and tragic ending of his previously ordered and secure way of life following his father's death and the authorities' decision to demolish the bath-house. At several points in the film, we also see altruistic love or compassion wordlessly manifested through the medium of water, as when Old Liu opens up the valves of the bath-house to allow his estranged elder son Da Ming to enjoy a shower, or when Er Ming unexpectedly intervenes with a garden hose at a local open-air variety show in the park to enable Miao Zhuang to overcome his shyness and finally perform 'O Sole Mio' in public. In a key scene half-way through the film, Da Ming is woken by a violent storm in the middle of the night, and goes to the aid of his elderly father who has climbed out onto the leaky glass roof in the torrential rain to try to stop the rainwater pouring into the bath-house with tarpaulin sheets, while in another important episode, Mr Zhang, a regular client who habitually takes refuge in the bath-house from his wife's constant nagging and scolding, eventually manages to overcome his impotence (or so we may infer) and be reconciled with his estranged wife in an after-hours tryst in the bath-house discreetly arranged by Mr Liu.

The story of Mr and Mrs Zhang is not without its comic side, but it also highlights the extent to which the bath-house and its culture of care have become a focal point for mutual aid involving both the staff and the clientele. In much contemporary discourse about the role of self-care in healthcare and medicine, self-care is implicitly contrasted with the hi-tech, capital- and labour-intensive forms of socialised medical and healthcare provision characteristic of most developed nations. But in *Shower,* self-care also goes hand-in-hand with relatively low-tech and spontaneous expressions of a communal lay tradition of mutual aid, which extends well beyond the sphere of physical health to include aspects of psychosocial and even spiritual well-being. Just as in Old Liu's bath-house, the care and maintenance of physical health go along with the nurturing and enhancement of emotional and spiritual well-being, so do self-care and mutual aid appear as two sides of the same coin. This is one of the most important 'messages' of the film, one which takes the discourse of self-care to a level seldom attained in modern Western discussions of the role of self-care in individual health maintenance or health policy for the 'community'.

Bodily and community care in 'Shower'

In *Shower,* 'self-care' is not a psychological process or psycho-therapeutic practice as such, nor is it a cure-all for the financial insolvency of healthcare systems, but rather, a system for maintaining bodily health and physical well-being through bathing, massage, cupping, tea-drinking, and other forms of relaxation, which indirectly serve to enhance the psychological and even spiritual well-being of the bath-house customers. The psychological benefits of the physical therapies offered by the bath-house are highlighted by wordlessly contrasting them with the hurried, highly impersonal and uncongenial experience provided by the fully automated 'Shower Station' which features so hilariously in the opening 'Human

Car Wash' sequence.[5] The 'self' in question is not the abstract entity of Western philosophy or psychoanalysis, but something much more like the 'body-self' described by Arthur Kleinman, Arthur Frank, and Havi Carel (Kleinman 1988: 11–13, 26–7; Frank 1995: 1–3, 27–52; Carel 2008: 13–14, 20, 22). Old Mr Liu takes great pride in the skill and professionalism with which he and his mentally challenged younger son Er Ming carry out their daily duties in the bath-house. But the type of care which their bath-house offers is about enjoying a physical place of refuge from the cares, worries, and responsibilities of the outside world in friendly company, and relieving anxiety and stress through creature comforts, gentle exercise, socializing, and informal mutual aid, and has nothing directly to do either with increasing the efficient use of scarce healthcare and nursing resources, defending vulnerable psyches from the overwhelming impact of traumatic memories, or even with the 'care of the soul' as such. Although there are moments when the register of the film shifts abruptly from the mundane level of daily life to the psychic realms of unconscious symbolism and spirituality, it does not directly engage in philosophical debates about the existence or nature of the 'self' or the soul. Rather, *Shower* is all about the dependence of everyday existential and emotional well-being on the shared cultivation and experience of certain traditional forms and practices of physical well-being, and the intimate connection between these forms and practices and a particular kind of therapeutic space and a certain old-fashioned Chinese way of urban living. This is the way of life characteristic of the old, now rapidly vanishing, inner city neighbourhoods with their low-rise, modest, cheek-by-jowl, single-storey houses and narrow, pedestrian-friendly streets and public open spaces which favour face-to-face contacts, neighbourhood gossip, mutual aid and the preservation of traditional forms of social relations and popular culture. In *Shower*, this is presented with some nostalgia, but not sentimentally or uncritically – the life of the old Beijing *hutong* neighbourhoods is portrayed with affection, but is not over-idealised or romanticised. Old Liu's bath-house is not proof against physical decay and death, and is largely powerless to prevent the violent intrusion of some of the worst aspects of contemporary Chinese life, including gangster violence, ruthless commercial exploitation, and the indifference of the Party and the state to the plight of ordinary people driven from their homes by wholesale redevelopment. But it does offer the regular customers (and, indeed, Old Liu and his sons) the reassurance of routine, companionship, and mutual tolerance, all of which allow the clientele to express themselves honestly, expose their frailties, ask for help, and sometimes even find relief from their woes in a shared semi-communal space.

However, the therapeutic and life-nurturing environment of the bath-house, with its deep though unspoken connection to nature and to the care and cure of the soul as well as of the body, is also shown as fragile, vulnerable to the forces of social and economic change, physical decay and death, severely limited by its exclusive homosociality, and doomed to extinction in face of the onslaughts of techno-modernity, rapid economic growth, and wholesale urban redevelopment. As one of the younger clients observes early on in the film, 'The pace of our lives is getting busier every day. Who can afford to spend the whole day in a bath-house?' It is scarcely a coincidence that Old Liu, who earlier has told his elder son Da Ming that he has devoted his whole life to the bath-house and at his age, is unwilling or unable to change his way of living, should himself die suddenly but quietly in the bath shortly after being given official notice of the bath-house's imminent destruction, together with that of the whole neighbourhood, to make way for some kind of intensive commercial or residential development.

Shower, Yangsheng and the digital world

Although this film was made barely 20 years ago, and while there are a few mobile phones in evidence (indeed, Mr Liu's sudden death occurs while Da Ming is momentarily out of the bath-room taking a call on his mobile from his wife in Shenzhen), mobile telecommunication is still clearly very much in its infancy in *Shower*, and we can be pretty sure that the bath-house has no Web site, let alone any social media presence. This is still very much a world of direct face-to-face contacts and exchanges – even the notice of the impending demolition of the bath-house is given in person by the local Party secretary. However, these facts also highlight the severe limitations of the old bath-house culture. It does not form part of any wider virtual network founded on shared interest and common therapeutic/*yangsheng* practice and is wholly dependent on the survival and physical integrity of the specific location, the bath-house itself, and the surrounding *hutong* quarter. In all these respects, in the digital world it could potentially be much stronger and more robust, attract a much larger and more varied clientele, bridge the age and gender gaps, and not be so dependent on the physical survival of the bath-house and the continued engagement of the Liu family in its day-to-day running. Indeed, such a shift has already happened to a considerable extent in communities like Hong Kong and in North America, where Web sites and E-magazines like http://*Yang-Sheng.com*, a very useful portal site for all manner of Chinese-derived or inspired health and healing practices, have attracted many followers not only among Chinese-Americans, but among seekers of a better way of living who have no specifically Chinese cultural heritage[6] (World Institute for Self-Healing, Inc.). But to return to the old Chinese bath-house culture so affectionately portrayed in *Shower*: while its amenities were only available to a fortunate few, the great beauty of the forms of care provided by Mr Liu's bath-house (and, indeed, of *yangsheng* culture generally) is that it was relatively sensitive and responsive to the needs and frailties of the individual, but without undermining the old communal values of social solidarity and shared responsibility for the welfare of all. It may well be argued that Zhang Yang's *Shower* presents a rather idealised, sentimental, and nostalgic view of traditional Chinese bath-house culture and urban living. But it also raises important questions not only about the nature and role of self-care and the values of mutual aid, but also about the relations between health and well-being, the urban environment, and human sociability which deserve more serious consideration and more concerted policy reflection and action than they have hitherto received either in China or in Western societies.

As has been noted elsewhere, the new and much-heralded 'Personalised Medicine' of tomorrow promises to individuate medical treatments to a much greater extent in accordance with the individual patient's particular strengths and weaknesses, especially those linked to genetic make-up, but at the cost of increasing the individual's sense of isolation and dependence on technical-medical experts, and of an accelerated loss of a sense of solidarity and shared community values and obligations (U.K. Academy of Medical Sciences 2015; Masters 2016; N.H.S. England 2016; Vollmann *et al*. 2016). Whether the large claims made for the potential future therapeutic benefits of Personalised Medicine will actually be borne out and, if so, whether this will mean a major shift of emphasis in healthcare practice away from generalised preventative measures towards ever more individuated hi-tech interventions at the cellular, genomic or molecular levels, remains to be seen. However, self-care is also a highly individuated form of healthcare, and even if the claims made for the new hi-tech version of Personalised Medicine should prove substantially justified, there will still be a great deal of scope for applying new and existing forms of self-care in areas such as health maintenance, accident and illness prevention, living with chronic disease and rehabilitation, while maintaining or enhancing well-being is also likely to require a more subtle and sustained approach in the medium and long terms than simply the application of hi-tech solutions. The great challenge for the future of healthcare will be to see whether the new forms of electronic and Web-based communication which characterise the digital world can increase the uptake of more traditional forms of self-care and *yangsheng* modalities and even boost the popularity of institutions like the Liu bath-house among all sections and age-groups of the community, thereby enhancing individual health and well-being, while at the same time effectively counteracting the tendency for the individual to become increasingly isolated and cut off from any sense of collective responsibility for the health of the whole community.

Notes

1 This paper began as a presentation to a joint Peking University-University College London Cross-Cultural Medical Humanities Conference-Workshop, *Self-Care in a Digital World*, held at the Institute of Advanced Studies, University College London, 7–9 November 2016. I am especially grateful to Dr Vivienne Lo (University College London) and Professor Chris Berry (King's College London) for helpful comments and suggestions on an earlier version, and to Dolly Yang and Penny Barrett (University College London) for invaluable assistance in the preparation of the manuscript.

2 The modern English-language literature on self-care in medicine and health care is very large and continually growing. The eight volumes to date of the international e-journal *SelfCare* (also known as *The Self Care Journal*), first published in 2010, give some idea of the scope and variety of recent theoretical and applied research and debates in the field (Self Care Journal 2010–).

3 I am especially grateful to Christina Yajin Lee (King's College London) for drawing my attention to this important dimension of 'self-care'.

4 *Shower* 洗澡 (*Xi Zao*), dir. Zhang Yang (Imar Film and Xi'an Film Studio, P.R. China, 1999); 92 mins. Zhang is also credited as principal author of the screenplay. Zhang Yang

张扬 (b. 1967) is usually regarded as one of the best-known members of the so-called 'Sixth Generation' or 'Urban Generation' of Chinese film-makers, a cohort characterised by a shared interest in the contemporary experiences of the Chinese urban population, especially individuals and groups disadvantaged or marginalised by rapid economic growth, urbanisation and changing patterns of family life. ***Shower*** was Zhang's second feature film following his debut with ***Spicy Love Soup*** 爱情麻辣烫 (*Aìqíng Má Là Tang*) in 1997. Though made on a very modest budget of US$350,000, with no very high expectation of domestic box-office success, ***Shower*** was favourably reviewed by many influential Western critics following its release at the Toronto International Film Festival in November 1999 and subsequently won a number of awards when screened in several Western film festivals in 1999–2001. For more details of the production, cast, box office, awards, etc., see https://en.wikipedia.org/wiki/Shower_(film) and http://www.imdb.com/title/tt0215369/

For Zhang and the 'Sixth Generation', see Zhang, Yinjin (2004): 291–92; Braester (2011): 179, and Berra (2014): 107. For generally favourable English-language reviews of ***Shower*** and interviews with Director Zhang, see Elley (September 1999); Porter (1999); Wilmington (July 2000); Palmer (July 2000); and Rayns (2001). For a more critical evaluation, see Chan (January 2009).

5 In the 'Chapters' menu of the multi-lingual DVD version of *Shower,* 'Chapter 1' is actually entitled 'Human Car-Wash'.
6 The monthly e-magazine *Yang-Sheng: Nurturing Life* is the organ of the 'World Institute for Self-Healing, Inc.' (WISH) which is based not in any Chinese-speaking territory, but in Ellicott City, Maryland, U.S.A. See http://yang-sheng.com/ and the related Facebook-mediated 'network for health, happiness and harmony' at www.facebook.com/YangSheng.net/.

Filmography

For Fun (*Zhao le* 找乐), dir. Ning Ying 宁瀛,1993.
Perpetual Motion (*Wu qiong dong* 无穷动), dir. Ning Ying 宁瀛,2006.
Shower (*Xi zao* 洗澡), dir. Zhang Yang 张扬, 1999.

Bibliography

Bell, J. (ed.) (2014) *Electric Shadows*: *A Century of Chinese Cinema*, London: British Film Institute.
Berra, J. (2014) Chinese Popcorn: Multiplex Cinema of the 2000s, in J. Bell (ed.) *Electric Shadows: A Century of Chinese Cinema*, London: BFI, pp. 104–11.
Braester, Y. (2011) Contemporary Mainstream PRC Cinema, in S.H. Lim and J. Ward (eds.) *The Chinese Cinema Book*, Basingstoke: Palgrave Macmillan, pp. 176–84.
Carel, H. (2008) *Illness: The Cry of the Flesh*, Durham, NC: Acumen Publishing.
Chan, A. (2009) Getting Home and Other Films of Zhang Yang, *Slant*, 15 January 2009, www.slantmagazine.com/house/article/getting-home-and-other-films-of-zhang-yang, accessed 27 March 2019.
China.org.cn (2003) *China Through a Lens: Director Zhang Yang Prepares for his Latest Flick*, www.china.org.cn/english/NM-e/82263.htm, accessed 27 March 2019.
Dear, D. (2012) Chinese Yangsheng: Self-Help and Self-Image, *Asian Medicine*, 7 (1): 1–33.
Easton, K.L. (1993) Defining the Concept of Self-Care, *Rehabilitation Nursing*, 18 (6): 384–7.

Elley, D. (1999) Review: 'Shower', *Variety*, 13 September 1999, http://variety.com/1999/film/reviews/shower-1200459104/, accessed 27 March 2019.

Farquhar, J. (2013) Chinese Medicine as Popular Knowledge in Urban China, in T.J. Hinrichs and L. Barnes (eds.) *Chinese Medicine and Healing an Illustrated History*, Cambridge, MA: Belknap Press of Harvard University Press, pp. 272–4.

Farquhar, J. and Zhang Qicheng (2012) *Ten Thousand Things: Nurturing Life in Contemporary Beijing*, Brooklyn, NY: Zone Books.

Foucault, M. (1990) *The Care of the Self: The History of Sexuality*, Vol. 3, trans. R. Hurley, London: Penguin Books.

Frank, A.W. (1995) *The Wounded Storyteller: Body, Illness and Ethics*, Chicago: University of Chicago Press.

Hartweg, D.L. (1991) *Dorothea Orem: Self-Care Deficit Theory*, New York: SAGE Publications.

Hibbard, J. and Gilburt, H. (2014) *Supporting People to Manage Their Health: An Introduction to Patient Activation*, London: The King's Fund.

Hinrichs, T.J. and Barnes, L. (eds.) (2013) *Chinese Medicine and Healing: An Illustrated History*, Cambridge, MA: Belknap Press of Harvard University Press.

Hsu, E. (ed.) (2001) *Innovation in Chinese Medicine*, Cambridge: Cambridge University Press.

Kalsched, D. (1996) *The Inner World of Trauma: Archetypal Defenses of the Personal Spirit*, London and New York: Routledge.

Kleinman, A. (1988) *The Illness Narratives: Suffering, Healing and the Human Condition*, New York: Basic Books.

Lim, S.H. and Ward, J. (eds.) (2011) *The Chinese Cinema Book*, Basingstoke, Hants: Palgrave Macmillan for British Film Institute.

Lo, V. (2001) The Influence of Nurturing Life Culture on the Development of Western Han Acumoxa Therapy, in E. Hsu (ed.) *Innovation in Chinese Medicine*, Cambridge: Cambridge University Press, pp. 19–50.

Local Government Association for England and Wales (2013) *Helping People to Look After Themselves: A Guide on Self-Care*, www.local.gov.uk/sites/default/files/documents/helping-people-look-after-a78.pdf, accessed 27 March 2019.

Local Government Association Press Release (2016) *Millions of 'Unnecessary' GP Visits Are for Coughs and Colds*, 5 November 2016, www.local.gov.uk/about/news/millions-unnecessary-gp-visits-are-coughs-and-colds, accessed 27 March 2019.

Lu Hongwei (2008) From Routes to Roots or Vice Versa: Transformations of Urban Space in China's "New Urban Films", *Asian Cinema*, 19 (2): 102–34.

Martin, F. and Heinrich, A.L. (eds.) (2006) *Embodied Modernities: Corporeality, Representation and Chinese Cultures*, Honolulu, Hawaii: University of Hawaii Press.

Masters, B. (2016) The Rise of Personalised Medicine, *Financial Times*, 18 August 2016, www.ft.com/content/4e825268-6432-11e6-8310-ecf0bddad227, accessed 27 March 2019.

Mind (2018) *Mental Health Problems – an Introduction*, www.mind.org.uk/information-support/types-of-mental-health-problems/mental-health-problems-introduction/self-care/#.WZSAMVGQzIU, accessed 27 March 2019.

——— (2018) *How to Improve Your Mental Wellbeing*, www.mind.org.uk/information-support/tips-for-everyday-living/wellbeing/wellbeing/?o=10135#.WZR_kFGQzIU, accessed 27 March 2019.

N.H.S. England (2016) *Personalised Medicine*, www.england.nhs.uk/healthcare-science/personalisedmedicine/, accessed 27 March 2019.

———— (2016) *Improving Outcomes Through Personalised Medicine,* www.england. nhs.uk/wp-content/uploads/2016/09/improving-outcomes-personalised-medicine.pdf, accessed 27 March 2019.

N.H.S. Self-Care Forum (2018) *Review of Self-Care Week 2018,* http://dev.selfcareforum. org/wp-content/uploads/2013/05/Rev_2018_SCW_final.pdf, accessed 27 March 2019.

Nursing Theory (2016) *Self-Care Deficit Theory,* www.nursing-theory.org/theories-and-models/orem-self-care-deficit-theory.php, accessed 27 March 2019.

Orem, D.E., Taylor, S.G. and Renpenning, K.M. (2001) *Nursing: Concepts of Practice,* St. Louis: Mosby.

Palmer, A. (2000) After "Spicy Love Soup", Zhang takes "Shower", *IndieWire,* 7 July 2000, www.indiewire.com/2000/07/interview-after-spicy-love-soup-zhang-takes-shower-81545/, accessed 27 March 2019.

Proctor-Xu, J. (2006) Sites of Transformation: The Body and Ruins in Zhang Yang's Shower, in F. Martin and A.L. Heinrich (eds.) *Embodied Modernities: Corporeality, Representation and Chinese Cultures,* Honolulu, Hawaii: University of Hawaii Press, pp. 162–75.

Random House Dictionary (2017) *Self-care,* www.dictionary.com/browse/self-care, accessed 27 March 2019.

Rayns, T. (2001) Shower (Review), *Sight and Sound,* 4 (58): 11–14.

Self-Care Forum U.K., www.selfcareforum.org/, accessed 27 March 2019.

————, *The Self-Care Continuum,* www.selfcareforum.org/about-us/what-do-we-mean-by-self-care-and-why-is-good-for-people/, accessed 27 March 2019.

Self Care Journal [SelfCare] (2010–), http://selfcarejournal.com/journal-archives/, accessed 27 March 2019.

Stedman, T.L. (2002) *The American Heritage Stedman's Medical Dictionary,* Boston, MA: Houghton, Mifflin & Co.

Theoretical Foundations of Nursing (2011) *Dorothea E. Orem: The Self-Care Deficit Nursing Theory,* http://nursingtheories.weebly.com/dorothea-e-orem.html, accessed 27 March 2019.

U.K. Academy of Medical Sciences (2015) *Stratified, Personalised or P4 Medicine: A New Direction for Placing the Patient at the Centre of Health Care and Health Education,* https://acmedsci.ac.uk/file-download/38266-56e6d483e1d21.pdf, accessed 27 March 2019.

U.K. Department of Health (2005) *Self-Care – A Real Choice: Self-Care Support – A Practical Option,* http://webarchive.nationalarchives.gov.uk/20090217000115/www. dh.gov.uk/en/Publicationsandstatistics/Publications/PublicationsPolicyAndGuidance/ DH_4100717, accessed 27 March 2019.

Vollmann, J., Sandow, V., Wäscher, S. and Schildmann, J. (eds.) (2016) *The Ethics of Personalised Medicine: Critical Perspectives,* Abingdon, Oxon and New York: Routledge.

Webbe, D., Guo Zhenyu and Mann, S. (2013) Self-Care in Health: We Can Define It, but Should We also Measure It? *Self Care,* 4(5): 101–6, http://selfcarejournal.com/article/self-care-in-health-we-can-define-it-but-should-we-also-measure-it/, accessed 27 March 2019.

Wikipedia Contributors (2019) Self-Care, *Wikipedia, The Free Encyclopedia,* https:// en.wikipedia.org/wiki/Self-care, accessed 27 March 2019.

World Institute for Self-Healing, Inc., *Yang Sheng (Nurturing Life),* http://yang-sheng. com/, accessed 27 March 2019.

Zhang Yingjin (2004) *Chinese National Cinema,* New York and London: Routledge.

4 Sentiments like water

Unsettling pathologies of homosexual and sadomasochistic desire

Derek Hird

East Palace West Palace (*Donggong Xigong* 东宫西宫), made in 1996, was the first explicitly gay film produced in the People's Republic of China. It examines the fluidity of desire, power, and sexual and gendered identities through the figures of A Lan 阿兰, a writer and night-time gay cruising regular in a central Beijing park, and Xiao Shi 小史, a policeman who arrests and interrogates him.[1] The film speaks to key concerns of the medical humanities, such as formations of gender and sexual identities, patient narratives, power dynamics between authority figures and ordinary people, and cultural histories of medical discourse. The film's director, Zhang Yuan 张元 (1963–), is a chronicler of alienated, subaltern groups: his films prior to *East Palace West Palace* explored the sensitive topics of mental illness, delinquency, and alcoholism, which led the authorities to ban him from film-making (Zhang 2002: 418). Zhang co-wrote the screenplay with Wang Xiaobo 王小波 (1952–1995), a pioneering writer and academic who wrote extensively on power and sexuality (Zhang and Sommer 2007: vii–xiv). Wang's short story 'Sentiments like Water' (*Si shui rouqing* 似水柔情) formed the basis of the screenplay. The stars of the film include amateur actor Si Han 司汗 (A Lan), and the now very famous professional actors Hu Jun 胡军 (Xiao Shi) and Zhao Wei 赵薇 ('Public Bus'). Produced by a French company, the film was financed by a grant of 900,000 francs from the French government and a 200,000 RMB grant from the Rotterdam International Film Festival (Lim 2006: 32, 192 n.19).

The story is rooted in early 1990s China, when the authorities took an overtly oppressive stance towards gay practices in public areas. At the centre of the plot is A Lan, a young gay man who frequently hangs out in the park with other gay men, looking for sex and companionship. One evening, he is arrested by Xiao Shi, a handsome, strapping police officer, who takes him to the park's police post for questioning. During the interrogation, which takes place over one whole night, A Lan 'confesses' his homosexuality to Xiao Shi. A Lan provides accounts of his sexual experiences with other men; these began in middle school, where he was also fascinated by a beautiful girl in his class, 'Public Bus'. Through these vivid recollections, A Lan's predilection for masochistic sex emerges. Xiao Shi condemns A Lan as sick and despicable (*jian* 贱), but A Lan refutes this, claiming that it is pure love that leads him to try to please his lovers. A Lan tells Xiao Shi the story of a female thief in ancient times who fell in love with her captor because she had no other choice: this story is depicted in the film through *kunqu* 昆曲 opera scenes. A Lan also reveals a childhood fantasy of being arrested by a towering policeman. Xiao Shi demands that A Lan show his 'real face' by dressing as a woman. A Lan does not wish to, since he conceives of his gay identity as distinct from cross-dressing. However, to please Xiao Shi, he dons women's clothes (confiscated by Xiao Shi from a cross-dressing park regular) and entrancingly enacts femininity. Through his stories and actions, A Lan spins a web of desire and seduction, drawing Xiao Shi ever closer, eventually succeeding – perhaps – in unsettling Xiao Shi's understanding of his own sexuality.

The title of the film can be read at several levels. Taken from Beijing gay slang, it refers to the public toilets in the Workers' Cultural Centre and Zhongshan Park to the west and east of Tian'anmen Square and the Forbidden City (Bao 2011: 115). More formally, the East Palace was historically the term for the residence of the crown prince. The West Palace was associated with the emperor's concubines, thus bearing a sexual connotation even before its use in gay slang. The title also hints at the developing mix of 'East' and 'West' in 1990s China. A Lan himself embodies 'Western' and 'Eastern' ideas and practices. On the one hand, he performs a gay identity; on the other hand, his wearing down of Xiao Shi's rigid ideas about sexuality equates to the role of water in Daoist philosophy, as the title of Wang Xiaobo's short story suggests. The *Daodejing* (*Tao Te Ching*) famously tells how the soft and the yielding can overcome the hard and the strong, just as water wears away rock (Lao-tzu 1993: 97).

Thematically, the film covers homosexuality, sadomasochism, cross-dressing, male femininity, and power relations between the rulers and the ruled. Uncertainty, ambiguity, and ambivalence are central to the film's depictions of sexuality. At the outset, the film pits two contrasting views against each other: A Lan holds that a man's love and desire for another man is justifiable and natural; Xiao Shi, representing the stance of the authorities, deems homosexuality morally despicable and a mental disorder. However, Xiao Shi's stance becomes progressively blurred during the film. The depictions of sadomasochistic practices present an ambiguous interplay of desire and punishment by showing that the hands that beat are also the hands that caress. Xiao Shi's view of cross-dressing proves ambivalent, moving between condemning and condoning it.

Xiao Shi's eventual desire to see A Lan as a beautiful woman, when considered alongside the *kunqu* opera scenes, is suggestive of late-imperial era opera patrons' desire for female-impersonating boy actors (*dan* 旦).[2] The feminisation of the younger male within same-sex erotic relationships locates same-sex desire within an overarching framework of *nannü* 男女 (literally 'man woman') relations, one of the foundational mechanisms through which power relations have been constructed in China, regardless of the 'sex' of the bodies involved (Liu *et al.* 2013). The historically influential *yin-yang* 阴阳 paradigm works together with the *nannü* framework. The disempowered man in Confucian superior-subordinate relations was labelled *yin*, enabling him to enact wifely virtue without being considered less of a man (Huang 2006: 2). The *yin-yang* paradigm helped legitimise same-sex relationships by placing them within the larger social order (Song 2004: 16–17). The *dan* boy actors took up feminine and subordinate *yin* positionings in their social and erotic relations with wealthy opera patrons.

The film's sympathetic portrayals of homosexuality, cross-dressing, and sado-masochism challenged their pathologisation in the 1990s. More than twenty years later, there has been progress in this direction. Nevertheless, widespread promulgation of conservative 'family values' still frequently results in the demonisation and pathologisation of identities and practices associated with these categories. In Xi Jinping's China, normative 'family values' promote universal marriage, and official media regulations define homosexual relations as abnormal, prohibiting their portrayal on television and in online audiovisual content; also banned is the depiction of any sexuality outside marriage (Zhang 2018). Gay venues and organisations remain relatively few in number, and the authorities keep them under close watch. Huge numbers of men and women conceal their sexual orientations and marry opposite-sex partners, often causing much distress and divorce further down the line (Jeffreys and Yu 2015: 88–9). Given the precarious environment in which sexual minorities find themselves, there is a pressing need to critique normative understandings of gender and sexuality. *East Palace West Palace* does this by illuminating the potential of queer identities and practices to undermine taken-for-granted gender and sexual norms and the power relations through which they are constructed.

From a masculinities studies perspective, the film shows the intertwining of historical and contemporary constructions of male sexuality and can be read as a contribution to discussions about what it means to be a man in contemporary China. Following the next section's discussion of the film's critical reception, I outline a brief genealogy of modern Chinese male sexuality, place the film in the context of late twentieth-century Chinese cinema, and use concepts from Chinese masculinities studies to examine the gender and sexual identities of the two main characters. Finally, I look at relevant examples of performance art in the wider context of cultural production in the 1990s. The chapter shows how notions of gender and sexuality make key contributions to debates about modernity in contemporary China.

Critical contexts

A Lan's masochistic love for his interrogator Xiao Shi, and the corresponding story he tells about the female thief's love for her jailer, suggest an allegory of the relationship between the Chinese state and people, or perhaps more specifically intellectuals. For some critics the film points towards the abject position of ordinary Chinese people and intellectuals vis-à-vis their rulers; for others, the film portrays the people's complicity in their own oppression and willingness to be disciplined. Still others emphasise the film's depiction of political struggle at a micro-level, in which power is not possessed and deployed coercively by one party alone, but is relatively diffuse, fluid, and open to manipulation, allowing for transformation of subjectivities and subversion of hierarchies.

Allegorical interpretations abound in the critical literature. For Chris Berry, the park is a 'heterotopic representation' of China, and A Lan's enjoyment of Xiao Shi's bullying implies that 'in a police state masochism is the only surefire road to fulfillment' (Berry 2000: 193). A heterotopic reading of the park also suggests the past haunting the present: the park design brings to mind the imperial pleasure gardens of the Summer Palace, or the fictional gardens of *Dream of Red Mansions*, which are marked by sexual desire and power (Yi 2004: 88). Berry (1998) also suggests that A Lan's articulation of a gay identity highlights a growing contest for access to public space and discourse in postsocialist China. For Song Hwee Lim (2006: 69–73, 89), A Lan's performance of femininity within the context of the *kunqu* opera scenes represents the Chinese state's structural feminisation of intellectuals and artists. Similarly, Shannon May (2003: 159) argues that Xiao Shi's forcing A Lan to dress as a woman is a symbolic castration that points to the Chinese state's emasculation of creative figures such as Zhang Yuan himself.[3]

But allegorical readings are not without drawbacks. Dai Jinhua 戴锦华 (1998, discussed in Shernuk 2012: 29–30) cautions that they may diminish the story's focus on the manipulability of power between individuals. More specifically, some commentators argue that interpreting A Lan's public 'confession' as an attempt to achieve public recognition for gay sexuality presupposes an already formed, yet constricted, Chinese gay subject, whose full realisation depends on him achieving more public visibility in the manner of his Western counterparts (Bao 2011: 117; Shernuk 2012). Duane Shernuk (2012: 58–63) points out that applying a Euro-American form of gay identity politics to a Chinese population for whom it is not wholly appropriate crowds out differently configured sexualities. Nevertheless, Shernuk (*ibid.*: 62) acknowledges that the film's Western-influenced sexual identities play to the values of its intended transnational audiences at international, independent film festivals. As such, the film partly panders to the notion of a 'global gay' identity premised on a Western model, popularised in Dennis Altman's (1997) portrayal of emerging gay Asian identities. Furthermore, metaphorical readings of the film run the danger of positioning the state as 'inherently normative' and artists as 'inherently queer' (Shernuk 2012: 30). A more nuanced perspective recognises the co-existence of queerness and normativity within the everyday practices of both the state and its citizens. Shernuk argues that the film (and the short story more so) reveals the state's complicity in enabling A Lan's masochistic pleasures; depicts the ease with which A Lan incorporates marriage, homosexuality, and cross-dressing into his gendered and sexual subjectivity; and shows the latent queerness in Xiao Shi's sexuality (*ibid.*: 40–55). To better illuminate the different strands of the lead characters' sexualities, I will now briefly outline the attempts to construct a 'modern' Chinese male sexuality.

Constructing 'Modern' Chinese male sexuality

Homosexual relations in premodern China were widespread and even celebrated (Hinsch 1990; Wu 2004). They were largely shaped by age, social status, and gender enactment. Older, higher-status men took the masculine penetrating role in relationships with younger, lower-status, and usually more feminine-looking and -acting men (Hinsch 1990: 9–13; Huang 2006: 149; Song 2004: 134). *Yin* and *yang* served to mark these unequal subject positions. Upon public exposure of the relationships, stigma, and the severest legal punishment, attached to the penetrated male, not the penetrant (Sommer 1997, 2000: 148–54; Song 2004: 134). The lively late Qing culture of homoerotic relationships between opera clientele (officials, literati, and merchants) and *dan* produced ornately composed 'flower guides' (*huapu* 花谱), in which the qualities of leading *dan* were discussed (Wu 2004: 16–17).

By contrast, ideas about gender and sexuality arriving in China from Europe in the late nineteenth century condemned homosexuality as immoral, effeminate, and sapping the vigour of a modern nation state. Thus, as national pride and male honour were at stake, 'to pursue modernity in China under the self-conscious semi-colonial gaze meant to abolish same-sex relations' (Kang 2009: 146). A 1912 Beijing police bulletin complained that the prostitution of young *dan* opera performers to wealthy patrons attracted 'the derision of foreign nations' (Kang 2009: 115–16; Wu and Stevenson 2006: 51–2). In the decades that followed, leading intellectuals such as literary reformer Hu Shi 胡适 (1891–1962) and sexologist Pan Guangdan 潘光旦 (1898–1967) condemned the 'abnormality' and immorality of *dan* actors, characterising homosexuality as a nation-weakening 'disease' that had to be eliminated (Chiang 2010: 648; Wu and Stevenson 2006: 53–4).

In this environment of open hostility towards homosexuality, the international opera icon Mei Lanfang 梅兰芳 (1894–1961) refashioned *dan* costumes so that they concealed the male body underneath. Mei generated 'a sartorially neutral, historically abstract, and politically uncompromised male body' that had nothing to do with femininity, unlike the seductively feminised and sexualised bodies of *dan* actors in the Qing theatre world (Zou 2006: 88). The de-feminised male bodies of Republican-era *dan* were premised on Western biomedical discourses of gender and sexuality. Howard Chiang argues that the reenvisioned *dan* can be seen as a prototype of the 'modern homosexual' (Chiang 2010: 648). The pathologisation of homosexuality continued into the socialist era. Sex education pamphlets from the late 1940s and 1950s described homosexuality as a pathological disorder – a viral infection in the brain – curable by heterosexual marriage (ibid.: 649–50). Although there was no specific law forbidding homosexuality, homosexual acts were often punished through the offence of hooliganism, with sentences sometimes extending to many years (Ma 2003: 124–5).

The state began to retreat from micro-controlling citizens' lives in the late 1970s, but it was not until the 1990s that more wide-ranging debates on homosexuality became nationally prominent. Increasing consumerism and participation in the global economy, coupled with the lessening of state interest in policing personal sexuality, facilitated the expression of non-normative sexual desires. Gay identity emerged in the context of postsocialist China's grand modernising project to imagine and build the new identities and practices suitable for China's entrance on the late twentieth-century global capitalist stage (Bao 2011: 133–4). Yet in the 1990s medical field, homosexuality was still largely constructed as deviant and/or an illness, alongside other forms of 'deviance' such as cross-dressing and transgender/transsexual identities (Bao 2011: 78). Books by medical scholars and physicians laid out taxonomies of homosexuality, and advocated psychological counselling, herbal medicine, and aversion therapy as 'cures' (ibid.: 78–9). In this discriminatory climate, prior to the revision of the penal code in 1997 that removed the offence of hooliganism, the police frequently raided gay cruising areas and bars (Ma 2003: 127). The opening scenes of *East Palace West Palace* depict such a raid on a park near the Forbidden City during a 1991 public health campaign. The film therefore serves as an important reminder of the hard-handed methods employed by the authorities at that time. Homosexuality continued to be classified as a psychiatric disorder in the *Chinese Classification of Mental Disorders* until 2001. The film also attests to the persistence of older patterns of discrimination: A Lan is beaten up and stigmatised as the insertee in same-sex relations, echoing attitudes expressed in premodern Chinese legal cases.

Late twentieth-century Chinese cinema

Contextualising *East Palace West Palace* also requires locating it within transformations in post-Mao Chinese cinema. Visual and literary culture shifted its focus from rural to urban and national to transnational in the last two decades of the twentieth century. By the 1990s, in the context of huge rural to urban migration and rapid urban development, the city, as a creator of new forms of hybrid identities, 'had become a subject in its own right' (Visser 2010: 9). In Zhang Yimou's 张艺谋 *Red Sorghum* (*Hong gaoliang* 红高粱 1987), for example, the countryside was the locus for the exploration of gender and sexuality. Films exploring sexualities from the 1990s, such as *East Palace West Palace*, Liu Bingjian's 刘冰鉴 *Men and Women* (*Nannan nünü* 男男女女 1999), and Stanley Kwan's (Guan Jinpeng 关锦鹏) *Lan Yu* (蓝宇 2001), depict urban Beijing as a generator of emerging gay lifestyles and communities. Such films have played a role in building gay identities and cultures in China (Bao 2011: 113). And whereas 1980s New Chinese Cinema was an experimental national cinema of 'cultural critique' unbeholden to the market economy, 1990s Chinese cinema became enmeshed in commercially driven 'transnational production, exhibition, distribution, and consumption in the world market' (Lu 1997a: 8–9; Lu 1997b: 130).

The shifts from rural to urban and national to transnational are often categorised in terms of film-making generations. Fifth-generation directors such as Zhang Yimou (b. 1951), Chen Kaige 陈凯歌 (b. 1952), and Tian Zhuangzhuang 田壮壮 (b. 1952), who graduated from the Beijing Film Academy in 1982, moved beyond socialist realism but did not completely let go of its themes, moral framework, and rural settings (Larson 2011: 113). Their early films were typically set in stark locations that put landscape and peasants together in a quest for the 'roots' of Chinese culture as a response to China's opening to the world (Cornelius and Smith 2002: 35–7). The marketisation process that Deng Xiaoping accelerated after the 1989 Tian'anmen protests increased economic liberalisation and urbanisation but did not erode CCP dominance. Zhang Yuan, Wang Xiaoshuai 王小帅, Jia Zhangke

贾樟柯, and other sixth-generation directors who came to prominence in this climate were often partly funded from abroad (Cornelius and Smith 2002: 107–8). They generally eschewed their predecessors' predilection for Chinese culture, national allegory, literary allusions, and social morality to focus on young people's perspectives of their own experiences in urban environments (Cornelius and Smith 2002: 108; Larson 2011: 113, 116).

While *East Palace West Palace* in many ways exemplifies this shift of attention to the lives of ordinary urban citizens, it also lends itself to allegorical interpretations, as discussed previously. A Lan's question to Xiao Shi – 'We love you; why don't you love us?' – to the backing of *kunqu* opera music, is suggestive of a cultural critique of Chinese state-society relations through the perspective of ordinary urbanites. The film thus points to the persistence of a sexualised and gendered power relationship between the governing and the governed in China. It therefore offers a political and cultural critique at the national level, yet at the same time explores the newly forming sexual subjectivities of postsocialist China's urban modernity. I will examine later how this plays out in the figures of A Lan and Xiao Shi, but first present an overview of relevant concepts from Chinese masculinities research.

Chinese masculinities

The *wen* 文 (cultural accomplishment) and *wu* 武 (martial prowess) dyad set out by Kam Louie and Louise Edwards is central to understanding the historical development of Chinese masculinities (Louie and Edwards 1994; Louie 2002, 2014). *Wen* qualities include excellence in poetry and calligraphy; *wu* qualities include physical strength and military acumen (Louie 2002: 14). Both *wen* and *wu* were regarded as masculine attributes. Men of standing possessed either or both, although *wen* generally enjoyed primacy over *wu* (Louie 2002: 11–12). Influential premodern literary models of masculinity include the *wen*-identified *caizi* 才子 (talented scholar) and *junzi* 君子 (cultivated gentleman). The *caizi* was the romantic male protagonist in *caizi-jiaren* 才子佳人 (scholar-beauty) romances. Femininely beautiful, frail, and emotionally vulnerable, the *caizi* was nonetheless seen as the ideal male lover (Song 2004: vii). The *junzi*, by contrast, was a model of emotional self-control, including containment of sexual passion (Louie 2015: 113; McMahon 1988: 50). The *junzi*'s status derived from his embodiment of Confucian virtue, observance of the rites, high level of learning, and political service to the nation (Louie 2002: 44–5; Song 2004: 88–97).

In the Confucian worldview, only men were free to aspire to full moral personhood by attaining a harmonious range of dispositions. This could be achieved through a relatively androgynous personality in which *yin* and *yang* circulated (Furth 1999: 46; Hall and Ames 1998: 81). Relatively 'ungendered' Confucian moral personhood enabled subordinate men to take up the subject position of wife or concubine in relation to their superiors to demonstrate their virtue (Huang 2006: 2; Song 2004: 12). In these instances, *yin* and *yang* marked positionality in particular instantiations of power relationships, not fixed gender identities (Song

2004: 13). The relatively androgynous male body also enabled ideal male beauty to be described in feminine terms (Huang 2006: 135–54).

The concept of *nannü*, in like manner, serves to mark power positionings, and is not limited to sexed bodies per se. During the Han dynasty, Confucian scholars mapped a cosmological theory of '*yang*-high and *yin*-low' onto conjugal relations (Liu *et al.*: 128 n. 27). Since then, in patriarchal and elitist fashion, *nannü* has been interwoven with *yin-yang* in classical Confucian scholarship, commentarial traditions, laws, rituals, and everyday practices between men, women, and men and women (*ibid.*: 19–20). As a marker and producer of hierarchical power, *nannü* is as relevant to the exploitation of non-elite boys as it is to the exploitation of non-elite women and young girls. He-Yin Zhen 何殷震 (c.1884 – c.1920), an early twentieth-century feminist, was the first to use *nannü* as an analytical tool to deconstruct patriarchal power relations and show how the concept organised and policed the value put on the work done in domestic and public domains (*ibid.*: 11–22).

The male sexualities of A Lan and Xiao Shi

Wen-wu and *yin-yang* traces are manifest in A Lan's relationship with Xiao Shi. As a writer, A Lan is associated with *wen*, and is clearly talented with words, for his 'confession' vividly weaves together narratives about his past and present. A Lan can be viewed in this light as a surrogate for China's literary and creative intellectuals such as Zhang Yuan and Wang Xiaobo. As a slender, young, attractive man (desired by women as well as men), A Lan also echoes the historic figure of the *caizi*. His relatively androgynous appearance recalls the premodern body in which *yin* and *yang* circulate. His demonstration of feminine virtue as womanly supplicant to Xiao Shi rehearses the subordinate male role in historical Confucian relationships. And while he may not reflect the full panoply of *junzi*-type moral cultivations that Bao (2018) perceives in the character of Lan Yu (including humanity, righteousness, knowledge, integrity, loyalty, honesty, kindness, and forgiveness), many of these qualities could be applied to A Lan.

A Lan's *yin* positioning towards Xiao Shi is further reflected in the film's frequent association of him with Daoist notions of water. The *Daodejing* recommends that by not contending or contesting, the weak – like water wearing down the hardest stone – can overcome the strong (Allan 1997: 47–8). A Lan's masochism, in which he yields, like water, empowers him, as his desire and ability to be punished undermines and ultimately defeats attempts to make him conform to heteronormative expectations (Shernuk 2012: 42). The trope of water thus represents sexual power as diffuse, fluid, and constitutive of subjects and subjectivities, enabling subversion and transformation of power relations. For example, A Lan recounts enjoying his emetic when undergoing gay cure therapy in hospital, and when he is slapped by Xiao Shi he remembers being filled with pleasure when one of his sexual partners slapped him in a bathtub (symbolically overflowing with water). In the final scenes, water is again flowing everywhere, implying that A Lan is succeeding in undermining Xiao Shi's authority and rendering his sexuality more fluid. In the *Daodejing*'s metaphorical depiction, all streams ultimately flow into a river, which, like a woman during coitus, takes a lower position; but the river – and therefore the female – ultimately subsumes and conquers all (Allan 1997: 45–6). From a Foucauldian perspective, power flows like water, diverts when meeting resistance; this in turn gives rise to further diversions and resistances (Lo and Barrett 2012: 25). As such, A Lan's masochism begins to undo the power hierarchy instantiated by the *nannü* framework.

A Lan's expansive view of sexuality includes but cannot be reduced to gay identity. He learnt from his wife, 'Public Bus', that everyone is born *jian* (despicable, base, cheap), yet as Shernuk (2012: 36) points out, Hongling Zhang and Jason Sommer's translation of *jian* as 'easy' in their English version of Wang's (2007) short story raises the possibility of positive and pleasurable associations. A Lan's 'aesthetic of beauty', which determines his choice of sexual partners, exceeds conventional hetero-homo divisions (Shernuk 2012: 14). The short story brings out very clearly the love and indeed sexual desire A Lan feels for his wife, thereby blurring his sexuality. A Lan's eventual transformation into a seductive, feminine 'woman', albeit at first reluctantly in the film, also shows an openness towards reconfiguring his gender identity. His belief that love can justify anything leads A Lan to accept the demands and cruel treatment of Xiao Shi and others. In this, A Lan is drawing on reform-era discourses that place love at the centre of the modern subject, which has helped legitimise gay relationships that are presented in terms of romantic love (Bao 2011: 103). The state (e.g. in the form of Xiao Shi) may not recognise same-sex love as 'proper love', but gay-identifying people such as A Lan appropriate the discourse of love to articulate their identity and empower themselves (*ibid.*). A Lan's 'easy' view of sexuality places him at odds with Xiao Shi's restrictive notion of appropriate sexual desire.

Echoes of historical masculine subjectivities can also be found in Xiao Shi. As a physically tough, uniformed policeman, he manifests *wu* qualities, and he also takes up an empowered *yang* positioning vis-à-vis A Lan's feminine *yin*. In the context of the film's *kunqu* opera theme, his insistence on routing his sexual desire for A Lan through the latter's feminine cross-dressing echoes the format of same-sex erotic relationships in the late Qing theatre world, which legitimised homosexuality through the feminine performance of the *dan* (Lim 2006: 72). In this sense, Xiao Shi aligns himself with the *nannü* paradigm and the normative, hierarchised, Confucian social order. The salience of the operatic scenes and music emphasise the ghosts of historic same-sex erotic relationships, although Xiao Shi's sexuality can also be interpreted through the lens of 'Western' heteronormativity.

At the start of the film, Xiao Shi is presented as straight identifying. He is disgusted by the 'despicable' sexual practices of A Lan, although his decision to interrogate A Lan overnight belies a curiosity in non-normative sexuality. Yet by the final scenes of the film, Xiao Shi's previous containment of his sexual desires, whether interpreted as heteronormative or *junzi*-like, has broken down. He appears to be on the verge of making love with A Lan and is transfixed when A Lan caresses him. In the short story, Xiao Shi's sexuality is transformed much more: he makes love with A Lan several times, comes to understand himself as gay, and is identified as such by his co-workers. As Shernuk and Dai both argue, this undermines the allegorical reading of intellectuals as queer and the state as non-queer, and shows the manipulation and fluidity of power and desire between individuals. 'It is hard to tell whether the policeman victimises the gay man, or whether the gay man corrupts the policeman' (Bao 2011: 128).

Gender and sexuality in 1990s performance art

1990s performance art offers another context of cultural production in which to analyse the feminine and/or suffering, masochistic male body. Performance art, like homosexuality, came to prominence in the 1990s. At this time, there was increasing circulation of Chinese and foreign artists and art literature in and out of China. The transgression of gender boundaries and the disciplining of the body in the formation of the postsocialist Chinese subject are the preoccupation of some works in this period (Lu 2007: 17). In particular, performance artists Ma Liuming 马六明 (b. 1969) and Zhang Huan 张洹 (b. 1965) engaged with themes that Zhang Yuan and Wang Xiaobo raised through the figure of A Lan.

Ma Liuming used his naked male body to express femininity, thus transgressing and challenging conventional gender boundaries. His performances 'defy the biopolitics of traditional patriarchal authority by opening up the questions of gender-bending, cross-dressing, and sexual ambiguity' (Lu 2007: 71). For doing so, Ma was detained by the state for two months. In the early 1990s, Ma created the persona of Fen-Ma Liuming 芬·马六明. Fen means 'fragrant' and carries feminine associations. Ma's purpose was to question and make ambiguous existing gender boundaries through a persona that was 'neither homosexual, hermaphrodite, transvestite, nor androgyne' (Ivanova 1999: 203). In Wang Xiaobo's short story especially, A Lan's capacious sexuality and feminine performance resonate with Ma's category-defying stance.

Through an effeminate face, flowing long hair, but an anatomically male body, sometimes naked, sometimes cross-dressed, Ma's work challenges the 'disciplinary regime' that monitors and regulates bodies, desires, and sexuality (Lu 2007: 76). Ma's 1998 performance, *Fen-Ma Liuming Walks on the Great Wall*, in which he walks naked along deserted sections of the most salient symbol of the Chinese nation, enacts a lonely yet stark challenge to deeply embedded ideas about masculinity, patriarchy, and authority (*ibid.*: 77–8). In doing so, Ma blurs not just gender boundaries, but also those between the creative intellectual and the state. His anatomically male body marks his belonging to the privileged gender in Chinese cultural tradition; yet by baring his body, and displaying a feminine face and hair, Ma raises questions about queerness and concealed desires inherent in the Chinese state. The inherent queerness of the state also manifests in Xiao Shi's growing awareness of his complicity in satisfying A Lan's masochism and his growing sexual desire for A Lan.

Whereas Ma's work transgresses conventional gender identity, Zhang Huan's art emphasises bodily suffering, endurance, cruelty, masochism, self-torture, and self-mortification: this renders it allegorical of the 'living condition of the artist-citizen in China' (Lu 2007: 72). Through three works in 1994 and 1995, Zhang exposed his naked male body to pain and torment. In *12 Square Meters* (Beijing East Village 1994), he sits naked covered in honey in a filthy public toilet, while insects crawl over his body and bite him. In *65 Kilograms* (Beijing East Village 1994), he is suspended from the ceiling in iron chains; a doctor draws blood from his body that drops onto a heated plate, releasing an acrid smell. In *25 mm Threading Steel* (Beijing 1995), he lies naked in front of a threading machine that shoots hot sparks onto his body, causing him to shake with pain (Lu 2007: 79). Zhang's immobilised and soundless bare body symbolises the silent endurance of artists, intellectuals, and the wider populace in the face of political oppression. Yet his very decision to torture his body in this way also suggests the possibility of masochistic pleasure. In sadomasochistic game-playing, the discipliner and the disciplined are engaged in a fluid dance of desires, which the apparently oppressed party can manipulate to shift the balance of power. In *East Palace West Palace*, A Lan's sexual masochism draws out Xiao Shi's own queer desires and suggests the possibility of a different tomorrow.

Conclusion

East Palace West Palace's unravelling of normative notions of gender, sexuality, and desire reveals the fluid construction of power hierarchies, subjects, and subjectivities. It highlights conflicting visions of what it means to be a modern Chinese man, and, most subversively, it lays open the inherent queerness of the state. Xiao Shi's dilemma is that if he accepts the legitimacy of A Lan's sexual desires, he also has to recognise himself as a queer subject. In the film, this is particularly hard for him to do; in the short story, he does admit to himself that he is gay, although that very admission plunges him into despair.

The film explores the Chinese state's response to the emergence of expressions of gay sexuality. On the one hand, the state/Xiao Shi seems almost seduced by a notion of modern male sexuality that includes same-sex desires; yet on the other hand, it/he denies the legitimacy of same-sex desire by preventing its representation. The state decriminalised homosexuality in 1997, stopped viewing it as a mental illness in 2001 (Mountford 2010), and allowed a circumscribed flourishing of gay cultures for more than a decade. Since 2015, the state's bans on portraying gay relationships in the media and its labelling of homosexuality as abnormal point to the struggle within the state about the kind of male sexuality it believes is suitable for a modern China (Zhang 2018). Informing this struggle are the historical spectres of the hierarchical *nannü* framework, the *yin* positioning of intellectuals vis-à-vis the state, and elite desires for the feminine beauty of androgynous young men.

Xiao Shi's pledge to 'teach A Lan a lesson' in the final scenes is saturated with deep sexual desire for A Lan. Xiao Shi's hands dispense both love and punishment. Normativity and queerness, like *yin* and *yang*, are shown to be co-existing, embodied components both within Xiao Shi and A Lan and within the metaphorical bodies of the state and the intellectual class. The seductive masochism and transgressive sexuality of the film and contemporaneous performance art pose a question to the state that is as pertinent today as it was over twenty years ago: At what point will you (the state) acknowledge your own inherent queerness? For only when the Chinese state accepts that it too can be queer, feminine, masochistic or 'easy' will it fully endorse and legitimise queer Chinese sexualities. Only then will it become possible for *nannü* hierarchies to become undone.

Notes

1　China-born Pai Hsien-yung's 白先勇 1983 groundbreaking Taiwanese gay novel *Crystal Boys* (*Niezi* 孽子), also located in and around a city centre park, explores homosexuality in the context of 1970s Taiwan. It was adapted as a film in Taiwan in 1986, and to great acclaim as a television series in 2003 (Huang 2010: 391).
2　In Jie Guo's (2011: 1059) reading of Pai Hsien-yung's *Crystal Boys*, the image of its gay characters is evocative of late imperial era *dan* actors and boy prostitutes.
3　Situated in a different sociopolitical context, Pai Hsien-yung's *Crystal Boys* is also suggestive of allegorical readings on the theme of power, most commonly discussed in terms of a fraught father-son relationship between a paternal China and its rebellious Taiwanese offspring (Guo 2011: 1056). Another interesting point of comparison is its metaphorical depiction of central Taipei's New Park as a kingdom of boy prostitutes and nation of motley citizens that possesses its own unorthodox histories and legends (*ibid.*: 1061–3). A 'site of flowing desire' (Huang 2010: 390), Pai's New Park is, in its own way, a sexualised, heterotopic representation of Taiwan.

Filmography

East Palace West Palace (*Donggong xigong* 东宫西宫), dir. Zhang Yuan 张元, 1996.
Lan Yu (蓝宇), dir. Stanley Kwan (Guan Jinpeng) 关锦鹏, 2001.
Men and Women (*Nannan nünü* 男男女女), dir. Liu Bingjian 刘冰鉴, 1999.
Red Sorghum (*Hong gaoliang* 红高粱), dir. Zhang Yimou 张艺谋, 1987.

Bibliography

Allan, S. (1997) *The Way of Water and Sprouts of Virtue*, Albany: State University of New York Press.
Altman, D. (1997) Global gaze/global gays, *GLQ*, 3: 417–36.
Bao, H. (2011) 'Queer Comrades': Gay Identity and Politics in Postsocialist China, PhD Thesis, The University of Sydney.
———. (2018) Haunted Chinese Gay Identity: Sexuality, Masculinity, and Class in *Beijing Story*, in D. Hird and G. Song (eds.) *The Cosmopolitan Dream: Transnational Chinese Masculinities in a Global Age*, Hong Kong: Hong Kong University Press, pp. 73–86.
Berry, C. (1998) East Palace, West Palace: Staging Gay Life in China, *Jump Cut*, 42: 84–9.
———. (2000) Happy Alone? Sad Young Men in East Asian Gay Cinema, *Journal of Homosexuality*, 39 (3–4): 187–200.
Chiang, H. (2010) Epistemic Modernity and the Emergence of Homosexuality in China, *Gender & History*, 22 (3): 629–57.

Cornelius, S. and Smith, I.H. (2002) *New Chinese Cinema: Challenging Representations*, London: Wallflower.

Dai Jinhua 戴锦华 (1998) Zhizhe xixue: yuedu Wang Xiaobo 智者戏谑: 阅读王小波 (The Banter of a Sage: Reading Wang Xiaobo), *Dangdai zuojia pinglun* 当代作家评论, 2: 21–34.

Furth, C. (1999) *A Flourishing Yin: Gender in China's Medical History: 960–1665*, Berkeley: University of California Press.

Guo, J. (2011) Where Past Meets Present: The Emergence of Gay Identity in Pai Hsien-yung's *Niezi*, *MLN*, 126 (5): 1049–82.

Hall, D. and Ames, R. (1998) *Thinking from the Han: Self, Truth and Transcendence in Chinese and Western Culture*, Albany: State University of New York Press.

Hinsch, B. (1990) *Passions of the Cut Sleeve: The Male Homosexual Tradition in China*, Berkeley: University of California Press.

Hird, D. and Song, G. (eds.) (2018) *The Cosmopolitan Dream: Transnational Chinese Masculinities in a Global Age*, Hong Kong: Hong Kong University Press.

Huang, H. (2010) From Glass Clique to Tongzhi Nation: Crystal Boys, Identity Formation, and the Politics of Sexual Shame, *Positions: East Asia Cultures Critique*, 18 (2): 373–98.

Huang, M. (2006) *Negotiating Masculinities in Late Imperial China*, Honolulu: University of Hawaii Press.

Ivanova, M. (1999) Ambiguity, Absurdity, and Self-Creation in the Art of Ma Liuming, *Positions*, 7 (1): 201–23.

Jeffreys, E. and Yu, H. (2015) *Sex in China*, Cambridge: Polity.

Kang, W. (2009) *Obsession: Male Same-Sex Relations in China, 1900–1950*, Hong Kong: Hong Kong University Press.

Lao-tzu (1993) *Tao Te Ching*, trans. S. Addiss and S. Lombardo, Indianapolis: Hackett.

Larson, W. (2011) The Fifth Generation: A Reassessment, in S.H. Lim and J. Ward (eds.) *The Chinese Cinema Book*, Basingstoke: Palgrave Macmillan, pp. 113–21.

Lim, S.H. (2006) *Celluloid Comrades: Representations of Male Homosexuality in Contemporary Chinese Cinemas*, Honolulu: University of Hawaii Press.

Liu, L., Karl, R. and Ko, D. (eds.) (2013) *The Birth of Chinese Feminism*, New York: Columbia University Press.

Lo, V. and Barrett, P. (2012) 'Other Pleasures'? Anal Sex and Medical Discourse in Premodern China, in R. Reyes and W.G. Clarence-Smith (eds.) *Sexual Diversity in Asia, c. 600–1950*, Abingdon, Oxon: Routledge, pp. 25–46.

Louie, K. (2002) *Theorising Chinese Masculinity: Society and Gender in China*, Cambridge: Cambridge University Press.

———. (2014) Chinese Masculinity Studies in the Twenty-First Century: Westernizing, Easternizing and Globalizing *Wen* and *Wu*, *NORMA: International Journal for Masculinity Studies*, 9 (1): 18–29.

———. (2015) *Chinese Masculinities in a Globalizing World*, Abingdon: Routledge.

Louie, K. and Edwards, L. (1994) Chinese Masculinity: Theorizing *Wen* and *Wu*, *East Asian History*, 8: 135–48.

Lu, S. (1997a) Chinese Cinemas (1896–1996) and Transnational Film Studies, in S. Lu (ed.) *Transnational Chinese Cinemas: Identity, Nationhood, Gender*, Honolulu: University of Hawaii Press, pp. 1–31.

———. (1997b) National Cinema, Cultural Critique, Transnational Capital: The Films of Zhang Yimou, in S. Lu (ed.) *Transnational Chinese Cinemas: Identity, Nationhood, Gender*, Honolulu: University of Hawaii Press, pp. 105–36.

———. (2007) *Chinese Modernity and Global Biopolitics: Studies in Literature and Visual Culture*, Honolulu: University of Hawaii Press.

———. (ed.) (1997) *Transnational Chinese Cinemas: Identity, Nationhood, Gender*, Honolulu: University of Hawaii Press.

Ma, J.W. (2003) From '*Long Yang*' and '*Dui Shi*' to Tongzhi: Homosexuality in China, *Journal of Gay & Lesbian Psychotherapy*, 7 (1–2): 117–43.

Martin, F. and Heinrich, L. (eds.) (2006) *Embodied Modernities: Corporeality, Representation, and Chinese Cultures*, Honolulu: University of Hawaii Press.

May, S. (2003) Power and Trauma in Chinese Film: Experiences of Zhang Yuan and the Sixth Generation, *Journal for the Psychoanalysis of Culture and Society*, 8 (1): 156–60.

McMahon, K. (1988) A Case for Confucian Sexuality: The Eighteenth Century Novel *Yesou Puyan*, *Late Imperial China*, 9 (2): 32–53.

Mountford, T. (2010) The Legal Position and Status of Lesbian, Gay, Bisexual and Transgender People in the People's Republic of China, *Outright Action International*, www.outrightinternational.org/content/china-legal-position-and-status-lesbian-gay-bisexual-and-transgender-people-people%E2%80%99s, accessed 18 April 2018.

Reyes, R. and Clarence-Smith, W.G. (eds.) (2012) *Sexual Diversity in Asia, c. 600–1950*, Abingdon: Routledge.

Shernuk, D. (2012) Queer Chinese Postsocialist Horizons: New Models of Same-Sex Desire in Contemporary Chinese Fiction, 'Sentiments Like Water' And 'Beijing Story', MA thesis, University of Oregon, https://search.proquest.com/openview/130803086e7533dd845633a86ebd6ac7/1?pq-origsite=gscholar&cbl=18750&diss=y, accessed 28 October 2017.

Sommer, M. (1997) The Penetrated Male in Late Imperial China: Judicial Constructions and Social Stigma, *Modern China*, 23 (2): 140–80.

———. (2000) *Sex, Law, and Society in Late Imperial China*, Stanford: Stanford University Press.

Song, G. (2004) *The Fragile Scholar: Power and Masculinity in Chinese Culture*, Hong Kong: Hong Kong University Press.

Visser, R. (2010) *Cities Surround the Countryside: Urban Aesthetics in Post-Socialist China*, Durham, NC: Duke University Press.

Wang Xiaobo 王小波 (2007) East Palace West Palace, trans. H. Zhang and J. Sommer, in Wang Xiaobo, *Wang in Love and Bondage: Three Novellas by Wang Xiaobo*, Albany: State University of New York Press, pp. 119–45.

——— (2007) *Wang in Love and Bondage: Three Novellas by Wang Xiaobo*, Albany: State University of New York Press.

Wu, C. (2004) *Homoerotic Sensibilities in Late Imperial China*, London: RoutledgeCurzon.

Wu, C. and Stevenson, M. (2006) Male Love Lost: The Fate of Male Same-Sex Prostitution in Beijing in the Late 19th and Early 20th Centuries, in F. Martin and L. Heinrich (eds.) *Embodied Modernities: Corporeality, Representation, and Chinese Cultures*, Honolulu: University of Hawaii Press, pp. 42–59.

Yi, J.J. (2004) *The Dream of the Red Chamber: An Allegory of Love*, Paramus: Homa & Sekey.

Zhang, H. and Sommer, J. (2007) Introduction, in Wang Xiaobo (ed.) *Wang in Love and Bondage: Three Novellas by Wang Xiaobo*, Albany: State University of New York Press, pp. vii–xiv.

Zhang, Y. (2018) Chinese Gay Apps Stop Short of Fighting Homosexual Ban on Social Media, *Global Times*, www.globaltimes.cn/content/1098382.shtml, accessed 18 April 2018.

Zhang, Z. (2002) Zhang Yuan, in Y. Tasker (ed.) *Fifty Contemporary Filmmakers*, London and New York: Routledge, pp. 418–29.

Zou, J. (2006) Cross-Dressed Nation: Mei Lanfang and the Clothing of Modern Chinese Men, in F. Martin and L. Heinrich (eds.) *Embodied Modernities: Corporeality, Representation, and Chinese Cultures*, Honolulu: University of Hawaii Press, pp. 79–97.

Part 2
Film and the public sphere

5　The fever with no name

Genre-blending responses to the HIV-tainted blood scandal in 1990s China

Marta Hanson

Among the many responses to HIV/AIDS in modern China – medical, political, economic, sociological, national, and international – the cultural responses have been considerably powerful. In the past ten years, artists have written novels, produced documentaries, and even made a major feature-length film in response to the HIV/AIDS epidemic in China.[1] One of the best-known critical novelists in China today, Yan Lianke 阎连科 (b. 1958), wrote the novel *Dream of Ding Village* (丁庄梦, copyright 2005; Hong Kong 2006; English translation 2009) as a scathing critique of how the Chinese government both contributed to and poorly handled the HIV/AIDS crisis in his native Henan province. He interviewed survivors, physicians, and even blood merchants who experienced first-hand the HIV/AIDS 'tainted blood' scandal in rural Henan of the 1990s giving the novel authenticity, depth, and heft. Although Yan chose a child-ghost narrator, the *Dream* is clearly a realistic novel. After signing a contract with Shanghai Arts Press he promised to donate 50,000 yuan of royalties to Xinzhuang village where he researched the AIDS epidemic in rural Henan, further blurring the fiction-reality line. The Chinese government censors responded by banning the *Dream* in Mainland China (Wang 2014: 151).

Even before director Gu Changwei 顾长卫 (b. 1957) began making a feature film based on Yan's banned book, he and his wife Jiang Wenli 蒋雯丽 (b. 1969) sought to work with ordinary people living with HIV/AIDS as part of the process of making the film. He publicly invited members of HIV/AIDS communities to participate in making a film based on Yan's *Dream* and conceived of a related documentary filmed on the set (Li 2016: 231). Some officials in the Health Ministry supported Gu's proposal to combine a feature film with a documentary as integral parts of a broader multimedia HIV/AIDS public health education campaign in conjunction with the Film Bureau State Administration of Radio, Film, & TV. At the time, Gu's wife Jiang Wenli was also a volunteer AIDS educator for the Ministry of Health. This may explain their proposal as well as why three other AIDS educators/performers played roles in the film (Qian 2016: 228, fn39).

Released in 2011, the resulting *Love for Life* (*Zui ai* 最爱) was the first feature-length movie to address the HIV/AIDS epidemic in Chinese popular culture. Its sympathetic portrayal of HIV+ characters attempts to counter the real-life stigmatization and discrimination against people living with HIV/AIDS in China.

As part of this state-sponsored HIV/AIDS public health education campaign, Zhao Liang 赵亮 (d. 1971), one of China's best-known independent documentary filmmakers, was invited to make the documentary.[2] The resulting *Together* (*Zai yiqi* 在一起) combines footage of the making of *Love for Life* and interviews with the film's HIV+ and non-HIV+ actors and extras with at-home interviews and online exchanges that Zhao Liang arranged through online social networks with people living with HIV/AIDS in China.

Zhao Liang clarified the intent of this multimedia collaboration with an introduction to his documentary in Chinese and the following English translation:

> In 2009, director Gu Changwei reached out to the public, seeking HIV positive people to participate in the making of the film *Tale of Magic*.[3] By having HIV+ people working and living with members of his cast and crew, he hoped it would strengthen the public's understanding of AIDS, and reduce discrimination against HIV positive people. We documented this process.[4]

Considered together, *Dream of Ding Village, Love For Life*, and *Together* offer a unique case study of the power of blending different cultural forms to tell new stories that have potential to improve epidemiological outcomes, affect social change, and possibly even transform individual lives.[5] The following chapter first examines the *Dream of Ding Village* as a novelist's direct response to the HIV–tainted blood scandal in rural Henan in the 1990s, secondly turns to Gu Changwei's *Love for Life* as part of a government-supported public-health campaign, and thirdly discusses Zhao Liang's documentary *Together* as navigating the related fine line between independent expression and government censorship.

These artists gave 'the fever with no name' not just a name but also a history with multiple stories, subplots, and fictional characters as well as actual human faces and testimonies. As the medical historian Charles E. Rosenberg succinctly wrote, 'In some ways disease does not exist until we have agreed that it does, by perceiving, naming, and responding to it' (Rosenberg 1992: xiii, xxii). Once a disease has been diagnosed, the disease concept itself can be used as a social diagnosis of broader social ills that contributed to the disease's manifestation and which the disease's presence brings into sharper focus (Rosenberg 1992: xxii). Naming the fever in China as HIV/AIDS makes it newly visible as an epidemic with a unique history comprised of complex narratives. People can then use this history to diagnose the broader social, economic, and political problems that contributed to its emergence, exacerbation, and failures to adequately respond.

The fever in the *Dream*

The concrete road linking Ding Village with the outside world was built ten years ago, when everyone in the village was caught up in the blood-selling boom. As Grandpa stood at the roadside looking towards the village, a gust of wind seemed to clear his head and restore order to his muddled thoughts. Things he hadn't understood before began to fall into place. For the first time since he'd left the village early that morning to meet with the county cadres, the fog seemed to lift. There, standing at the roadside that linked Ding Village to the rest of the world, realization dawned on him. The realization that with clouds comes the rain. That late autumn begets winter's chill. That those who had sold their blood ten years ago would now have the fever. And that those with the fever would die, as surely as the falling leaves.

> – *The fever hid in blood; Grandpa hid in dreams.*
> – *The fever loved its blood; Grandpa loved his dreams.*
>
> (Yan 2009: 7–8)

So begins the *Dream of Ding Village*. The definite article 'the' refers to an unspecified fever that parallels the central protagonist 'Grandpa'. The blood where the fever hides is analogous to the dreams within which Grandpa hides. What is this fever that loved blood as much as this Grandpa loved his dreams?

The narrative continues in italics with the dream Grandpa had over several nights:

> *the cities he'd visited –* Kaifeng and Wei County, *with their underground networks of pipes likes cobwebs – running thick with blood. And from the cracks and curvatures of pipes, from the l-bends and the u-bends, blood spurts like water. A fountain of brackish rain sprays the air; a bright-red assault on the senses. And there, upon the plain, he saw the wells and rivers all turned red, rancid with the stench of blood. In every city and every township, doctors wept as the fever spread. But on the streets of Ding Village, one doctor sat and laughed. Bathed in golden sunlight, the village was silent and peaceful, its residents behind locked doors. But, day by day, the doctor in his white lab coat, his physician's bag at his feet, would sit perched upon a rock beneath the scholar trees and laugh. Ha-ha-ha-ha-ha. The sunshine would be filled with the sound of laughter. A big loud belly-laugh, ringing out as clear as a bell, strong enough to shake the trees, and make the yellow leaves rain down, as surely as the autumn breeze.*
>
> (Yan 2009: 8)

The water in the plumbing infrastructure of Kaifeng and Wei county as well as 'the wells and rivers' have all turned to blood, implicating state governance in the widespread contamination of what was once clean water. It's the same blood that has carried 'the fever' to 'every city and every township' through the 'networks of pipes' in humans as well as cities. Everywhere else physicians weep in despair; only the doctor in Ding Village appears to have gone mad. This short dream sequence signals the nightmare that will weave through the novel.

As soon as Grandpa awakens, he is summoned to meet with the local 'bigwigs' or county officials. Because Ding Village's mayor has died from the fever, Grandpa remains the only senior person in the village left to deal with the outside world. He learned several things from this meeting about the fever that has ravaged Ding Village. First, and likely most important, 'was that the fever wasn't really a fever at all. Its proper medical name was Acquired Immune Deficiency Syndrome, or AIDS' (Yan 2009: 9).

The scandal behind the Dream

This fictional opening matches well the historical reality in Henan province of the 1990s that Chinese villagers had no idea what was the 'strange illness' or 'nameless fever' that was killing them (Gittings 2001a: 15; Renwick 2002 377 fn2). After the post-Maoist 'reform and opening' policies in the late 1970s unraveled the commune system underlying the rural healthcare system, the state had to develop new ways to generate revenue for rural healthcare. Building on the blood donation systems established during the Second Sino-Japanese War in Southwest China (Soon 2016) and since the 1950s in Henan province, state and health officials sought to deal with their financial shortfall in the 1990s by encouraging poor villagers to sell their blood and plasma for profit (Hayes 2005: 14; Jun 2011: 78). The local Henan government developed what they called a 'blood economy' (*xuejiang jingji* 血浆经济) in order to 'shake off poverty and attain prosperity' (*tuopin zhifu* 脱贫致富) and so 'make people rich and the nation strong' (*minfu guoqiang* 民富国强) with minimum state investment or infrastructure required (Chan 2016: 189).

At the time, this was considered a win-win situation for poor farmers as well as state, medical, and pharmaceutical institutions. Serious problems arose, however, when greed for profits from blood products took precedence over safe blood and plasma donation practices. Many people donated plasma multiple times in a day when once in two weeks is what the Red Cross recommends. But worse, after extracting the plasma many collection stations pooled the blood before re-injecting it into the donors, thereby dramatically increasing possibilities of HIV infection. It's no surprise then that by 1995 medical workers first detected cases of HIV/AIDS among Chinese living in rural Henan and linked them to the recent surge there in blood-selling practices (Hayes 2005: 14–15).

Despite these findings, in 1995–96 the Henan Provincial Health Department director still stated that 'There is no HIV/AIDS in Henan Province'. Five years later in 2000, however, the government could no longer deny that there was HIV/AIDS in Henan. In fact, by then some estimated that between 500,000 to 700,000 people had contracted HIV/AIDS in Henan province alone (He 2000; Hayes 2005: 12). Some even estimated upwards to 1.2 million cases of HIV infection by then in Henan (Eberstadt 2002: 30; Hayes 2005: 13). As with the fictional Grandpa's realization that all those with the fever who had sold their blood ten years previously would eventually die, a decade after the Henan provincial scheme had begun for farmers 'to get rich quick' (*kuaisu zhifu* 快速致富) via selling their plasma, evidence was finally made public that there was a major HIV/AIDS epidemic deep within rural Henan.

The early history of HIV/AIDs in China from 1985 to the present can thus be summarised in three infection stages: 1) from the first diagnosis in 1985 to 1988 when most cases were found among foreigners or Chinese who had been overseas and mostly in coastal cities; 2) from 1989 to 1993 when cases continued in coastal cities but most new ones were found among intravenous drug uses (IDUs) in Yunnan and started to appear as well among sex workers, those seeking treatment for sexually transmitted infections (STIs), and Chinese who had been employed abroad; and 3) from 1994 on when HIV/AIDS spread far beyond the coastal provinces and Yunnan to all of China's regions and provinces (Hayes 2005: 12–14). Due to the unique Chinese situation of unregulated markets for blood-based products, by 2004 the most distinctive flare up was predictably in Henan province within central China (see map in Volodzko 2016: http://media.economist.com/sites/default/files/cf_images/20050730/CAS911.gif).

By 2001, the enormous region stretching from the far southwestern town Ruili in Yunnan Province toward the northeast through Sichuan province to Henan province and on to Beijing was being called the 'road of death' (Renwick 2002: 378). The estimates from 500,000 to 1.2 million in Henan could have been even lower than actuality since '[p]eople either don't know that they have it or don't want to make it public' (Renwick 2002: 378). The numbers could have been higher because those in power participated in a cover-up. Should knowledge of the extent of HIV/AIDS infection rates in Henan become more widely known, Henan officials evidently feared more the loss of investment in their province than the continued loss of Henanese lives. Furthermore, Chinese government officials and Henan health authorities had promoted the largely unregulated blood trade in the first place. For fear of possible litigation, among other reasons, they chose silence and censorship over transparency (Hayes 2005: 16).

During the international uproar over China's lack of transparency during the SARS pandemic of 2002–3, which compelled the government to take unprecedented action to control it, entire villages were dying from AIDS (Epstein 2003). Instead those in power arrested and beat HIV+ villagers trying to draw attention to their suffering; harassed, sued, and carried out surveillance on health officials who spoke out; and fired journalists who tried to publish anything about the epidemic (Watts 2003: 1). International reportage from *The Guardian* and *The New York Times* instead contributed to a more proactive public-health shift in the Chinese government's approach to epidemics (Volodzko 2016). The important cultural responses to Henan's HIV-tainted blood scandal via Chinese fiction, film, and documentaries are best understood within this context of abuse of power through official silence, aggressive censorship via intimidation, and disregard for the welfare of the most vulnerable victims of the state's own unregulated for-profit blood-selling schemes.

The story within the Dream

Although journalists had done considerable work to expose China's HIV-tainted blood scandal by the early 2000s, the Hong Kong director Ruby Yang (Yang Zeye 楊紫燁) was first to use documentary to draw attention to the human cost of China's HIV–tainted blood scandal. Instead of taking on the decimation of entire HIV/AIDS villages, she focused on the orphans who lost not just their parents to AIDS but also the support of their extended families due to both stigma and poverty. Filmed in 2003 in Fuyang village, Anhui province, *The Blood of Ying-zhou District* 颖州的孩子 (2006) won the Academy's Best Documentary Short in 2007 with its compassionate portrayal of rural China's AIDS epidemic through its most vulnerable victims (Wong 2014). Within the next decade, Yang's *The Blood of Yingzhou District Revisited* (2013) focused on a new charitable boarding school where many of the same children featured in the earlier documentary either worked or lived and studied.

When Ruby Yang was researching and filming *The Blood of Yingzhou District* in the early 2000s, Yan Lianke was conducting fieldwork among villagers about their experience of the AIDS epidemic in his hometown north of Anhui in neighboring Henan. He visited repetitive at least seven times to carry out the research and closely consulted with Dr Gao Yaojie 高耀潔 (b. 1927) the AIDS activist-physician who spoke out publicly about the epidemic (Chan 2016: 190). She started working on the AIDS epidemic in Henan in 1996, only to experience harassment from local officials and be confined to house arrest because of her AIDS activism. Exiled in Manhattan since 2009, she turned her attention to finishing her memoires and other publications on HIV/AIDS in China (Liu 2010).

Dr Gao referred to the 'blood economy' as the 'blood disaster' (*xuehuo* 血禍) and 'national calamity' (*guonan* 國難) to bring attention to its severity. She also pointed out that although many HIV/AIDS cases in China were caused by the 'blood economy', people still thought of it as a 'moral disease' (*daodebing* 道德病) connected to homosexuality and sexual promiscuity for which the government need not be responsible (Chan 2016: 189–90; Gao 2010: 177, 342). Dr Gao's medical insights helped Yan use the novel form more effectively to switch the false 'moral disease' narrative that functioned to absolve government responsibility toward a more accurate 'blood economy' narrative that many Chinese HIV/AIDS patients are in fact victims of the government's own economic and public health policies (Chan 2016: 191).

Even the book's title contains cultural significance that helps shift this narrative. The family name Ding 丁 also means a man. In combination with other characters it can mean 'population' (*rending* 人丁) or 'man and woman' (*dingkou* 丁口). Ding Village is thus every man's village; its fate that of the larger population. The full title also quotes the eighteenth-century *Dream of the Red Chamber* (*Honglou meng* 紅樓夢), suggesting a parallel decline of Ding Village and tragic ending for the central lovers as occurs within the extended family in the original Qing novel.

Dream of Ding Village focuses on a family surnamed Ding – Grandpa or 'Professor Ding', his two sons, and his two grandchildren from the eldest son. The Ding family members' life fortunes take very different courses as a consequence of Ding Village being one of the 'model blood selling' villages in a fictional Wei county. His first son, Ding Hui, is the 'bloodhead' (*xuetou* 血头) villain who ran the village blood collection station, the epicenter of the fever now raging throughout the region. The younger son, Ding Liang or 'Uncle', became HIV+ by selling his blood at a blood station before the novel starts. He will fall in love with an HIV+ woman named Lingling whose husband as well as in-laws have rejected.

When the story begins Grandpa's only grandson, Ding Hui's 12-year-old son Ding Qiang, has already died, poisoned to revenge the deaths due to the fever in the village his unrepentant father has caused. The literary device of the child-spirit facilitates narration of emotional dimensions of the story that don't fit well into dialogue, keeps the dead child's character present through to the end, and haunts the village's eventual dénouement with an omniscient moral perspective.

Dream of Ding Village has an eight-part (*bufen* 部分, translated as 'volumes') structure that is bookended by dreams. The one-page volume 1 opens with three short dreams – The Cupbearer's, The Baker's, and The Pharaoh's Dreams – all of which reference producer-consumer and unequal-power relations related to the Pharaoh, an obvious synecdoche for the Chinese state. The chapters of volume 2 use Grandpa's dreams, narration of his recently murdered grandson, dialogue, and description to bring the reader into the complex microcosm of Ding Village the autumn before its demise. The chapters in the next volumes 3–7 cover the following year of inextricable decline.

Grandpa sets up the old village school outside of town as the quarantine for HIV+ villagers. The lovers Uncle and Lingling meet and have their first tryst there. Yet even that small community falls apart by the end of volume 3. Although the HIV+ villagers decide to regroup in the village school in volume 4, a new Maoist-era style management of fellow HIV+ residents takes over Grandpa's benevolent custodianship. Their Maoist-style new rule allows the selling off of most everything in the school as well as the cutting down of all the trees in the village to make coffins for the deceased. Defying social norms, Uncle and Lingling nonetheless move in together, get married, and die in volume 5, which concludes with their funeral. In volume 6, Ding Hui has an extravagant burial chamber created for both but only on the condition that Grandpa says that his younger brother and not he was the village bloodhead. Shortly after he moves his remaining family to the city, and meanwhile Ding's extravagant burial chamber, intended more for displaying his own wealth than expressing grief or remorse for their deaths, is ransacked.

By way of conclusion, volume 7 details how the new city-dweller Ding Hui carries out a matchmaking scheme to marry his deceased son to the much older deceased daughter of a 'powerful man', thereby creating new 'family ties' to ensure his political mobility within the metropolis. He ostentatiously returns to Ding Village to exhume his son's remains to be reburied in the new wife's hometown. Enraged with his son's behaviour, Grandpa kills Ding Hui with one blow to the back of the head while his grandson's funeral procession is still in full swing. Thus the *Dream of Ding Village* is bookended by two murders within one family – first villagers poison the grandson to avenge his father's crimes and then Grandpa kills his son as a form of redemption for his crimes against the village – and dreams. After having been arrested and then released for this murder, in the concluding volume 8 the book ends with Grandpa's final dream: with a flick of her willow branch in the mud, the mythical primogenitor Nüwa resurrects the devastated, depopulated, and barren landscape the fever has left in its wake with tiny mud people.

Yan used the novel form to launch a serious indictment of state complicity in this scandal from the lowest to highest levels of Chinese government. Modeling *Dream of Ding Village* on the catastrophe of AIDS villages in rural China in the 1990s allowed Yan to highlight the cost of China's capitalist development for innocent villagers and the unequal power at all levels between them and their government. Yet he also acknowledged self-censorship related to other matters he observed – especially disturbing are his accounts of how cavalier the bloodheads were with handling the donors' blood – about the HIV/AIDS epidemic in Henan in order to publish in Mainland China (Zhang 2006).

Nonetheless, the Chinese government still banned the original version of *Dream of Ding Village* for what the censors alleged were descriptions that exaggerated the AIDS crisis in rural China. The full version was published in Hong Kong (2006). The English translation (2009) is based on it. The movie script had to be modified further for *Love for Life* to accommodate the Chinese government's censorship demands (Qian 2016: 204).

The fever in *Love for Life*

One of the reasons the Chinese government likely supported making *Love for Life* is because of its focus on sick villagers who contracted HIV, considered an 'innocent' or 'legitimate' way from the 'moral disease' perspective.[6] No gay people, sex workers, or intravenous drug users enter the narrative of either the novel or the film. *Love for Life* also reduced the higher levels of government complicity in the HIV/AIDS epidemic detailed in the *Dream* down to just the county-level bloodhead, represented by the eldest son. By contrast, most Anglo-American films devoted to the HIV/AIDS epidemic were located in major cities and focused on the gay population, prostitutes, intravenous drug users, and other people considered to engage in high-risk behaviours (Li 2016: 235; i.e., Philadelphia Story 1993; Rent 2005; Dallas Buyers Club 2013). The television film on the American teenage hemophiliac expelled from a suburban middle school in Kokomo, Indiana in the late 1980s is the one exception (Ryan White Story 1989).

Although AIDS is mentioned in the beginning of the film as well as the *Dream*, the villagers call it *rebing* 热病 (lit. 'Hot diseases') throughout both the novel and film. As one scholar has argued '*Rebing* not only refers to the fever associated with AIDS, but also signifies people's irrational and crazy materialistic desire, hence an absurd and ill-practiced modernization' (Chan 2016: 191). The first character *re* 热 (heat, hot) in combination with other characters, for instance, can also mean 'bustling with noise and excitement' or 'lively' (*renao* 热闹), 'zealous', 'ardent', and 'enthusiastic' (*rexin* 热心), and 'passionate' (*reqing* 热情). These phrases support the argument that a social fever for gaining wealth went hand-in-hand with mounting medical cases of the fever.

Giving the umbrella term *rebing* for the 'fever' also effectively emphasises the unspecified spectral quality of the fever as a character haunting both novel and film. The *Yellow Emperor's Inner Canon: Basic Questions* (ca. first[t] c. BCE) originally distinguished two types of Hot diseases related to different types of climatic *qi*.

The first included acute-onset febrile disorders caused by external pathogenic *qi* related to changing seasons or local weather. The second was a type of 'Cold Damage' (*shanghan* 傷寒) acquired in the winter but which went dormant until the heat of the spring or summer manifested it as excessive heat and internally impairing dryness. The first *Inner-Canon* definition that Hot diseases could be due to other types of pathogenic climatic *qi* also facilitated conceptualising epidemics as due to pathogenic environmental *qi* unrelated to the winter cold or local climate (Hanson 2011: 16–17).

The rendering of the shared symptoms the characters experience in Chinese as *rebing* also domesticates the foreign-sounding medical neologism for AIDS, *aizibing* 爱滋病 (or 艾滋病, the spelling used in the novel) into a more familiar Chinese disease concept. The second character in the compound *aizi* for AIDS, *zi* 滋 (to grow, multiply, spurt, or burst), however, can also have an aptly negative sense. This is expressed in the character combinations *zishi* 滋事 and *zirao* 滋扰 meaning 'to cause trouble' or 'to provoke a dispute'. On the other hand, the homonym for the barely mentioned medical term – *aizi* 爱滋 (a transliteration for 'AIDS') – is *aizi* 爱资 (meaning 'love of capital'), as one scholar has argued captures how the post-socialist Chinese government's promotion of capitalism directly contributed to the spread of HIV/AIDS in China (Tsai 2011; Qian 2016: 220). Yet in the *Dream*, Yan did not use the character *ai* 爱 meaning 'love' but rather the character *ai* 艾 meaning 'Chinese mugwort', 'end, or stop', or 'pretty, handsome'. Although the phrase *aizi* 艾滋 is only used for transliterating AIDS, Yan's choice over the other option suggests both the version with which his informants may have been more familiar and a call 'to end the growth' (*aizi* 艾滋) of this disease. The peasants followed the government's policy 'to get rich quickly' (*kuaisu zhifu* 快速致富) only to receive ephemeral cash in exchange for permanently contaminated blood and a state that turned its back on them.

The family within Love for Life

In transforming the novel *Dream of Ding Village* into the film *Love for Life*, Gu Changwei chose not to include Yan's literary use of Grandpa's premonitory dream sequences but rather to amplify his choice of the child-spirit as narrator. One of the most powerful techniques of the film version is to accompany the child's haunting narration with aerial scenes of the village's surrounding countryside as if he's a spirit watching the scene below. This narrative device also reflects how many Chinese continue to believe in the afterlife (Wang 2014). The child-spirit thus states in the opening narration:

> Let's say our village is called Goddess Temple,
> High up in the mountains.
> Don't know from when,
> A Fever that the world called AIDS,
> Snuck into our village quietly from outside.
> With the Fever, life perishes like the fallen leaves (Chan 2016: 220).

In contrast to the novel's opening with Grandpa's dream and his revelatory meeting with local officials about the true nature of the fever, the film opens with the dead child identifying the fever as AIDS as the camera pans widely across the Henan mountains within which his family's 'Goddess Temple' village is nestled. This visual device coupled with the choice of an HIV+ non-professional child actor to play the grandson further amplifies the literary foundation Yan's *Dream* established with new visual possibilities the film medium allows.

The story is framed within two major relationships: those within and related to the three generations of the Zhao family (i.e. the Ding family in the novel) and the adulterous love affair between the younger of the two Zhao brothers, Zhao Deyi (played by Aaron Kwok Fu-shing 郭富城) and a married woman, Shang Qinqin (played by Zhang Ziyi 章子怡). Choosing lead actors who are household names in Mainland China to be the lovers appears to have been a strategy to evoke audience sympathy toward the HIV+ lovers. By extension, it's a strategy seeking greater compassion for people living with HIV/AIDS in China that the fever epidemic in the village epitomises.

The couple meet at the abandoned village school that Deyi's father, Lao Zhuzhu 老柱柱 (lit. 'venerable pillar', played by Tao Zeru 陶泽如) has converted into a hospice for all afflicted members of the village to live together free from the stigma and rejection of the healthy villagers. As the moral centre, the senior Zhao seeks to right the wrongs of his unrepentant older son, Zhao Qiquan 赵齐全 (played by Pu Cunxin 濮存昕), who as the now wealthy blood merchant is primarily responsible for the fever epidemic in the village. As the fever frays the ties binding the multi-generational Zhao family to the breaking point, it tightens the bond between the ill-fated lovers.

The plot revolves around three family relationships: the central conflicts within the Zhao family between Grandpa and his eldest bloodhead son; the love affair between Zhao Deyi 'Uncle' and Shang Qinqin (and the resulting tensions with their family members); and breaks in trust within the alternative family living in the school compound when several cases of theft are discovered. For example, Shang Qinqin arrives to the school wearing a bright red silk jacket that traditionally symbolises good fortune. Here it may symbolise the contaminated blood that unites her with those also residing at the school, the blood ties that the fever has forever frayed, and the passion she will soon reciprocate. But the jacket is stolen shortly after she arrives, the lifelong diary of the former Village Head also goes missing, and a bag of rice from the compound's kitchen is found hidden within the pillow case of the cook. These breaches in trust function as plot devices to flesh out the other characters whose families have rejected them. Within the school family, however, the transgressors are mostly exonerated of their crimes out of empathy that their tragic stories elicit among their surrogate family members living in the school.

Public-health quarantine in Love for Life

In addition to the aerial register that often accompanies the child-spirit's narration, the other visual register is in the streets, homes, and public gathering space of the village where the film vividly portrays how the healthy and sick villagers respond to the epidemic. The abandoned school that Grandpa has turned into a hospice receives most film time as the microcosm within the village microcosm. Historically, the school-turned-hospice represents a typical response to epidemic outbreaks to separate the sick from the healthy in quarantine, usually outside communities, and called variously in European medical history a lazaretto, leper colony, plague house, or pest house. Such spaces allowed a sense of normality to continue where the healthy resided while the eventual mortality from the epidemic played out separately in the segregated place.

This segregated space also allows a safe space for the exiled beyond the social constraints of the village where both the affair and some levity among the outcasts can occur as well. One of the funniest scenes is when a pig escapes the school's kitchen with the cook running in close pursuit through the village until the pig turns around and under her legs managing to take her for a ride on his back. The village school functions more to provide a space for an alternative family to develop among those living there expelled from their own families than a cordon-sanitaire to protect those same families from their infected exiles. This affection is expressed during the funeral procession for the cook who has died soon after the pig chase from a fever that broke out from her anger toward the pig. One of the most moving scenes in the film is when Qinqin and Uncle are roaming in the hills surrounding the school. Uncle attempts to outrun a moving train high above the mountains, a metaphor for both his soon-approaching death and 'love for life' as they've chosen to live what's remaining of their lives together free from social constraints (Qian 2016: 208–10).

Genre-blending in Love for Life

Although *Love for Life* fits well into a multimedia HIV/AIDS anti-stigmatization public health campaign, it is also fundamentally a love story told within a family melodrama. The genres of Hollywood love story and medical docudrama are combined in the final dénouement of the lovers' lives and so too the house of Zhao. Melodramas are characterised by an appeal to emotions over subtle characterization and so tend to have stereotyped instead of nuanced figures. Thus the villainous profit-driven eldest son markedly contrasts with the victimised carefree younger son. Their father is the stalwart moral centre that neither son comes close to emulating. Melodramas tend also to be situated in the private sphere with some kind of challenge from without. With a medical twist, the fever takes on the role of the typical seductress, malefactor, or villain challenging from without the family's harmony within. Thus the euphoria of the HIV+ lovers' beginning matches the pathos of their final hours together. Some viewers may find these kinds of black-and-white contrasts unconvincing, even corny and simplistic, but they nonetheless fit well into the genres within which they participate. One scholar analysed 'the sentimental touch', or the melodramatic dimensions, of this film as cinematic strategies intended to touch people emotionally in the right way, 'by "moving people to *tears*" rather than to other physiological responses'. Related to the genre choice of melodrama for *Love for Life*, she further argues that 'such generic excesses attempt to address the cultural problems brought on by both HIV/AIDS and China's newfound capitalism' (Zuo 2015: 216).

Much of Uncle and Qinqin's love affair centres on how to make their commitment to each other legitimate by divorcing from their spouses, sharing living spaces, and eventually getting married. When Qinqin's husband, tipped off by two non-infected villagers, catches the new couple when they first get together, she is forced to return home against her will. Eventually chased out, her mother-in-law asks her to return only once her husband has found a new wife so that then they can get divorced. Upon her second return to the school, despite resignation, Uncle convinces her to resist her decent into depression, love openly together, and move into an abandoned one-room cottage high on a hilltop.

When they decide to get married, Uncle seeks help from his doubtful father to help with Qinqin's divorce. Related to the theme of profit-making off of an other's misery, Qinqin's husband agrees but only on the condition that Uncle wills him the house he once shared with his first wife. Uncle and Qinqin move into Uncle's original house and seek help from the elder brother for political legitimation through a marriage license from the state.

The day they receive their marriage certificates they dress in celebratory red and proudly announce their new status to everyone in the village, passing out lucky candies to all they meet, but the villagers turn away from them. With incomparable fortitude, they live openly as husband and wife in their new home.

Distraught by all of these events, Grandpa implores his surviving son to redeem himself with the villagers and finally make amends for the fever's increasing death toll. Despite his father's moral example and ethical arguments, the wayward son has switched from blood banks to one profit-making scheme after another. Profiting off the villagers' misery, he sells coffins to the families of the dead and organises ghost marriages between the deceased. Ghost marriages occur between the unmarried deceased in part as a means to pacify their spirits in the afterlife. Clearly profiting off the still common Chinese belief in the afterlife, a villager nonetheless praises Ding Hui for solving problems for the living by selling coffins at a low price and arranging ghost marriages for their lonely dead (Wang 2014: 146).

The ancient practice of ghost marriages has been observed in Singapore in the 1950s to resolve several social problems such as acquiring a grandson to carry on the family name when the birth son has prematurely died without heir or securing the relationship (and responsibilities) of a living daughter-in-law after the premature death of an unmarried son, (Topley 1955, 1956). Not only is there a popular culture film niche about ghost marriages in modern China[7] but also a market for unmarried women's corpses and bones that has led to grave robbery and even murder. The practice has been observed recently in contemporary Shanxi, Shaanxi, and Henan provinces as well as Hong Kong (Tsoi 2016). These marriages are sometimes simply a means of emotional compensation for bereaved families of prematurely deceased offspring. However, they also can function to solidify new relations among the living just as in the ghost marriage of the young boy, which is intended to strengthen his father's own political ties with a man more powerful than him that is part of the conclusion of the *Dream of Ding Village* and *Love of Life*.

Love of Life significantly does not conclude with Grandfather's murder of his profit-driven eldest son. Rather it concludes with the lovers' final night. At the heat of the summer, Uncle is struck down by a severe fever that will not break. Understanding what his delirium means, Qinqin succeeds in cooling him down by immersing herself in an outdoor stone basin of cold water and covering his body with her chilled flesh. Upon waking cured of his fever, he reaches for her to no avail. The camera pans to where she lay on the floor beside their bed, where she has passed away after completely exhausting her own energy to restore his during the night. Rather than live out the rest of his remaining life without her, he takes his own life by allowing himself to bleed to death by cutting his flesh.

The final scene returns to the day when they had received their marriage certificates, dressed up, and went out to share their good fortune with fellow villagers. Now alone in a stone-stepped corridor of the village, Qinqin emotionally reads out loud several times the formal People's Republic of China's statement legitimating their marriage. This underscores the film's narrative that the top-level of the state came through for the lovers before their end. It reminds reviewers that the film itself was a product of the Chinese state trying to present itself in the best possible light. As a part of a broader HIV-AIDS public health campaign, the film provides some information on how HIV is transmitted and confronts HIV stigmatization head on, but the Chinese state's central role in the HIV-tainted blood scandal that tragically exacerbated the AIDS epidemic in rural China is strategically reduced to just the greed of one local-level cadre with no moral compass.

HIV/AIDS in *Together*

Similar to *Love for Life*, *Together* also visually opens with panoramic views of rural Henan Mountains before it settles down on the film set. Several members of the film crew and extras are surprised to learn that there are HIV+ people working as actors and working on the set. Zhao also used online chat rooms for people living with HIV/AIDS to portray a wider range of such people than did either the novel or film. In interviews he says that he made considerable effort to first establish friendships before discussing participation in his documentary. Only six people agreed to be on the film set, two in face-blurring interviews and three as full participants. Another four agreed to be interviewed off the set but again without fully showing their faces. The following four subsections move first from the on-set family that develops between three of the HIV+ participants in the film to scenes of the young boy HIV+ actor off set with his family. The discussion then expands further to the wider HIV/AIDS community Zhao was able to reach via online chat rooms and face-to-face interviews and, finally, to the documentary's multimedia dimension as part of the Health Ministry's public-health campaign.[8]

The on-set family in Together

Much of *Together* focuses on three of the six HIV+ people who agreed both to participate in the film's production and be filmed in the documentary. First, there is Hu Zetao, the 12-year-old HIV+ boy who plays the child-spirit in *Love for Life*. His mother died from AIDS when he was just four years old. During the filming of the documentary, he lived with his grandmother, father, and stepmother and attended the AIDS Rose childcare at the Red Ribbon School in Shanxi province, which then had 16 children living with AIDS.

One of the caretakers at the school, Ms Liu Liping (known online as AIDS Rose), agreed while taking care of Hu Zetao to be filmed on set. She had been HIV+ for a decade after receiving a contaminated blood transfusion at a hospital when she was in a coma-state from an ectopic pregnancy. The third featured HIV+ person is the middle-aged Mr Xia from Shanghai who agreed to work as the stand-in for the main actor Aaron Kwok. Out of shame, he never revealed how he contracted HIV but nonetheless stated that 'If my face can change people's attitudes toward the disease even a bit, then let it be uncovered'.

Mr Xia's online name, 'Mr Down and Out', captures well how negatively he perceived his HIV+ status. Although he shared that his wife died in a car accident, he never revealed how he contracted the disease. We learn more about him obliquely when he expresses the typical 'moral view' that some means of transmission are innocent – such as the child's in-utero transmission and Ms Liu's contaminated blood transmission – and other means – such as however he acquired it – are illegitimate. Among the 'guilty' cases, he portrayed his HIV+ status as a 'punishment'. He testified to his experiences with discrimination, living a closeted life regarding his status, and having a mostly single anonymous life within a monastery. Yet he nonetheless spoke frankly in interviews both on set and in front of the monastery where he lived. Before the filming was complete, Mr Xia became sick with a rash requiring him to leave to adjust his medications. When thanking everyone for their kindness toward him, by acknowledging that 'nobody here discriminated against me', he appears also to convey a transformation in his self-esteem and sense of self-worth stemming directly from his participation.

Despite the separate lives of these three HIV+ participants – the young boy actor Hu Zetao, his care-giver Mrs Liu (online AIDS Rose), and Mr Xia (online Mr Down and Out) – formed a tight-knit nuclear family on the *Love for Life* set. The documentary's main story line centres on them talking amongst themselves about their lives and aspirations in their rooms, outside, and on set. One particularly moving scene captures them having a picnic in the shade of a flowering tree discussing what they would like to return as if reincarnated. Their presence in *Together* demonstrates how participation in a documentary can itself be a catalyst for individual self-awareness and change through such intimate conversations. These three HIV+ participants appear to be presented within the documentary genre as possible models for new ways of living with HIV/AIDS and acting toward HIV+ people for future viewers of the documentary.

The film crew represented a preliminary 'test audience', in fact, since some of the crewmen quit the film at the beginning when they learned they would be working with HIV+ people on the set. Other crewmembers expressed their concerns about being among HIV+ people and admitted their lack of knowledge about transmission, effectively representing the reservations of the wider non-HIV+ audience the documentary also intended to reach. Recreating an on-set family within the frame of the documentary functioned to create a social unit immediately recognizable to a potentially skeptical audience. This family-centred strategy appears to be a deliberate one within the Chinese context to transform potential viewers' negative views of and interactions with people living with HIV/AIDS into more positive humane ones.

The off-set family in **Together**

Similar to the children portrayed in *The Blood of Yingzhou District*, the most compelling figure in Zhao Liang's *Together* is the HIV+ child actor Hu Zetao. Like Yang, Zhao also allows the boy to discuss his experiences living with HIV/AIDS separate from his family. He also films scenes within his home where he lives with his grandmother, father, and stepmother. Zhao's portrayal of Hu Zetao is as compassionate as Yang's earlier portrayals of HIV+ children. It is just as honest about discrimination from their own family members as well as other children and adults in their villages. Both artists bring the problem of HIV/AIDS stigma and discrimination down to the most intimate family level. By portraying individuals within their social worlds, they reveal how stigma often sets its first and most painful wounds through familial interactions.

The viewer sees how subtle discrimination still played out within young Hu's family members despite their understanding of how HIV/AIDS is transmitted. In one of the most moving scenes, his father selected food for him rather than have his chopsticks touch shared dishes. Although Hu was told he could select his own food, he was clearly uncomfortable with the action and, at first refusing, only tentatively tries to find some remaining noodles. Before filming, in fact, the rest of the family ate separately from him. That had changed in the process of making the documentary, but they still had a washbasin set aside for him. Zhao Liang also films him washing his own basin and utensils. Particularly uncomfortable are scenes that reveal tensions with his stepmother who resents that his father did not inform her of his son's HIV+ status before getting married and remains unconvinced that the father is not also infected. She also requested that her face be blurred. It is clear that she has not fully embraced her stepson and regrets that his HIV+ status is public knowledge in the village. Nonetheless, her discomfort and unease likely mirrors well how some potential Chinese viewers may also feel about people living with HIV/AIDS both within and outside their families.

In contrast to his relative silence in his own household, Hu Zetao is notably more relaxed and talkative within his on-set family. Back with them, he opens up about his experiences with fellow villagers, which resemble the discrimination the children of Yingzhou District also described. Since many of the villagers know he is HIV+, they also keep their distance from him. When they socially ostracise him in this way, he admits to sometimes going closer toward them and saying that he would infect them. He does this just to antagonise them. He poignantly remarks that if they were also infected they would no longer have reason to discriminate against him. Although Zhao's *Together* clearly builds upon Ruby Yang's focus on vulnerable HIV+ children who still face related tensions within their own families, he cast a broader net to capture the experiences of a wider range of HIV+ people in China.

The wider net cast in Together

In an interview Zhao stated that he initially hesitated to accept Gu Changwei's offer to film a documentary about people living with AIDS in China on the film set of what became *Love for Life*. He eventually agreed to do it largely because of the wider audience within China that working with the state's Health Ministry would allow his work to reach. But in the beginning it was quite difficult to find HIV+ people who were willing to participate, much less be filmed in the joint film-documentary and public health campaign project. Nonetheless, in addition to the six who agreed to work on the set (including the on-set family of three), it also features segments of interviews with four of the 60 AIDS patients he successfully reached through live-chat exchanges.

Together illustrates this searching process via the web by typing out conversations on screen as if live onto film footage of various towns and cities in China where his interviewees (i.e., Invisible Angel, Eternal Love, etc.) presumably lived closeted lives. This visual strategy effectively captured the human intimacy of these exchanges over deeply personal matters while simultaneously conveying the painful isolation many of these same people discussed experiencing in their daily lives.

In these scenes Zhao also integrated the experiences of those people living with HIV/AIDS who engaged in more high-risk behaviours such as unprotected heterosexual and homosexual intercourse and sharing needles for intravenous drug use. Since most of these people did not agree to be part of *Love for Life*, reproducing the social media 'live chat' means he used to interact with them on screen reveals how they've used both the web to create their own online HIV/AIDS communities and the new documentary genre (as far as they were comfortable) to make their voices heard.

There were some notable exceptions of HIV+ people – a woman who contracted it through sexual intercourse, a former drug-using single mother, a divorced woman, and a sexually active man – some of whom allowed themselves to be filmed within their own homes. Snow, a 32-year-old women, sits in what appears to be the reception room in a restaurant or possibly a 'house of entertainment'. She confesses that she didn't realise that she needed to protect herself when she had sex but 'now I won't do it without a condom'. Although she recounts that the guys say, 'What fun is washing your feet with socks on', nonetheless she recounts that when she explains carefully the risk to them and their wives, they are now able to accept using a condom. Although her mother knows that she is sick, she has not informed her what kind of illness it is because she finds it shameful. This shame is mirrored in the censoring of her status as a sex worker, perhaps because she appears to be continuing to work as one without any noticeable sense of shame.

Censoring explicit acknowledgement of the sex industry context within which Snow contracted HIV contrasts with the next woman interviewed who acquired the HIV virus through intravenous drug use. This fact may have passed China's censors precisely because she has since renounced drugs and demonstrates guilt for her current situation. Furthermore, her son's father has abandoned them and, being too sick to care for him alone, they now live with her parents where she furthermore expresses remorse for contributing to their burden. She movingly admits to nearly killing herself and son with rat poison. Yet although she shields her face and that of her son while expressing fear that her condition will influence his kindergarten friends' opinions of him, she allowed Zhao to film them together at home. This scene shows her not only choosing life over death, but also making a shift in her life course by agreeing to the one-on-one interview itself.

A college-aged woman who appears to have been interviewed in her dorm room was infected by her first boyfriend. She only found out through a college blood drive. She expresses despair that she has become HIV+ in this way before even entering the world. Similarly, another woman named Ms Zhao was infected by her husband who was also her sole sexual partner. He had not previously informed her that he was HIV+ when they married. Both of these women express feelings that their lives have been destroyed before they had truly begun. Filmed discretely without fully revealing her face, the interview itself appears to be helping Ms Zhao come out of her shell. She thus performs another possibility of how to live with her status, if not openly among her co-workers, at least more honestly among those who belong to the same online community through which she responded to Zhao.

On the other side of the spectrum from these women related to acceptance of HIV+ status, Zhao also interviewed a sexually active gay man. Zhao lingers on many details of the simple one-room apartment as a way of portraying the man whose face is otherwise not revealed. A single bed, desk for computer, some dressers, and a chair comprise his small apartment. The most moving part of the exchange is when the man explains that most of the gay men he knows use condoms. Sometimes with a trusted partner, however, they choose not to, which is how he admits that he thinks he contracted HIV. Although he suspects who passed the HIV virus on to him, he is not completely sure. Also he chose not to contact him about it, suggesting a deeper sense of betrayal as well as shame. This life-changing fact, however, neither deterred him from seeking further male partners nor from being active as a leader in the online gay community.

As a result of such open nonjudgmental personal interviews, *Together* not only testifies to the range of people living with HIV/AIDS in China today but also demonstrates the power of the documentary genre itself as a means for them to find their own voices to effect positive change in the broader society as well as within themselves.

The public-health campaign dimension of Together

The different narrative genres of fiction, film, public health message, and propaganda all come into play most clearly in *Together*. Three government agencies – the Health Ministry, Central Propaganda Department, and the State Administration of Radio, Film, and Television's film bureau – were involved in financially backing as well as censoring the final results of *Together* and *Love for Life*. *Together* made this collaboration transparent by filming the board meeting scene when representatives of the Health Ministry have been brought together with those in the State Administration of Radio, Film, and Television and also the Peking Union Medical Hospital. The public health officials used this board meeting as a platform within the documentary medium to explain how HIV/AIDS is transmitted and treated and what the government is doing about it. This is clearly a direct public health message to prevent its further spread, get people to seek treatment, and encourage compassion of non–HIV+ people toward people living with HIV/AIDS in China.

The documentary then shifts into a completely different visual mode that follows a straightforward style of a public-health message. Against a moving image of one slightly larger green cell amongst several other grey cells, the text summarises important years in China's AIDS history according to this documentary's state sponsors: 1) 1985 China reports its first case of AIDS; 2) 2003 The Chinese government implements the 'Four Free One Care' Policy; 3) 2006 The State Council approves and implements 'AIDS Prevention Regulations'; and 4) 2010 China lifts travel restriction on foreign visitors with AIDS, STDs or Leprosy.

Just as the single green cell begins to enter one of the gray cells, suddenly an explanation appears that clarifies that the background film is 'The first time scientists photographed the process of the AIDS virus spreading inside a human body'. This excerpt of a scientific film within the documentary film effectively amplifies the message of the next two statements that summarised the then-current situation of the Chinese AIDS epidemic: 1) Of an estimated 740,000 people with HIV/AIDS, approximately 400,000 do not know that they have it; 2) of 48,000 new cases of transmission in 2009, there were 43.3% heterosexual, 32.5% homosexual, 24.3% injection drug use, and 1.0% mother-to-child forms of transmission; 3) sexual transmission remains the main vector; 4) homosexual transmission is increasing; and 5) although overall HIV/AIDS in China is at low levels and slowing down, certain areas remain serious and numbers of people there are still increasing due to diverse means of transmission.

In the concluding minutes, Zhao shifts from the four registers that have mostly structured his documentary – the on-set family centred around the boy Hu Zetao, his actual off-set family life, the direct interviews, and the online exchanges with HIV+ people – to film an AIDS activist on a busy street corner. Rather than close *Together* with the utopian world of 'family' and ideal of 'togetherness' the community established on the *Love for Life* film set represents, one scholar argues this shift to the city street forces viewers back to the cruel reality of the present and all the problems that remain. The activist is Liu Jiulong 刘九龙, a PWA street artist, who tells people that although he is an *aizi bingren* 爱滋病人 (an AIDS patient), he would like to hug them (Li 2016: 248–9). Although most people walk past him, an 80-year old woman allows him to hug her and then a younger woman gives him a hug. The documentary functions here as an explicit public-health message: hugs don't transmit AIDS. But the street scene also enacts the acceptance of one HIV+ person that the documentary-cum-film hopes to achieve for all people living with HIV/AIDS in China.

This example of AIDS public health education on the street segues into final interviews with members of the film crew and the two main stars of the movie – Zhang Ziyi and Aaron Kwok. They both reassert the overall message of *Love for Life* that HIV+ people deserve to be loved, to connect, and to experience happiness just like everyone else. Kwok concludes 'don't let them be isolated' and Zhang states that she 'wants society to be like our movie crew'. Speaking directly to the camera, Zhang Ziyi encourages fellow Chinese to put an end to the social exclusion, stigmatization, and discrimination of people living with HIV/AIDS in China. Their testimony clarifies that the intention of this film-documentary project was to create a model community on the film set of HIV+ and HIV– people living harmoniously together that could be followed everywhere China. *Together* documents an artistically conceived and yet Chinese government-backed media experiment intended to transform how HIV/AIDS people are treated broadly in Chinese society.

Together, *Love for Life*, and *Dream of Ding Village* are revealing examples of how some of China's most socially engaged contemporary artists navigate the line between independent expression and critical thinking, on the one side, and access for their creative works to the government-controlled distribution networks to audiences within mainland China that requires government approval, financing, and thus censorship within China's authoritarian system, on the other side. As one scholar concluded, Zhao's documentary 'is neither conservative, caving to State pressure, nor liberal, striving to legitimise gay rights. It is primarily pragmatic. The core effort of *Together* lies in 'demystifying' the popular imagination of AIDS by bringing out a full range of coming-out stories' (Li 2016 249).

Zhao Liang has been criticised for selling himself out by working with the Chinese government on *Together*. He admits, for example, that he accepted some official censors' requests for changes, such as deleting mention that one of the women he interviewed (i.e., Snow) contracted HIV/AIDS through sex work. *Together* also notably did not address how the government's lack of transparency about, and attempts to conceal, the extent of the HIV/AIDS epidemic in China contributed to exacerbating it (Wong 2011).

Nonetheless, Zhao included marginalized people who contracted HIV/AIDS through sex work, homosexual sex, and taking drugs in the first Chinese government supported documentary about HIV/AIDS discrimination. *Together* is an illuminating example of how one of the most fearless documentary makers confronting injustice in early twenty-first-century China has carved out a space within China's authoritarian system for a wider spectrum of HIV+ Chinese individuals to share their life experiences. *Together* demonstrates the documentary's greater potential power than either film or fiction to allow subaltern peoples to speak for themselves.

Conclusion

The preceding analysis shows how in the immediate post-SARS moment from 2003 on the Chinese government took a new multimedia approach to a public health campaign to counter prejudice, stigma, and discrimination against people living with HIV/AIDS. This required compromises from all the artists involved: Yan Lianke's banned novel was further adapted to an accepted film script by reducing its critique of government complicity down to the local cadre; Gu Changwei and his wife Jiang Wenli had to develop a proposal for the film and documentary that officials in the Health Ministry would support; and though asking Zhao Liang to make a documentary on the making of the film gave the project more credibility, he suffered considerable public shaming as a 'sell-out' for his participation (Wong 2011; Li 2016: 232–3).

Although the *Dream of Ding Village* is arguably closest to the dystopian reality of the actual situation in rural Henan villages, it is the feature film *Love for Life* that has likely had the most public exposure through both the fame of its actors and its genre's form. Although *Together* was released in 17 Chinese cities on World AIDS day, 1 December 2010 and selected the following February for the 61st Berlin International Film Festival (Li 2016: 232 fn5), it now likely has the smallest audience consisting of AIDS activists and foreign film enthusiasts. *Together* remains accessible online abroad with all its revelations about risky behaviours and yet compassionate portrayal of homosexuals and drug users in China.

Those who feared that Zhao has sold his soul to the Chinese state by collaborating with the Chinese government to make *Together*, however, need look no further than his recent muckraking documentary on the environmental destruction of Inner Mongolia wrought by Chinese toxic coal mining and iron works in *Behemoth* (*Beixi moshou* 悲兮魔兽 2015). This has lead one reviewer to call him a modern-day Dante (Weissberg 2015). Although Zhao has returned to his originally independent modus operandi, we may well see him straddling the independent-mode and government-sponsored mode of documentary making depending on the messages he chooses to convey and the audiences he wishes to reach in the future.

The other Chinese documentary filmmaker on HIV/AIDS in China, Ruby Yang, has taken a different approach since she filmed *The Blood of Yingzhou District* in 2003. A decade later Yang returned to Yingzhou to document what had become of the same children she featured earlier. The original documentary was a heart-wrenching entry into the intersections of poverty and disease, social stigma, and child abandonment. *The Blood of Yingzhou District Revisited* (2013), by contrast, presents a heart-warming account of the social and institutional transformations that occurred within just a decade that facilitated the taking care of, educating, and integrating of these children into Chinese society as they matured into students and adults. This makes one wonder if Yan Lianke, Gu Changwei, and Zhao Liang returned to rural Henan would they be able to report back that their collective effort to put human faces on the HIV/AIDS epidemic in China had comparable effects?

Their collective storytelling via fiction, film, and documentary nonetheless put a human face on the HIV/AIDS epidemic in rural Henan in China in the 1990s and actual people living with HIV/AIDS across China. Once named HIV/AIDS, the fever *rebing* could then become a social diagnosis of failures in government transparency due to complicity, an unfettered capitalist market that encouraged unregulated blood selling, and a rural healthcare system that had essentially collapsed. Framing the particular history of the HIV/AIDS epidemic in China in such ways also makes it possible to inspire participants, moviegoers, and readers as well as people living with HIV/AIDS themselves to take action that could affect change in their lives, communities, and institutions far beyond their initial inspiration from the novel, film, and documentary. As importantly, such cultural responses have the power to compel the Chinese government to respond and by so doing take responsibility for the care of some of their most vulnerable citizens.

Notes

1 Other independent documentaries and cultural responses to HIV/AIDS in China not discussed here include Zhuang Kongshao's *Huri* 虎日 (*Tiger Day* 2002); Chen Weijun's *Hao si buru lai huozhe* 好死不如赖活着 (*To Live is Better Than to Die* 2005); Ai Xiaoming's *Zhongyuan ji shi* 中原纪事 (*The Epic of Central Plains* 2006); and *Guan'ai zhi jia* 关爱之家 (*Love and Care* 2007). See Zuo (2015: 206).
2 For his filmography see his website: http://zhaoliangstudio.com/about, accessed 24 March 2019.
3 *Tale of Magic* was one of several names being considered before Director Gu settled on *Zui ai* (lit. most loved, but translated as 'Love for Life' for the movie). The 'drama of changing titles' was mentioned but other titles not specified in Qian (2016: 204). The English Wikipedia page gives two other English alternatives by which the film was known: *Life Is a Miracle* and *Til Death Do Us Part*. https://en.wikipedia.org/wiki/Love_for_Life, accessed 19 September 2018.
4 The original Chinese and English translation opens the documentary. www.youtube.com/watch?v=hu8H4jju3oA, accessed 14 March 2019.
5 During the early 2000s, photojournalist Hu Guang 户广 (b. 1961) produced unflinching photographs of AIDS victims in rural Henan, for which, in 2004, he won a First Prize World Press Photo award (World Press Photo 2004; China Underground 2017).
6 In 2011, the Chinese director Zhang Miaoyan also released a Sino-French made film about the AIDS villages in Henan shot in black and white titled *Black Blood* (*Heixue* 黑血). It focuses on a poor couple that tries to make ends meet by selling blood and then by starting a blood-collecting business (Adams 2011).
7 Xref Peng Tao's Cremator Xref also Meng Ong's *A Fantastic Ghost Wedding 2014*. See link www.imdb.com/title/tt3460062/?ref_=ttpl_pl_tt, accessed 19 March 2019.
8 The opening credit to the 'Film Bureau State Administration of Radio, Film, & TV' underscores this connection.

Filmography

Filmography for Gu Changwei

And the Spring Comes (*Li chun* 立春), dir. Gu Changwei, 2007.
Love For Life (*Zui ai* 最爱, also known as *Tale of Magic*, *Life Is a Miracle* and *Til Death Do Us Part*), dir. Gu Changwei, 2011.

Love on the Cloud (*Weiai zhi jianru jia jing* 微爱之渐入佳境), dir. Gu Changwei, 2014.
Never Abandon, Never Give Up, dir. Gu Changwei, 2009 (Short film for the International
    Labour Organization's ILOAIDS program).
Peacock (*Kongque* 孔雀), dir. Gu Changwei, 2005.

Filmography for Zhao Liang

Behemoth (*Beixi moshou* 悲兮魔兽), dir. Zhao Liang, 2015.
Crime and Punishment (*Zui yu fa* 罪与罚), dir. Zhao Liang, 2007.
Farewell Yuanmingyuan (*Gaobie Yuanmingyuan* 告别圆明园)), dir. Zhao Liang, 1995.
Paper Airplane (*Zhi feiji* 纸飞机), dir. Zhao Liang, 2001.
Petition the Court of Complainants (*Shang Fang* 上访), dir. Zhao Liang, 2009.
Return to the Border (*Zai jiang bian* 在江边), dir. Zhao Liang, 2005.
Together (*Zai yiqi* 在一起), dir. Zhao Liang, 2010.

Bibliography

Adams, M. (2011) Black Blood, *Screen Daily*, 6 February 2011, www.screendaily.com/black-blood/5023345.article, accessed 19 September 2018.
Adams, V., Erwin, K. and Le, P.V. (2006) Public Health Works: Blood Donation in Urban China, *Social Science and Medicine*, 68 (3): 410–18.
Asia Pacific Arts (2017) *Interview with Director Zhao Liang*, www.youtube.com/watch?v=Sk_NB0coRII, accessed 7 October 2017.
Berry, C., Lu Xinyu and Rofel, L. (2011) Alternative Archive: China's Independent Documentary Culture, in C. Berry, Lu Xinyu and L. Rofel (eds.) *The New Chinese Documentary Film Movement*, Hong Kong: Hong Kong University Press, pp. 135–54.
Chan, S.W. (2016) Narrating Cancer, Disabilities, and AIDS: Yan Lianke's Trilogy of Disease, in H. Chow (ed.) *Discourses of Disease*, Leiden: Brill, pp. 177–99.
China Underground (2017) *The Shocking Images of the "AIDS Village in Henan"*, 4 July 2017, https://china-underground.com/2017/07/04/shocking-images-aids-village-henan/, accessed 19 September 2018.
Chow, H.Y.F. (2016) *Discourses of Disease: Writing Illness, the Mind and Body in Modern China*, Leiden: Brill.
Davison, N. (2011) The Men Who Gave Aids to China: The Scandal That Saw 'Blood Merchants' Infect Thousands of People with HIV Has Always Been a Taboo Subject. But a New Film Hopes to Change That, *The Independent*, 22 May 2011, www.independent.co.uk/news/world/asia/the-men-who-gave-aids-to-rural-china-2287825.html, accessed 4 October 2017.
Eberstadt, N. (2002) The Future of AIDS, *Foreign Affairs*, 81 (6): 22–45.
Edwards, D. (2015) *Independent Chinese Documentary: Alternative Visions, Alternative Publics*, Edinburgh, Scotland: Edinburgh University Press.
Epstein, G.A. (2003) While Battling SARS, China neglects AIDS, *The Baltimore Sun*, 4 May 2003, http://articles.baltimoresun.com/2003-05-04/news/0305040318_1_people-with-aids-luo-china, accessed 29 September 2018.
Gao Yaojie 高耀潔 (2010) *Gaojie de linghun: Gao Yaojie huiyilu* 高潔的靈魂: 高耀潔回憶錄 (*A Noble and Unsullied Soul: Gao Yaojie Memoirs*), revised and enlarged ed. Hong Kong: Ming Pao.
Gittings, J. (2001a) The Aids Scandal China Could Not Hush Up: Health Officials' Blood-for-cash Scheme Breeds HIV Tragedy, *The Guardian*, 11 June 2001, www.theguardian.com/world/2001/jun/11/china.internationaleducationnews, accessed 4 October 2017.

————. (2001b) China Finally Wakes Up to Aids Timebomb: Epidemic Fear Forces More Openness, but Stigma Remains, *The Guardian*, 13 November 2001, www.theguardian.com/world/2001/nov/13/aids.china, accessed 4 August 2018.

Guo Jinhua and Kleinman, A. (2011) Stigma HIV/AIDS, Mental Illness, and China's Non-persons, in A. Kleinman *et al.* (eds.) *Deep China*, Berkeley: University of California Press, pp. 193–212.

Hanson, M. (2011) *Speaking of Epidemics in Chinese Medicine: Disease and the Geographic Imagination in Late Imperial China*, London: Routledge.

Hayes, A. (2005) AIDS, Bloodheads & Cover-Ups: The 'abc' of Henan's AIDS Epidemic, *AQ: Australian Quarterly*, 77 (3): 12–16, 40.

Hays, J. (2008) *Zhao Liang and His Films Petition, Crime and Punishment, and Together*, October 2011, http://factsanddetails.com/china/cat7/sub42/item1835.html, accessed 7 October 2017.

He Aiping (2000) Revealing the "Blood Wound" of the Spread of HIV/AIDS in Henan Province, *US Embassy (Beijing)*, www.usembassy-china.org.cn/english/sandt/henan-hiv.htm, accessed 7 October 2017.

International Labour Organization (2008) *The First Targeted HIV/AIDS Prevention Campaign in China Featuring Migrant Workers for Their Hometown Fellows*, Press release 25 November 2008 about Gu Changwei's short film *Never Abandon, Never Give Up*, www.ilo.org/beijing/information-resources/public-information/press-releases/WCMS_142075/lang – en/index.htm, accessed 12 March 2019.

Jing, J. (2011) From Commodity of Death to Gift of Life, in A. Kleinman *et al.* (eds.) *Deep China*, Berkeley: University of California Press, pp. 78–105.

Katz, A. (2011) A Dark Reimagining of Chinese Blood-Selling Scandal, *The Boston Globe*, 9 January 2011, http://archive.boston.com/ae/books/articles/2011/01/09/a_dark_reimagining_of_chinese_blood_selling_scandal/, accessed 6 October 2017.

Kessel, J.M. (2011) *Filming China's Dark Side*, 13 August 2011, www.nytimes.com/video/world/asia/100000000844065/filming-chinas-dark-side.html, accessed 11 February 2018.

Kleinman, A., Yan Yunxiang, Jing Jun, Lee, S., Zhang, E., Pan Tianshu, Wu Fei and Guo Jinhua (eds.) (2011) *Deep China: The Moral Life of the Person: What Anthropology and Psychiatry Tell Us About China Today*, Berkeley: University of California Press.

Li Li 李力 (2016) Together: Contagion, Stigmatization and Utopia as Therapy in Zhao Liang's AIDS Documentary Together, in H.Y.F. Chow (ed.) *Discourses of Disease: Writing Illness, the Mind and Body in Modern China*, Leiden: Brill, pp. 231–51.

Liu, J. (2010) Exiled China Aids Activist Mourns Her Former Life, *BBC News*, 20 October 2010, www.bbc.com/news/world-11446636, accessed 16 August 2018.

Qian, K. (2016) Reluctant Transcendence: AIDS and the Catastrophic Condition in Gu Changwei's Film Love for Life, in H.Y.F. Choy (ed.) *Discourses of Disease: Writing Illness, the Mind and Body in Modern China*, Leiden: Brill, pp. 203–30.

Renwick, N. (2002) The 'Nameless Fever': The HIV/AIDS Pandemic and China's Women, *Third World Quarterly*, 23 (2), Global Health and Governance: HIV/AIDS (April): 377–93. Published by Taylor & Francis, Ltd.

Rosenberg, C.E. (1992) Introduction, Framing Disease: Illness, Society, and History, in C. Rosenberg and J. Golden (eds.) *Framing Disease, Studies in Cultural History*, New Brunswick, NJ: Rutgers University Press, pp. xiii–xxvi.

Soon, W. (2016) Blood, Soy Milk, and Vitality: The Wartime Origins of Blood Banking in China, 1943–45, *Bulletin of the History of Medicine*, 90 (3) (Fall): 424–54.

Topley, M. (1955) Ghost Marriages Among the Singapore Chinese, *Man*, 55: 29–30.

———. (1956) Ghost Marriages Among the Singapore Chinese: A Further Note, *Man*, 56: 71–2.

Tsai, C. (2011) In Sickness and in Health: Yan Lianke and the Writing of Autoimmunity, *Modern Chinese Literature and Culture*, 23 (1) (Spring): 77–104.

Tsoi, G. (2016) China's Ghost Wedding and Why They Can Be Deadly, *BBC News*, 24 August 2016, www.bbc.com/news/world-asia-china-37103447, accessed 17 August 2018.

Volodzko, D. (2016) China's Looming AIDS Epidemic from Globalpost, *The Week*, 8 July 2016, http://theweek.com/articles/632926/chinas-looming-aids-epidemic, accessed 4 August 2018.

Wang Jingwei (2014) Religious Elements in Mo Yan's and Yan Lianke's Works, in A. Duran and Y. Huang (eds.) *Mo Yan in Context*, West Lafayette, IN: Purdue University Press, pp. 139–52.

Watts, J. (2003) Hidden from the World, a Village Dies of Aids While China Refuses to Face a Growing Crisis, *The Guardian*, 24 October 2003, www.theguardian.com/world/2003/oct/25/aids.china, accessed 4 August 2018.

Weissberg, J. (2015) Film Review: 'Behemoth' Zhao Liang acts as a Modern-day Dante Exploring Inner Mongolia's Environmental Destruction by Toxic Mining, *Variety*, 25 October 2015, https://variety.com/2015/film/festivals/behemoth-review-1201625962/, accessed 11 February 2018.

Wong, E. (2011) Chinese Director's Path from Rebel to Insider, *The New York Times*, 13 August 2011, www.nytimes.com/2011/08/14/world/asia/14filmmaker.html, accessed 11 February 2018.

———. (2014) Q. and A.: Ruby Yang on Hong Kong Youth and Identity, *The New York Times*, 15 October 2014, https://sinosphere.blogs.nytimes.com/2014/10/16/q-and-a-ruby-yang-on-hong-kong-youth-and-identity/, accessed 30 August 2018.

World Press Photo (2004) *Contemporary Issues, Stories, 1st Prize, Lu Guang*, www.worldpressphoto.org/collection/photo/2004/31427/10/2004-Lu-Guang-CIS1-JL, accessed 30 March 2019.

Yan Lianke 阎连科 (2009) *Dream of Ding Village* (*Dingzhuang meng* 丁庄梦), trans. C. Carter, New York: Grove Press 2009.

Yang, Zeye Ruby 楊紫燁 (2006) The Blood of Yingzhou District (*Yingzhou de haizi* 颍州的孩子), produced by Thomas F. Lennon, on Youtube, www.youtube.com/watch?v=Gt_TxXGhTTY, accessed 12 March 2019.

———. (2013) The Blood of Yingzhou District Revisited (*Yingzhou de haizi houji* 颍州的孩子后记), produced by Thomas F. Lennon, on *Youtube*, www.youtube.com/watch?v=CkZMJIAz3ec, accessed 12 March 2019.

Zhang Ying 张英 (2006) Being Alive Is Not Just an Instinct, *ESWN Culture Blog*, 23 March 2006, interview with Yan Lianke online, http://zonaeuropa.com/culture/c20060327_1.htm, accessed 4 October 2017.

Zhao Liang 赵亮 artist website in English and Chinese, http://zhaoliangstudio.com/about, accessed 4 October 2017.

———. (2011) *Together*, on Youtube, www.youtube.com/watch?v=hu8H4jju3oA, accessed 29 September 2018.

Zuo, M. (2015) Bodies, Blood, and Love: The 'Touching' Politics of HIV/AIDS Film *Love for Life*, *Journal of Chinese Cinemas*, 9 (3): 204–22.

6   *Fortune Teller*

The visible and the invisible

Lili Lai

This chapter is about a certain vision of what makes for marginality and invisibility in the city's peripheries. It aligns itself with Xu Tong 徐童, director of the documentary film *Fortune Teller* (*Suanming* 算命 2009), and his project of making disabled people (among others) more visible in a nuanced way to mainstream society, by highlighting the film's argument that physical/intellectual disability is only one reason for social invisibility and exclusion from the 'civic'. There are many forms of marginality, but all of them are made more or less invisible in everyday urban social practice. When the filmmaker's gaze turns to these lives, it can show that many different kinds of lives are understandable as ordinary ways of coping with life's challenges despite exclusions and injustices.

In particular, this chapter explores the way in which *Fortune Teller* portrays socially-marginalized characters – disabled people, prostitutes, and elderly homeless people – in contemporary China. It first discusses how the people represented in this film are largely invisible in mainstream society. Then four major aspects of the film will be analysed: first, the often neglected issues of desire and intimate feelings of the disabled; second, their poignant experiences growing up with family members; third, the 'bitterness' (*ku* 苦) of their encounters with the county official who is in charge of their state welfare; and finally, the ways in which they achieve dignity in their lives. As part of Xu Tong's *Vagabonds Trilogy* of documentary films (*Youmin sanbuqu* 游民三部曲, 2009–2011), *Fortune Teller* features Li Baicheng 厉百程, a man who is partially disabled with chronic weakness and pain in his legs, and his wife Pearl Shi 石珍珠, who has a hearing and speech impairment as well as an intellectual disability. Living in an urban village about 35 kilometers from Beijing and 283 kilometers from Li's hometown in Qinglong County, Hebei Province, Li and his friends' lives are invisible to most people. This documentary, however, seeks to make visible that they share much everyday life and many of the same ordinary concerns, family relationships, responsibilities, and challenges as the able-bodied face every day. Meanwhile, the lack of public facilities for disabled people in the county office for civic services highlights the irony of the current situation for the disabled in China. In many senses of the word, Li and Shi and their friends stumble along, but with dignity.

People

Disability in China, as elsewhere, is often synonymous with marginality. Indeed, *youmin* 游民, the Chinese equivalent of vagabond, a term that appeared as early as in the *Liji* 禮記 (Book of Rites, comp. Late Warring States-Han dynasty), is a classical Confucian term that refers to the people who wander outside the ancient Chinese well-field system (*jingtian zhidu* 井田制度) and are therefore considered a potential threat to social stability. The derogatory sense of *youmin* persists in contemporary Chinese. *Fortune Teller* opens with a scene in Yanjiao Town, an urban village outside Beijing. The shabby houses, the puddles after rain, and the narrow muddy streets all convey the marginality of the place and its people, on a rural-urban fringe. The film starts when Li, a fortune teller, receives a customer, Miss Tang, who runs a brothel in the neighbourhood. The people featured in this documentary are mostly migrants who left their home towns long ago. Li is from Qinglong county, Hebei province, while Tang is from a province in the northeast of China. It seems that Li never attended any school, a common condition for many disabled people.

As a matter of fact, street fortune tellers in China are mostly disabled people. One reason for this is that there are very limited resources for education for disabled people in China. As Deng and Harris point out, historically a sympathetic social attitude toward people with disabilities in China had been carefully nurtured, but they were also kept at the bottom of the hierarchical feudal pyramid in a culture of compassion instead of education (Deng and Harris 2008: 196). Special education institutions began to be established by American and European missionaries after 1840, but there were only 42 special schools serving just over 2,000 students in 1949 when the People's Republic of China was established (*Ibid.*). According to a research report by Jeffrey Kritzer, in 1980 teacher training for special educators began but it was not until the 1990s that teacher training institutions were required to offer special education courses (Kritzer 2011: 57–63). Although the 1986 Compulsory Education Law mandated that every child should be given the right to nine years of free public education, educational opportunities for disabled Chinese are still lacking, not to mention those who are of older generations like Li and his friends. But Li is very articulate throughout the film. As a professional fortune teller, he has to read classical Chinese and be familiar with ancient divination texts such as *Guiguzi* 鬼谷子 (Master of Ghost Valley, comp. Warring States to Han period, 475BCE–220CE).

In the first scene, the camera lingers on Li as he mutters incantations in front of a statue of Buddha that stands on his desk. Then the camera pans outside to see Pearl Shi, Li's wife, who is evidently disabled but whose gait is less impaired than that of her husband. Her husband requires two walking sticks but is agile in his movements. As the film unfolds revealing the couple's life, the viewer is introduced to Li's two brothers, who are both physically impaired too. His younger brother is also a fortune teller in the Beijing area, while his elder brother lives alone in their home village in Hebei. Other members of Li and Shi's social network include Miss Tang's fellow sex workers, a prisoner's wife who comes to Li for help in identifying ways to alter her and her husband's fortune, and Li's old friends in his home county, who have been homeless for most of their lives. All of these people, most of whom are invisible to mainstream society, are gradually made more visible to the viewer through their everyday practices, mundane feelings and expressions, and ordinary relationships with each other and with the world, despite what would seem to be an 'abnormal' way of life.

Desire, intimacy, family

The question of sexual desire, expression, and activity among disabled people has recently become an important topic in disability activist projects as well as in critical, historical, and empirical studies (Rapp and Ginsburg 2013: 53–68). Li, as the film's protagonist, does not shy away from this topic. In the documentary, he makes it clear that he was annoyed by the director's 'ignorant' assumption that he would not be capable of enjoying a sexual life due to his congenital disability. With both his hands gesturing tongue movements, he gives an elaborate description of how deep kisses should be, his face glowing with vivid memories. In one of the most moving moments in the film, the deliberately low camera position captures expressions of rather 'normal' desire in a man, despite his age and impairment. He is not the only person in the film to assert their sexuality: Li's homeless pals in Hebei county town also tell of their unfortunate experiences of going to the brothel and being mocked by the girls.

The film's message is that there is no need to be shy about human desire. Li tells the camera that he married Pearl precisely because of sexual attraction, while at the same time he openly admits some regret about marrying a disabled woman. But since they are a family now, he carries on with her as his life companion. The documentary shows us how Li cares for Pearl: he washes her hands, gives her painkillers, and puts her to bed. As they walk together hand-in-hand, Pearl is always leaning against Li, despite his compromised gait. With such palpable intimacy between this disabled couple, it is clear that they are sticking it out together, or to adopt a Chinese phrase, they rely on each other's fate: *xiangyi weiming* 相依为命.

Pearl, we learn, had been badly treated by her own family before marrying Li in her forties. She was born with hearing and speech impairments and faced discrimination throughout her life. Her parents died when she was eight years old. We are not given details of how she was raised but when the couple go back to their home county for a visit, we are shown a shelter that now houses goats. According to Li, that is where Pearl lived for 16 years. It is clear that Pearl had been treated as a kind of monster and she was kept at a distance from the other family members. As a child and a young woman she remained invisible, not being allowed to intrude upon 'normal' family life. Pearl's elder brother, now a grandfather of three, tells the camera how in an effort to prevent the birth of future 'anomalies' like his sister Pearl, he cleaned up the family graveyard to change the family *fengshui* 风水, the geomantic influences on their lineage, or simply their fate. Still, he could not accept the fact of Pearl being born disabled but nevertheless also human. Instead, he blames the family *fengshui*.

Li did not have a happy experience with his own family either. He was driven out when it was found out that he would not be able to walk due to problems with both legs. However, all four brothers including Li developed impairments as time went on. Similarly to Pearl's family, Li's elder brother claims that their house had bad *fengshui*, on account of having an evil and inauspicious orientation to their family graveyard. But they were too poor to do anything about it and so had to accept the inevitable fate of being a disabled family. Disability is here understood as the visible effect of an invisible fate or of hard-to-read *fengshui* dispositions. As Pearl's elder brother comments during their visit, Li and Pearl have managed to be good people in their lives and so it is thought that, through meritorious deeds, they will accumulate positive *karma* and be 'healthy' in their next life: a yet invisible fate that wraps around and shapes their future. Apparently, even Li and his brother and their fortune telling (*suanming* 算命) customers believe that disability is an expression of an evil and inauspicious fate, which is why they have learned to 'tell fortunes' and perhaps why their customers also believe that these disabled men might have special access to the as yet invisible future.

Bitterness

How is disability framed through the social organization of daily life, and in the techniques of governmentality? Many close-ups of Li the fortune-teller in the film clearly show his physical difficulties. The most ironic scene is the couple's visit to the Qinglong County office of the China Disabled Persons' Federation, which has many steep stairs that the couple must climb to reach the office. Many countries, including China, have implemented policies that ensure that public facilities enable access for disabled people. According to the World Health Organisation:

> Disability is thus not just a health problem. It is a complex phenomenon, reflecting the interaction between features of a person's body and features of the society in which he or she lives. Overcoming the difficulties faced by people with disabilities requires interventions to remove environmental and social barriers.
>
> (WHO, *Disabilities*)

It has become a matter of common sense in much of the world that public facilities are expected to provide means to reduce – if not remove – environmental barriers. This trend is also closely associated with changing social attitudes toward disabled people. However, research has found that China is one of the most unfriendly countries toward the disabled in the world (Samuel *et al.* 2018: 83–97). For example, although it is required to set up tactile paving on the sidewalks of major urban roads, people often find the blind tracks being occupied by bikes, motorcycles, or even kiosks selling magazines, not to mention that these tracks often lead to a dead end or a tree (Wu *et al.* 2017: 485–7). Few buses provide wheelchair access in Beijing, certainly none in Qinglong County. It is no wonder that disabled people are invisible in most public spaces, despite state policies that aim to prioritize integration (Samuel *et al.* 2018: 83–97). There is still limited public planning and public use of resources for disabled people (Wu *et al.* 2017: 485–7). The invisibility of disabled people becomes even more striking given reports that the number of disabled people in China reached 85 million in 2013 (*Zhonghua xianfeng wang* 中华先锋网 2013), compared to over 39 million in the US (Cornell University Disability Statistics 2013).

The purpose of Li and Pearl's visit to the county office was to claim their subsistence allowances as disabled citizens. This is why, as vagrants or 'vagabonds', they had to return to Qinglong. However, the official in charge declined their request, saying that they were not among the neediest applicants since they could still come to the office by themselves. Li came on crutches because his right leg is of no use at all; he has to rely on the crutches to support his body while moving forward with the left leg alternately. A long shot captures Li labouring up a rugged and rough road up a hill in his hometown, his body moving rhythmically up and down, one leg dragging the other along. Li remonstrates to the county official: 'It's extremely hard for me to keep going like this. I come here only for the basic living needs. I don't have any children to rely upon'. He is told to apply to the township government for a basic living allowance, the minimum subsidy that the state provides for rural residents who live in poverty. This response ignores any disability benefits that Li may be entitled to claim. Li challenges the official, 'So what is the Federation for?' The answer comes: 'You should work hard yourself, there are about 30,000 disabled people in this county, you can't rely on the government'.

Li makes his living by fortune telling. If this is a case of him being self-reliant, it does not solve all his bureaucratic problems. His business suffers frequent disruption on account of his physical challenges. He recalls occasions when the local government has mounted campaigns against 'illegal' practices such as fortune telling, and how his reduced physical capabilities have made him the one who is always grabbed by the police. A poignant vicious circle forms here for people like Li in their old age. As they grew up without access to education, many do not have access to legal jobs. They are encouraged by the China Disabled Persons' Federation to be self-reliant, but practicing fortune telling is seen as an illegal business. In other words, Li and his friends' lives are beyond the purview of state services but not of policing. When they go to ask for help, the government urges them to rely on themselves, but when they try to be self-reliant, the government attacks their business (fortune telling or begging on the street) by declaring it illegal. This is an onerous citizenship at best.

Nussbaum has argued that:

> Any decent society must deal adequately with the needs of citizens with impairments and disabilities for care, education, self-respect, activity. And a satisfactory account of human justice requires recognizing the equal citizenship of people with impairments, and thus the very great continuity between 'normal' lives and those of people with lifelong impairments.
>
> (Nussbaum 2007: 98–9)

What the film attempts to convey is that for Li and his friends the 'bitterness they eat', or *chiku* 吃苦, comes not from their impairments but from a denial by the 'normal' world of their right to a livelihood and human dignity.

Life and dignity

Xu Tong's documentary makes it clear that Li and Pearl live a very basic life, with their needs barely met. Nevertheless, Li never seems to consider himself to be 'abnormal'. On the contrary, we see in him what Nussbaum describes as the 'great continuity between normal lives and those with lifelong impairments' (*ibid.*). *Fortune Teller* does not just content itself with 'speaking for the subaltern' by silently critiquing the state's inadequate attention to the disabled, emphasizing only their 'miserable' lives. Instead, it highlights the moments filled with joy in their rather normal everyday lives. One scene, for example, captures Pearl's effort on a sunny afternoon to make a bed for a cat, albeit with difficulty. Everyone watching would be moved by her joyous laughter upon seeing the cat jumping into the bed she builds. In fact, there are quite a few occasions in the documentary that portray Li and his friends' love of animals. When commenting on his brother's hobby – he is also a fortune teller with crippling leg pain – of buying sparrows and goldfish from a market and then setting them free in the suburbs, Li insists 'it's better to raise animals than to release them, you do more good'. To Li and his friends, the world also contains many different types of animal dignity, all of which deserve care and respect. As Li states, 'When a stray cat comes to your door, it's a gift. With so many households in this courtyard, why did the cat choose your home? Because it has been evaluating everyone's moral conduct, it chose you due to your good fortune. Don't look down on small animals'. Animals too deserve respect and dignity and are in turn able to dignify human life.

This remark illustrates not only Li's respect but also his care for animals, or 'ten thousand things' (*wanwu* 万物), to use his own words. *Wanwu* connotes the heterogeneity of things in the world, but difference can never be treated as inequality. As he states firmly, 'Human beings should have ability to accept, understand, and enjoy *wanwu*. If you make a living from fortune telling, it is also your duty to persuade people to do good deeds'. Li believes in and practices what he preaches. This distinguishes him from bogus fortune tellers who only tell fortunes to make a living. It gives him a higher morality, and is something that moves the audience and makes them recognize the hidden virtues of these 'invisible' people. Here Li goes further to show an even greater demand that he makes of himself as a fortune teller, in spite of his disability, to lead a life in this world, conscientiously.

Conclusion

Throughout *Fortune Teller*, the camera is deliberately positioned lower than most of the characters' bodies and the subjects' awareness of the camera is openly demonstrated. The film's approach to everyday life is rather anthropological, in that it pays attention to fine details, such as the puddles after rain in the opening scene. Special attention is paid to the language used by the fortune teller and his friends, their body images and movements, and other background details. There are important scenes revealing the ways in which medicine, health, and well-being are intertwined. For example, when we see how every evening Li has to administer to Pearl the painkiller that she needs, the camera patiently records how he first pours hot water into a big bowl and inserts a pill into Pearl's mouth. This attention to the detail of everyday care demonstrates the couple's intimacy and deep mutual reliance, undeniably a form of happiness and well-being. In addition, the film narrative adopts the genre of traditional Chinese novels, providing subtitles for each chapter in classic Chinese manner. This is meant to remind us of the alternative societies formed by marginal groups in China, namely the 'brothers of the rivers and lakes' (*jianghu* 江湖), often showcased in those traditional novels. Perhaps the implication is that the invisible *jianghu* society is in some ways more egalitarian than the visible modern mainstream society. Once the disabled and the marginal are treated as equals – a condition that has not yet been achieved in China, as *Fortune Teller* reminds us – we can all learn how to appreciate other lives, with full respect for what they can teach us.

Filmography

Vagabonds Trilogy (*Youmin sanbuqu* 游民三部曲), dir. Xu Tong:
Wheat Harvest (*Maishou* 麦收), 2008.
Fortune Teller (*Suanming* 算命), 2009.
Shattered (*Lao tangtou* 老唐头), 2011.

Bibliography

Cornell University Disability Statistics (2013) *2013 Disability Status Report: United States*, www.disabilitystatistics.org/reports/2013/English/HTML/report2013.cfm?fips=2000000&html_year=2013&subButton=Get+HTML#prev-all, accessed 28 August 2018.

Deng, M. and Harris, K. (2008) Meeting the Needs of Students with Disabilities in General Education Classrooms in China, *Teacher Education and Special Education*, 31 (3): 195–207.

Kritzer, J.B. (2011) Special Education in China, *Eastern Education Journal*, 40 (1): 57–63.

Nussbaum, M.C. (2007) *Frontiers of Justice: Disability, Nationality, Species Membership*, Cambridge and London: The Belknap Press of Harvard University Press.

Rapp, R. and Ginsburg, F.D. (2013) Disability Worlds, *Annual Review of Anthropology*, 42: 53–68.

Samuel, K., Alkire, S., Zavaleta, D., Mills, C. and Hammock, J. (2018) Social Isolation and Its Relationship to Multidimensional Poverty, *Oxford Development Studies*, 46 (1): 83–97.

World Health Organisation (WHO), *Disabilities*, www.who.int/topics/disabilities/en/, accessed 25 July 2018.

Wu Yue, Xue Pingju, Wu Mengzhu *et al.* (2017) Analysis on Current Situation of Urban Barrier-free Facilities and Suggestions for Improvement, *Zhongguo kangfu lilun yu shijian* (China Journal of Rehabilitation Theory and Practice), 23 (4): 485–7.

Zhonghua xianfeng wang 中华先锋网 (Vanguard of the Chinese Nation Website) (2013) *Zhongguo gelei canjiren zongshu da baqian wubai wan* 中国各类残疾人总数达 8500 万, 20 May 2013, www.zhxf.cn/info/1788/155357.htm, accessed 25 July 2018.

7 *Longing for the Rain*

Journeys into the dislocated female body of urban China

Vivienne Lo and Nashuyuan Serenity Wang
With Chen Jiahe, Ge Yunjiao, Li Weijia, Liu
Hanwen, George Yao, Yang Qihua, Yang
Xingyue, Yang Yi, Zhou Dangwei

There is a quiet revolution going on in director Yang Lina's 杨荔纳 Beijing: you can sense it lurking in the supermarkets, in the thick toxic air, in between the towering thighs of Big Pants China Central TV tower, driving down the Avenue of Eternal Peace and under the plastic Rainbow to Tiananmen square. It is unsettling the city right down to the last remaining traditional courtyard houses, where Fang Lei's 方蕾 mother- in-law is about to ascend to the realm of the spirits.

Caught in between the busyness of men, with too much time on their hands and money to spend, middle class housewives are doing it for themselves – quite literally. As the camera pans in on the protagonist, Fang Lei, masturbating on her sofa to a pornographic DVD, we simultaneously look out over the emptiness of Beijing. Fang Lei is 'longing for rain' – for the love, sex, and passion of the euphemistic Chinese title of the film *Chunmeng* 春梦 'lit. spring dream'. We soon discover her apparently amiable husband hiding under the sheets with his games console, too frenetically engaged with the digital world to notice his wife's growing alienation. The film subsequently charts the breakdown of the couple's relationship and the husband's abduction of their daughter as Fang Lei loses her way in a world where she cannot differentiate the phantasms of day and night.

In the cold, subdued light of her high-rise solitude Fang Lei's desire dissipates into the atmosphere, into everywhere. She inhabits the flipside of the phallic cityscape itself, playing the pervasive *yin* (the ever-present dark) to the hyperactive bright *yang* of life in the capital. Cold water, cognate with *yin*, is the element which flows through all of the scenes where Fang Lei experiences emotional intensity: rain, tears, showering, lakes, sea, and snow. But Fang Lei is also nowhere, aimlessly pushing a shopping trolley, lost in her own reflection behind the glass window of her high-rise apartment, following the sirens on the street, on a journey dislocated in time and space.

As Fang Lei's dislocation from her family and the world around results in both her behaviour and state of mind transgressing all boundaries of normalcy, *Longing for the Rain* invites us to enter into her spiritual crisis and follow her itineraries through the cityscape and her own inner landscape in search of what is, ultimately, an uncertain healing process (Figure 7.1). In an interview I (Lo) conducted in 2016 Yang Lina confided,

> I can only talk from my personal experiences and my observations. Friends around me, women of my age . . . everyone's situation is different, and everyone is in a different state. I don't think I can say anything on their behalf, *but one thing is certain, that is, the rhythm of life is so fast that we can't keep up. It is not so much sexual confusion as it is a spiritual confusion.* In the film, sex is just a vehicle. What I mainly want to express is our spiritual dilemma, our spiritual condition, and the spiritual conditions of these women.
>
> (our emphasis. tr. Guo Liping)

There are many points of Medical Humanities interest in this film about the embodiment of spiritual confusion in contemporary China. Merleau-Ponty (1945, tr. Smith (1965): 112–70) described the body as a symbolic object, not something that ultimately belongs to us as we might assume, but as representative of our relationship to the totality of what surrounds us. Our bodies are not, however, just a corpus of symbols or a silent container inscribed with metaphors; they are constructed through ever-emerging processes where they lived and connected body itself participates actively in its own formation. Most obviously the film communicates these processes as it visualises a culturally specific illness narrative and a quest for healing. Illness narratives presented as ways of journeying towards health and well-being are nothing new, but Yang Lina's filmic tale acknowledges that people do not always get better. As Fang Lei's world falls apart and her grasp on reality gets ever more fragile, we also discover the spiritual geography of her sensual body as a reflection of the plural medical landscape of Beijing, and by

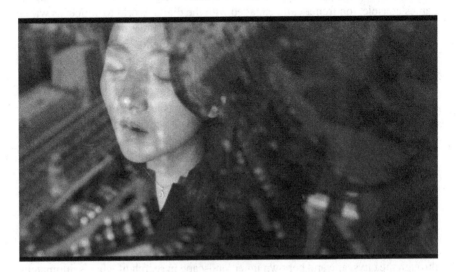

Figure 7.1 The emptiness of Fang Lei's mood merges with the cityscape

implication that of the psycho-spiritual condition of urban middle-class women themselves. As a narrative of, and in, the capital city of China, it is also a feminist critique of the state of things.

Through the insight of film theorist Zhang Yingjin we see in the film three phases of space-making: 'space as product; space as process; space as productive' (Zhang 2010: 1).

Through intersecting Fang Lei's fragmented body, her psychopathology, and her disturbing fantasies, with both the plural urban and religious landscapes of Beijing, Yang Lina animates a visual culture that is unique to China and China's medico-spiritual traditions. The productive space that Yang Lina creates between Fang Lei's body and the city of Beijing processes together historical and contemporary space: it borrows narrative journeys from tales of the supernatural that date to the Tang period, medieval religious pilgrimage, and geo-emotive body landscaping traditions from much before that and shows how they pervade the present. Fang Lei constantly shapes her own environment to these traditions, and journeys through them as a riposte to the dissatisfying urban domestic landscape that she finds herself in. In contrast to historic itineraries, however, the space that Yang Lina articulates is resolutely female, and therefore serves to comment on the disconnect between China's supersonic economic and political rise onto the global stage and those lost in the spiritual maze of its urban underbelly.

Neither author was born a Beijinger or identifies as wholly 'Han' Chinese, so we tested the film's success in representing the experiences and frustrations of those closer to the lives portrayed in the film. As in Chapter 10 (Vuillermin) we used students' subjective viewer-responses with the help of eight UCL postgraduate students, mostly women in their 20s, younger than the fictional protagonist, although brought up in similar urban contexts. Most were registered on the UCL postgraduate module Chinese Film and the Body in the Chinese Medical Humanities programme (2017–18). They were therefore well aware of the module's aims to 'to analyse representations of social and cultural issues related to health, medicine, and the body in twentieth and twenty-first century China'.

The student-centred teaching setting was my own home (Lo) and I prepared them a lavish Chinese meal to get them in the mood to share their responses to the film. *Longing for the Rain* has not been given the Dragon Seal of Film Bureau censorship approval, so it is not the kind of feature that they would be accustomed to seeing in mainland China. They were therefore curious about the experiment, agreeing about the plight of unhappy urban housewives, and engaging in heated discussion about honour in marriage and whether or not one can cheat with a spirit lover, and the merits and morality of having a lover at all as a woman.

The ghost lover

Ostensibly, all is well. Fang Lei is a loving mother and wife, makes excellent dumplings, and is primary carer for her charmingly demented mother-in-law. But when her computer game obsessed husband and beloved child have left for work and school, an eerie quiet comes over the apartment. Left to her own devices she begins to observe herself as if in a dream. So, when a ghostly figure turns up in her dreams-cum-daydreams, first violently and then in a full-on seduction, we ask who is looking at whom? Who is the subject of the dream? Are we looking at her looking at twenty-first-century life in Beijing, or at the spectral life of her own body? Are these subjects and objects one and the same thing?

The sensuous touch of the stranger's body turns the dark nightmare of the initial intrusion into pleasure as the attacks become erotic rather than solely violent – awakening new passions within her body. As Fang Lei begins to give in to the seductions of the spectral lover, he emerges slowly in fragmented close up shots of his first violent and then seducing body. A montage of extreme close-ups of his nipples, long hair, and fleshy drooping bottom lip combine to create a shadowy, quasi feminine, figure who is at first clad all in black. As he slowly becomes the lover she cannot live without, he transforms into a romantic white-robed chevalier riding at the edge of the sea, suggestive of the lover's tryst of historical drama (Figure 7.2). In her darkening fantasies she begins to appear in a long black hooded cloak, as if swapping roles.

The image is, as George Yao, one of the students, points out

> a completely opposed vision of her husband . . . her husband has short hair, this man has long hair; her husband always wears very casual outfits, this man wears the very fancy and historical outfit; her husband is kind of passive during the sex while this man was kind of dominating and very aggressive.

Yang Lina intends to draw on the hugely popular *liaozhai* 聊斋 or *zhiguai* 志怪 tradition. This is a genre that began in the Tang dynasty and grew out of the

Figure 7.2 Fang Lei, now robed in black, watches her spectral lover riding towards her like a romantic hero dressed in white

recording of 'abnormal' omens, often providing a supernatural commentary on political events, turning stories of the strange, 'uncanny' phenomena outside normal experience, into a literary form (Zeitlin 1993). These stories are inhabited by transmogrifying female fox spirits, snakes, dragons, and reptiles of all sorts that prey on upright scholarly men. But women on the edge are also prone to supernatural hauntings. Ming dynasty (1368–1644) medical histories have included a category that explains the propensity for sexual madness in women as 'dreaming sex with demons' (Chen 2003: 188–99). Although Yang Lina professes not to know of the medical tradition, she says:

> this topic is not a strange topic in ancient Chinese society and classical literature. [but] what I intend to express is not related to the past or the ancient times. This film is about the anxiety of modern people. I intend to explore our current rhythm of life and people's state of mind.
>
> (tr. Guo Liping)

The disturbing intrusion of the ghost-like figure into Fang Lei's life disrupts what appears to be the perfectly modern nuclear family, challenging the sanctity of her home and her own willingness or ability to perform the normal social duties of wife and mother – in this way it mimics the conventional Chinese family drama where the family as a collectivity is in crisis centred around social duty (Berry 2008: 235). In Chinese terms of hierarchical but reciprocal responsibility, the husband is also not performing his duties and Hollywood films too put the blame on the weak or ailing patriarch figure. But in this case our heroine is not a misunderstood virtuous heroine – notwithstanding all the women in our student audience feel a deep sympathy for her – she is the destroyer of the Chinese family, rather than the victim. As Fang Lei becomes incapable of separating reality from dream, she loses her mind, as well as her body, and drives herself further and further away from her family, ultimately forfeiting both husband and child.

Yet, while profoundly disturbing for these reasons, the film is also strangely and instantly reassuring for its familiarity, for anyone who knows the atmosphere of twenty-first-century Beijing. While clearly a social and political critique it also speaks of the director's love for the city and its women.

Yang Lina says:

> For me, this woman expresses her physical condition and spiritual condition through dreams. It is a beautiful way of expression for me. Dreams can represent dissatisfaction with reality, longing for something which one doesn't have in reality. Dreams can help us understand the conditions of this woman.
>
> (tr. Guo Liping)

How does Yang Lina create this troubling, yet familiar reality?

I (Lo) first met Yang Lina at the end of a long motorbike ride chasing her and her teenage daughter around the riding schools of the north east suburbs of Beijing.

After a series of misunderstood WeChat directions, we ended up meeting at a bank in town. But since it was a warm Saturday afternoon in late summer, and those suburbs remained green and rural, it was very pleasant. And I share the daughter's love of horses, which was an immediate bond. Yang Lina knows this elite Beijing inside out and our students confirm her success in bringing this Beijing and its social dysfunction to the screen.

One of the students, Yang Yi, is a traditional medical practitioner from Beijing and roughly the same age as the fictional Fang Lei:

> So, these characters and the screen scenes are, really, really like people's life in Beijing. The smog, and the building, the CCTV building. And all these Hutong (traditional alleyways), and the kind of taxi and buses, the traditional kind of squares. And also the Temple of Heaven park within it. It's like a trip back home. All those landscapes, those characters . . . the relationship between the couple are also familiar. They don't have really deep, intellectual, conversations. They don't really talk. They just live together, like . . .
>
> George Yao adds: Roommates.

Yang Lina's personal relationship with the Beijing environment and social networks are evidenced in the use of non-professional actors for all but two of the parts in the feature film. She told me:

> Except for the heroine and her husband, all other people in the film are non-professional actors and actresses. The supporting actress is played by one of my friends and this is her first foray into acting. In addition, *the Daoist priests are professional priests; monks in the temples, the fortune-teller, and all other actors are non-professional actors.* The temple in the film is the temple where I made my documentary in 2008. Not all Chinese temples are open for filming. I am on good terms with the masters and monks in the temple, so I could shoot this film there. China's censorship system has restrictions regarding temples, eroticism, and ghosts. *It does not matter if fox spirits are portrayed in the film, but ghosts are taboo.* This film has not passed censorship and has not been shown in China yet.
>
> (our emphasis. tr. Guo Liping)

Yang Lina was originally a documentary film maker, now turned feature film maker. As a fictional account of the sexual audacity and awkwardness of the life of the nouveau riche *Longing for the Rain* is enriched by her own early autobiographical documentary style developed through *Old Men* (*Laotou* 老头, 1999), about her elderly neighbours, and the ironically titled drama of her parents' divorce and its devastating effects on her little brother, *Home Video* (*Jiating luxiangdai* 家庭录像带, 2001). She is therefore very comfortable with the transitions between attempting to record reality, and the fantasies of narrative:

> Because I started by shooting documentaries, therefore there are many elements of documentaries in my films. I've always been committed to

aesthetically or methodologically making my films fusions of documentaries and feature films. . . . So my documentaries are much like feature films, and feature films like documentaries.

(tr. Guo Liping)

This technique is clear from the outset when the shots of Fang Lei in the supermarket are interlaced with her interviews of housekeepers and carers from among the middle-aged female migrant workers in Beijing, highlighting the dissonance between the urban and rural female experience in the capital. In these shots there is a clear sense that the protagonist herself is the documentary filmmaker, interviewing her subjects in a self-reflexive manner. This has the effect of multiplying the spectator's points of view, and foreshadows that as the narrative unfolds, Fang Lei, like the migrant workers who talk of leaving their children at home in the countryside, will lose her child.

In the cityscape scenes, we see a docu-cinematic style of cinematography: the camera follows the fluid movement of our protagonist just as it captures the vibrant energy of Beijing, its every cell in constant motion. The three entities, city, protagonist, camera, move in parallel but they also deliberately fail to negotiate with one another. All the elements of the city and its population move with intent towards pre-destined ends; yet, in fact, we cannot tell why everything is constantly in transit or where we are supposed to be going. The most real sense of the city is therefore underexposed. The city seems hardly bothered by the existence of the camera and does not seem to cooperate. The space, the people, and the camera's eye all have an independent fluidity that fosters a sense of mutual irrelevance. The disinterested reality that Yang Lina skilfully frames through this failed negotiation between dramatic tensions reflects two distinct tendencies in her work. First, her own inclination is to use interview and person-to-person intimate narrative. Second, these scenes invoke the observational documentary style that Chinese independent film makers have a long history of preferring, and which has exerted a deep influence on her work.

As the frenetic *yang* energy of the outward facing city surrounds Fang Lei's growing trauma and disorientation, inside the house the lively haunting *yin* force – for ghosts like women and water are also of *yin* – begins to dominate the landscape of the film (Allan 1997: 35–54). The fragmentation of his body is therefore also a fragmentation of hers, both seen in interactive close ups during their sexual encounters. The *yin* nature of the female body is most powerfully presented through multiple scenes involving water: the sexual 'rain' of the euphemistic title, turns into flood water as Fang Lei submerges herself fully clothed to cool her ardour. An excess of *yin*, so lusciously and lasciviously portrayed in the film, has always mounted both political and sexual challenges to male power in Chinese literature. Depraved and dangerous beauties, from Dan Ji 妲己, wife of the last king of Shang 商纣王, to Bao Si 褒姒, consort of King You of Zhou 周幽王, to Lü Zhi 吕雉, wife of the founder of the Han dynasty, Liu Bang 刘邦, to the self-styled female 'Emperor' Wu Zetian 武则天 and her grandson's unforgettable concubine, Yang Guifei 杨贵妃, were blamed in the standard histories for endangering or bringing down their respective dynasties; and their corruption of political power was naturalised through a cosmic transgression framed in terms of yin-*yang* imbalance (Raphals 1998: 61–86; Liu 2014).

Itineraries through a plural medical landscape

As Fang Lei embarks on a journey to heal herself of her soulless life and gothic fantasies, she takes us through the maze that is the dysfunctional emotional and medico-spiritual architecture of Beijing and its environs, to glitzy clubs full of gigolos, solemn Tibetan-Buddhist temples where her aunt from out-of-town agonises over salvation; to Daoist priests down hidden alleyways whose talismans will protect her from the evil spirits – evil spirits that are residing in her torso – to suburban fortune tellers with whom she prays and whose spiritual empathy brings her to tears. Their sexual and spiritual quests for healing illustrate a very female 'relation between the spatial structures and their inhabitants' and the ways in which space and architecture identify the human body (Boumeester 2011: 247; Landy 2010: 121).

Poignantly, despite a swift descent into what would certainly be labelled an emergency in psychiatric terms, an inability to distinguish dream from reality, Fang Lei never consults a psychiatrist. The male students in our audience were outnumbered 2:1 by the women, but they had strong opinions about the solutions to Fang Lei's problem. Liu Hanwen stated, 'she should have some communication with her husband or seek some psychological help'. Another, a professional male psychiatrist, Zhou Dangwei, was the only person in the audience to proffer a psychiatric interpretation of Fang Lei's condition:

> I believe that, from a psychological standard the woman in that movie became more and more psychotic. Because before she was a bit neurotic but not so . . . bad. But after a lot of wrong treatments she became more and more psychotic. Because, she treated the [ghost] figure as real, equal to the fantasy figure in her dream. This is very dangerous, for her real life. I think she will become schizophrenic. She will become more and more paranoid.
>
> (tr. Guo Liping)

Despite her girlfriend's advice, however, Fang Lei never visits a psychiatrist or therapist. The director says:

> Around me, in Beijing, as far as I know, there are many professional women, artists, and intellectuals who will choose to consult Buddhists, Rinpoche and other religious masters to solve their own psychological problems. The reason for this is first that psychiatry in China is not very developed. Secondly, talking with Daoist or Buddhist masters can give these people psychological comfort.
>
> (tr. Guo Liping)

The field of Health Humanities has long embraced study of all the broader ways in which healthcare involves those other than professional medical communities.

It has, however, been commonplace to believe that religious healing and traditional medicine survive only in remote and impoverished places where modern medicine cannot reach. But *Longing for the Rain* represents a plurality of medical care that is fashionable in elite and privileged urban circles.

Fang Lei first turns for help to her outrageously lascivious and well-heeled girlfriend, whose name always remains a mystery, and with whom she first tries shopping therapy. On one trip her friend suggests that her fantasies are simply sexual frustration and gives her sex toys and advises taking a young lover. China reputedly manufactures 95% of the world's sex toys and women are a large part of that customer base (ShamelessCh 2019). Medicalised sex play on offer from female assistants dressed in clinical coats has been a feature of China's high street *chengren shangdian* 成人商店 (adult shops) for a decade or more. The naked body started appearing again in the 1980s in magazines with titles like *Jiankang zhi you* 健康之友 (Our Health) and *Jiating Yisheng* 家庭医生 (The Family Doctor), always under the guise of offering medical advice. Often on show were genitalia with hideous cankers and so on. No doubt all of this is part of the long history leading to this fetish figuring so strongly in Chinese sex shop trade.

The students were divided along gender lines as to whether Fang Lei was a good mother or had destroyed her credibility by cheating with her spirit lover. They were particularly animated by the sex boys and toys for women in urban commercial districts, although there was some confusion about what exactly was for sale: sex or just alcohol and companionship, and its legality.

YANG XINGYUE: Men have multiple lovers and mistresses and you can see there is lots of prostitution in China. But it's not public knowledge that women can also say to each other 'why couldn't you get a lover like everyone else'. What's your impression? Are women are just covering the fact that they are having just as free relationships as men in China?

GE YUNJIAO: I'm not sure what's going on in Beijing, but in Shanghai there are more and more male prostitution clubs, the *niulang dian* 牛郎店. And these men are earning lots of money, even more than the superstars. It's got great career potential for men. I think these things must also happen in Beijing although I haven't lived there. . . . There are even some women prostitution clubs for lesbians in Shanghai, and in Hangzhou. I have talked with my friends who live in Hangzhou. I don't think this is an underground phenomenon, it is increasingly blatant, and accepted.

They do not offer sex, they offer company, and they sell food and wine, well it's just like someone to talk to you.

GEORGE YAO: In some places they are having sexual intercourse and that's illegal; in others they are just masturbating, and that's legal.

GE YUNJIAO: You can just regard these men as waiters, who talk to you more.

YANG XINGYUE: Just like the princesses in the KTV, right?

GE YUNJIAO: Yes, and that doesn't break the law . . . at first the sex tools were only sold to the men, but now they are even more sex tools for the women.

As Fang Lei's older girlfriend laments the inconstancy of men, the drunken scenes in the toy boy clubs increase the sense of isolation for both women. Despite the touching trust that is evident between the women, Fang Lei is not happy there and so together they embark on a deeper quest through the astonishing twenty- and twenty-first-century religious revival in China with the friend initially playing tour guide (Goossaert and Palmer 2011: 201–392; Johnson 2017).

Their stroll together to visit the Daoist priest is no more comfortable than the foray into the night clubs. The camera follows the women down a traditional Ming-dynasty walled lane such as one finds within the Forbidden City to a rather ordinary living room. The very real priest, clad in full ritual robes, first takes her pulse, and then identifies the ghost as mid-30s, five foot seven, and living within Fang Lei's chest area. Intoning a scripture, he calls on the Daoist guardian spirits, waves a ritual sword and beats her gently with a Daoist whisk (Strichmann 2002). Next, he produces his calligraphy brush like a magic weapon and scribes a protective talisman in Daoist magic design which she must fold in three and carry in her pocket. Her ghost is an evil spirit out to harm her.

Exorcism of ghosts and evil spirits has been a core part of the Daoist repertoire for nearly two thousand years. Powerful Daoist communities, such as the *Tianshi dao* 天师道 (Celestial Masters), emerged during the political fragmentation of the end of the Han dynasty (second century CE) with distinctive scriptures, institutions, and hierarchies, as well as complex pantheons of deities. They practised communal confession, forms of meditation, moral self-cultivation, followed dietary and medicinal regimens to prolong their lives, and visualised *qi* with specialised breathing techniques. Their ritual masters uttered incantations and gave doses of water infused with the ashes of talismanic writing; they performed sacrifices and exorcised ghosts and demons that took up residence within the body (Kaltenmark 1979: 41–4). Some of the millenarian Daoist cults even believed that through these techniques they would become the immortal chosen people who would survive a coming apocalypse. Living Daoist traditions testify that all of these practices have survived into the twenty-first century, in some form or other, despite 70 years of Communist campaigns against 'superstition'. Daoist priests and shamans still follow shamanic rituals that conflate travelling out-of-body through the universe with itineraries through the pathways of the inner body. The iconography and topographies of the Daoist body therefore overlap in their detail with physiological maps: the acupuncture points sparkle with names of rivers, stars, and constellations, with temples and gates to heaven and alchemical furnaces (Fava 2018: 51–73).

This visualisation of spiritual itineraries is first evidenced in the *Shanhai jing* 山海经 (Classic of Mountains and Seas; latest date first century BCE), a compilation that has been described as 'a manual on prodigies, a geographical gazetteer or explanatory notes on illustrations or maps' (Sterckx 2018: 39). Therein we find what Dorefeeva-Lichtmann speculates are 'mapless maps', itineraries at the origins of geomancy that navigate the mountain locations of divine powers and guardian spirits, and thereafter ground a tradition of spirit quests or out-of-body journeys of shamans (Dorefeeva-Lichtmann 2007: 53–62). Over the succeeding two millennia this tradition of spirit quests, pilgrimages, out-of-body and inner body, produced multiple imaginaries in both Daoist and Buddhist contexts. Manuscript images of Xuanzang's 玄奘 (602–664) pilgrimage to India to collect the Buddhist scriptures survive from medieval Dunhuang. His journey (together with the main protagonist, his companion and protector, the Monkey King Sun Wukong 孙悟空) was later immortalised in Wu Cheng'en's Ming novel *Xiyou ji*, 西游记 (Journey to the West, c. mid-sixteenth century), stories from which survive in practically every visual media from poster and advertisement to cartoon and film. *Journey to the West* embodies enduring and creative tensions in China's religious landscape: the state, Daoist, Buddhist, and more local practices for religious adepts. But the journeys recounted in the film are uniquely female itineraries which, perversely, have no happy or transcendental ending. Yang Lina charts a series of troubled displacements through the plural medico-religious landscape of urban Beijing that match the similarly troubled filmic landscapes of Fang Lei's inner body, her anguish and the fluidity of her passions, taking her on a pilgrimage into the suburbs, first to a fortune teller and then to a Buddhist monastery in the mountains.

The way to the female fortune teller tracks the two friends as they leave behind the glitzy urban nightclub, and its false promise of escape from Fang Lei's nightmare, to a less familiar, bleak rural reality. The trembling hand-held camera accompanies their car to the run-down village where the fortune teller lives. With the camera positioned in the back seat we follow the travellers in rear view so that the viewer is 'an observer ideally mobile in space and time' (Pudovkin 1949: 71; Branigan and Buckland 2014: 328) and then strolling behind them through deserted roadways full of building rubble (Figure 7.3). The contrast between the dull hues of the fortune teller's shabby village and the high saturated interior jars.

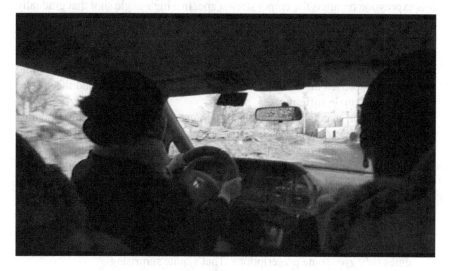

Figure 7.3 Driving with Fang Lei and her friend to the fortune teller

This time the glitz is that of the makeshift temple and religious paraphernalia of the fortune teller's crowded shrine. The welcoming spirit medium and the virtuoso mix of Buddhism and Daoism enchants Fang Lei. It is strange yet appealing to her. As the spirit medium channels the ghost's voice and reveals him as her husband in a former life who will save her and her family, Fang Lei finally breaks down in tears of relief.

In the next out-of-town journey Fang Lei's daughter goes missing from the car while she herself is somnambulant, running between the trees with her ghost lover. Waking from a scene of wild sex in the car she runs frantically around in the same deadly woods looking for the little girl. We are led through her terror to an unknown lake. As she throws herself into the chilly waters, clutching her daughter's inflatable toy, we experience that terror as both that of the distraught parent, and also the guilt of ambivalent mothering – an ambivalence almost unthinkable in Chinese culture. This monologue of maternal desperation is sandwiched between the scenes of the two men in her life, juxtaposing passionate sexual intimacy and passionless marriage. Between the two men she has not only lost her child, but she is also being punished by the weight of Chinese culture, for her own selfish desire and sensory indulgence. The child, in fact, does not die, but ends up in A & E, where the husband finally loses all patience with his wife's 'infidelity' rejecting totally her mad confession and pleadings for forgiveness. He whispers that she is nothing but a 'dirty whore' and that is the last we see of him or the child.

Desperate with grief and left on her own, Fang Lei scours the city looking for her child, wherein we meet Yang Lina herself playing director of the Women's Federation. But it is the Buddhist aunt, with whom Fang Lei has a natural affinity, who initiates the final journey which takes them out of town to a Tibetan Buddhist monastery. By this time, she is no longer curious or hopeful. Her pale emotionless expression parallels the empty snowscape. In a high-angle shot that gradually tracks backwards, we see the coach moving further and further into the distance, almost vanishing, engulfing Fang Lei's loneliness. At this point the majestic red pillars of the temple sparkle in the distance, a momentary respite from the film's monotonous palette. The all-female passengers get off the coach, silently forming two lines to approach the temple, seemingly muted by its gravity and the spectre of communal female suffering.

There we find a community of semi-deranged women consulting Buddhist monks, and participating in ecstatic group sessions. The participants are again not actors, so the scenes of the faithful and their consultations use semi-documentary footage of the use of Buddhist healing for real distress. How representative is it of actual medical and patient practice and how are the plural practices articulated and intersecting in the film? Yang Yi, the TCM practitioner, is astonished by the religious appropriation of her skills:

> The Daoist priest, and also the Buddhist priest, they both take pulses. Sometimes they give some prescriptions. That's quite surprising.

Buddhists have, in fact, always provided many forms of healing in the temples (Salguero 2014; Wang Jinyu 2018). We see an enigmatic abbot in the distance, a lone figure in the snow, seemingly, a celibate authority who offers salvation. The stages of Buddhist healing typically describe a narrative journey which includes curing illness, sharing those benefits with others, purifying the body and speech to prepare for death, achieving rebirth in the presence of the Buddha and finally enlightenment (Teiser 2019). At night amid women chanting *oh mane padme hu'm* (ཨོཾ་མ་ཎི་པདྨེ་ཧཱུྃ༔ [唵嘛呢叭咪吽]), an address to the bodhisattva of the same name, Manipadma 'Jewel Lotus' (aka the bodhisattva Avilokitesvara; Lopez 1988: 131), Fang Lei gives birth to a baby dressed in red. Has her ghost been exorcised, re-born as the abbot tells her? Or is the child a reincarnation of her own self? In Pure Land Chinese Buddhism (*Jingtu zong* 净土宗), the healing narrative ultimately ends in a pure birth, quite unlike blood-tainted human reproduction, a birth sym-bolised by a baby emerging wrapped in a Lotus flower (Yulin Cave 25 Pure Land mural).

Yet, at least in the view of one of our student respondents, the enigmatic Bud-dhist monk 'really has all the physical features, of the man in her dream' (George Yao). Whatever the director's intention, the final scenes of the film, as Fang Lei's lingering gaze rests on the abbot in the snow and she gently strokes her under-belly, are charged with the same quality of unfulfilled sexual desire that the film begins with. They undermine any audience desire to see our anti-heroine find an easy peace. Or in the words of the director:

> As far as I'm concerned, I think neither psychiatrists nor religions can solve people's psychological problems, because I think in the contemporary soci-ety, nobody can be another person's redemption. Therefore, I offer no con-crete answer to end the film. This is my observation of reality.
>
> (tr. Guo Liping)

For this audience member, however, Yang Lina does provide another kind of homecoming.

Female intimacy: to the heart of Beijing

If there is a final journey for Fang Lei it is not taken in one chronological sequence but emerges throughout the film linking all the moments of pleasure when women delight in each other's company and escape pre-destined female roles. Whether bathing and feeding children, playing with sex toys or sucking lollipops, in shop-ping malls, in prayer or ecstatic dancing, the care-connection between the women in the film, friends, mothers and children, and the older women in the family, is expressed through physical objects and practices – the source of the most joy-ful and intimate scenes in the film. The 'curious and telling correlation between the mobility and visual and aural sensations' brings an intimacy to the film that transcends the temporal, and even death, and takes us to the heart of Beijing, creating female inter-generational spaces between the city's old and new architectures (Shiel and Fitzmaurice 2001: 1). Li Weijia says:

> I feel it, the female in this film. The main character, she is kind of, like, isolated . . . it seems she only has one friend, and her only relative in this film is her auntie. Her parents do not appear in this film.. the husband does not pay attention to his own mother. And it is the wife, the mother, who really cares for the conditions of the grandma. Like she helps her to take the shower.

When Fang Lei gets called away from the Yonghegong 雍和宫 temple, she has to beg leave of her auntie from out of town who is praying for salvation from some emotional distress that we never get to know about. Granny has had a fall. In the homely, human comfort of the compound, far away from the madding streets of Beijing, they share a shower because Granny smells bad. Despite the fact that Granny doesn't even recognise her daughter-in-law, the soft intimacy that is created as Fang Lei gets naked to encourage her to wash, and playfully tweaks Granny's nipples, turns tragic mental decline into gentle humour.

The claustrophobic privacy of Granny's indoor life is cluttered with caresses, the joy of sweets, and the extra-sensory communication that the women share. The architecture of Granny's compound humanises the visual and sensory quality already identified for Fang Lei's sexuality, countering the emptiness of her illicit desire with tenderness. The brightness of the sun-filled courtyard illuminates just the two of them and creates a mutuality that others cannot access. Granny's growing dementia parallels Fang Lei's growing madness, and together they transcend social convention through a kind of mad-to-mad communing. Relief comes, in this way, through 'expansion from direct concentration on the character to his [her] immediate world' (Kolker 1983: 7). Like the Buddhist monks and nuns who do not really require faith or complete belief and understanding, these irrational moments are a source of spiritual sustenance.

Fang Lei is prescient of the exact moment that Granny dies and intuits the location of the shoes that Granny wants to wear at her funeral. It alarms her husband. But the film is unquestioning of the power of supernatural communication between women, and the comfort that it can bring. Our students related similar stories of family members, including men, who knew instinctively of the death of their loved ones before they were told (Zhou Dangwei). Non-verbal or written communications also extends to connections maintained over distance with children. Yang Qihua, our only undergraduate respondent, was wearing a Buddhist charm around his wrist. The youngest male participant in the experiment, he had been away from home for a long time and felt a bond of attachment through the religious paraphernalia sent to him by his mother:

> My mom strongly believes in it [religion]. Actually, throughout my life, my life choices are guided by this spiritual stuff. . . . Whenever there is trouble or a problem with my life, my mom will ask Daoist priests, or like monks from

the temple for help first. So, like, she puts their advice as a top priority. I feel more connection with my family. I've been abroad for so many years. I still keep the Buddhist scripts my mom sent to me recently. I don't like, believe in it completely.

Yang Qihua's mother is not the only Buddhist presence in the room. Yang Yi, our Beijing student, is also a Buddhist. For her, Buddhism is a 'way of explaining the world, the universe convinces me and brings me peace'. As Fang Lei drifts through various locations of Beijing, the city is presented as native space, as well as a site of multiple, polylocalised identities: both homeland and homelessness. She does not find peace. But it is in the intimacy with which women and their locations are consistently portrayed that we feel the greatest sense of homecoming. And this quality fills what otherwise would be a totally depressing film with a tangible sense of optimism, whether or not that was intended by the director.

Conclusion

Revisionist histories will tell us that there have been many routes to power for women in China with wealth and connections. Yet China's economic miracle means that the numbers of women with education, time on their hands and spending power has grown exponentially (Chen 2018). Apart from being there and experiencing the new forms of social dislocation that these new freedoms bring *en masse*, it is hard to appreciate the problem without Yang Lina's direction.

> One of the difficulties, including the last scene in the temple, seems to be the way out. But there is actually no way out. I am very pessimistic. I do not think this present era has any positive effect on me.
>
> (tr. Guo Liping)

Yang Lina's docu-drama intends to portray the experience of a national spiritual crisis through the lens of China's urban middle-class women. There is no doubt that the women students in our class recognised the director's vision as a reflection of their own experience of urban housewives in China, and the essential emptiness of Fang Lei's condition. The film constantly measures these empty spaces – not only collapsing the inhuman urban architecture into the emptiness of her soul but emphasising the lonely distance between each scene and the beholder (Bordwell 2013: 6).

As the filmic journey unravels a process that is both psychologically dysfunctional and destructive, as much as it provides a release from Fang Lei's boredom and frustration, it may be, as Yang Lina herself suggests, that there is no way out. Yet running through this spiritual chaos is a series of endearing moments of peace, hope, and humour, unfettered by patriarchal social or religious hierarchies. They serve to connect all the tender moments of maternal, sisterly, and womanly care, from the middle-aged girls playing with dildos to visions of Granny beyond the grave shining above Fang Lei's dreams like a demented bodhisattva.

Filmography

Filmography for Yang Lina

Home Video (*Jiating luxiangdai* 家庭录像带), dir. Yang Lina, 2001.
Let's Dance Together (*Yiqi tiaowu* 一起跳舞), dir. Yang Lina, 2007.
Longing for the Rain (*Chunmeng* 春梦), dir. Yang Lina, 2013, www.youtube.com/watch?v=XOhh_sS7ZPU, accessed 07 April 2019.
My Neighbors and Their Japanese Ghosts (*Wode linju shuo guizi* 我的邻居说鬼子), dir. Yang Lina, 2008.
Old Men (*Laotou* 老头), dir. Yang Lina, 1999.
The Love of Mr. An (*Lao An* 老安), dir. Yang Lina, 2008.
Wild Grass (*Yecao* 野草), dir. Yang Lina, 2009.

Bibliography

Allan, S. (1997) *The Way of Water and Sprouts of Virtue*, Albany: SUNY Press.
Berry, C. (2008) Wedding Banquet: A Family (Melodrama) Affair, in C. Berry (ed.) *Chinese Films in Focus II*, New York: Palgrave Macmillan, pp. 235–42.
Bordwell, D. (2013) *Narration in the Fiction Film*, Abingdon, Oxon: Routledge.
Boumeester, M. (2011) Reconsidering Cinematic Mapping: Halfway Between Collected Subjectivity and Projective Mapping, in A. Lu and F. Penz (eds.) *Urban Cinematics: Understanding Urban Phenomena Through the Moving Image*, Bristol: Intellect Books Ltd, pp. 239–56.
Branigan, E. and Buckland, W. (eds.) (2014) *The Routledge Encyclopedia of Film Theory*, London and New York: Routledge.
Bray, F., Dorofeeva-Lichtmann, V. and Métailié, G. (eds.) (2007) *Graphics and Text in the Production of Technical Knowledge in China: The Warp and the Weft*, Leiden: E.J. Brill.
Brownell, S., Wasserstrom, J. and Laqueur, T. (2002) *Chinese Femininities/Chinese Masculinities: A Reader*, Berkeley: University of California Press.
Chen, H. (2003) *Medicine, Society, and the Making of Madness in Imperial China*, unpublished PhD thesis, SOAS.
Chen, M. (2018) Wealth Report Asia 2018: Shanghai Reclaims the Top Spot, Julius Bär, www.juliusbaer.com/insights/arising-asia/wealth-report-asia-2018-shanghai-reclaims-the-top-spot/, accessed 23 February 2019.
Croll, E. (2013) *Feminism and Socialism in China*, Abingdon: Routledge.
Cui, S. (2008) *Women Through the Lens: Gender and Nation in a Century of Chinese Cinema*, Honolulu: University of Hawai'i Press.
Dai, J. (2002) *Cinema and Desire: Feminist Marxism and Cultural Politics in the Work of Dai Jinhua*, New York: Verso.
Dorefeeva-Lichtmann, V. (2007) Mapless Mapping: Did He Maps of the *Shan hai jing Ever Exist?* in F. Bray, V. Dorfeeva-Lichtmann and G. Métailié (eds.) *Graphics and Text in the Production of Technical Knowledge in China*, Leiden and Boston: Brill, pp. 217–94.
Fava, P. (2018) The Body of Laozi and the Course of a Taoist Journey Through the Heavens, in V. Lo and P. Barrett (eds.) *Imagining Chinese Medicine*, Leiden: Brill, pp. 351–72.
Goossaert, V. and Palmer, D. (2011) *The Religious Question in Modern China*, Chicago: Chicago University Press.
Johnson, I. (2017) *The Souls of China: The Return of Religion After Mao*, London: Penguin.
Kaltenmark, M. (1979) The Ideology of the T'ai-p'ing Ching, in H. Welch and A. Seidel (eds.) *Facets of Taoism*, New Haven: Yale University Press, pp. 19–52.

Kolker, R. (1983) *The Altering Eye: Contemporary International Cinema*, Oxford: Oxford University Press.

Landy, M. (2010) *Italian Film (National Film Traditions)*, Cambridge: Cambridge University Press.

Liu, X. (2014) *Exemplary Women of Early China*, trans. A. Kinney, New York: Columbia University Press.

Lopez, D.S. (1988) *Prisoners of Shangri-la: Tibetan Buddhism and the West*, Chicago: Chicago University Press.

Merleau-Ponty, M. (1945) *Phenomenology of Perception*, trans. C. Smith, New York: The Humanities Press.

Pudovkin, V.I. (1949) *Film Technique and Film Acting: The Cinema Writings of V.I. Pudovkin*, New York: Lear.

Raphals, L. (1998) *Sharing the Light: Representations of Women and Virtue in Early China*, Series in Chinese Philosophy and Culture, Albany: Suny.

Salguero, C.P. (2014) *Translating Buddhist Medicine in Medieval China*, Philadelphia: University of Pennsylvania Press.

Shameless, C.H. (2019) To Some Chinese Men, Sex Toys Can Become Full-fledged Girlfriends, *WeChat Feed*, 09 January 2019.

Shiel, M. and Fitzmaurice, T. (eds.) (2001) *Cinema and the City: Film and Urban Societies in a Global Context*, Oxford and Malden, MA: Blackwell.

Sterckx, R. (2018) The Limits of Illustration: Animalia and Pharmacopeia from Guo Pu to Bencao Gangmu, in V. Lo and P. Barrett (eds.) *Imagining Chinese Medicine*, Leiden: Brill, pp. 133–50.

Strickmann, M. (2002) *Chinese Magical Medicine*, ed. B. Faure, Stanford, CA: Stanford University Press.

Tatz, M. (1985) *Buddhism and Healing: Demiéville's Article "Byō" from Hōbōgirin*, Lanham, MD: University Press of America.

Teiser, S.F. (2019) Varieties of Religious Healing in Medieval Chinese Buddhism (lecture), Brunei Gallery, SOAS.

Wang Jinyu 王進玉 (2018) Images of Healing, Hygiene and the Cultivation of the Body in the Dunhuang Cave Murals, in V. Lo and P. Barrett (eds.) *Imagining Chinese Medicine*, Leiden: Brill, pp. 133–50.

Zeitlin, J. (1993) *Historian of the Strange: Pu Songling and His Chinese Classical Tale*, Stanford: Stanford University Press.

Zhang, Y. (2010) *Cinema, Space, and Polylocality in a Globalizing China*, Honolulu: University of Hawaii Press.

Part 3

Improving the education and training of health professionals

8 The gigantic black citadel

Design of Death and medical humanities pedagogy in China

Guo Liping

At Peking University Health Science Center, there are two elective courses that use films to guide discussions in topics of Medical and Health Humanities. One started in 2011 and is designed for graduate students, called 'Western Culture in Films', which mainly focuses on the culture of western medicine as practised in English-speaking countries. The other course, 'Films and the Medical Humanities' which started in 2014, is for undergraduate students. The instructors for the two courses come from a variety of disciplines: English, bioethics, health law, and the history of medicine. Both courses use western films, especially films of the English language. The language of instruction for the undergraduate course is Chinese; for the graduate course, English. The dominance of English-language films in these courses somehow worries the instructors. They have started the exploration of using Chinese films in such courses. This chapter proposes the use of a 2012 Chinese film *Design of Death* (*Shasheng* 杀生) by a 'sixth-generation' director Guan Hu 管虎 to explore the 'shady' aspects of modern medicine: the hierarchy in the medical establishment, the pressure to conform, the relentless pursuit of longevity (or rather, the delay of death), and the coldness, detachment, and deception of the doctor trained in western medicine (versus the doctor of Chinese medicine). This chapter will also explore the choice to die taken by the maverick hero Niu Jieshi 牛结实 (whose name literally means 'as strong as an ox') – can we empathise with him and if yes, how? Finally, discussing metaphors in the film with medical students will be a rewarding 'aesthetic route' to train their 'narrative competence' (Charon 2006: vii). Given the students' enthusiastic response to the screening and the subsequent Q&A session with director Guan Hu in December 2013 at Peking University Health Science Centre, there is all the more reason to recommend this film for the medical humanities classroom in China.

The film

Design of Death tells the story of 'a crowd working together to kill someone who refuses to conform' (Li 2012: 46). Niu Jieshi is regarded as a ruffian in the remote village called 'The Village of Longevity' where he lives, in a Southwestern province of China in the remote 1940s, in the Republican era. The distance from any direct criticism of the current administration undoubtedly made it easier for a film that represents a hero who challenges the prevailing authority to pass censorship. Both the minor and major 'crimes' he commits challenge the rules by which the villagers live – rules established by their ancestors. He takes preserved meat from the butcher without paying him, constantly peeps at the painter making love to his wife and makes fun of him. He saves the sexy Widow Ma who is to be sacrificed (drowned) for Great-Grandfather at his funeral (water cremation) and has sex with her (the village blacksmith has always coveted Widow Ma but doesn't dare do anything). He bathes in the 'Holy Water' of the village and digs up treasures from the villagers' ancestral graves, giving them as gifts at a villager's wedding. His most heinous crime is scattering 'the powder of lust' in the water system, making the entire village fall into frenzy. This is the last straw. The villagers decide that they have to get rid of him, 'This ruffian has destroyed all rules left by our ancestors. The gods will punish us. If we don't come up with a plan, we'll be doomed!' When several of their attempts to 'discipline' him end in failure, Dr Niu, who has left the village to attend medical school (probably in a western country) is asked to come back to design a death plan. Dr Niu uses 'mass psychological warfare' to deceive Niu Jieshi into believing that he has cancer just like his father – with everybody's strange reaction when they see him, the drinking tricks at the wedding, the ceremony of celebration in the rain, and the 'evidence' of a fabricated chest x-ray. When Niu Jieshi learns that Dr Niu is persuading the villagers to kill his unborn son as well by forcing Widow Ma to abort the fetus, 'to eradicate the weed with its root', he decides to die instead and pleads with the villagers that 'the baby is innocent'. He drags his blue coffin toward the death spot he has chosen on the mountain, returning all things he has taken from the villagers along the way. Just as he is approaching his death spot, he hears the cries of the newborn. . . .

At a closer look, this film fits in with what Chris Berry calls 'the Chinese family melodrama' (*Zhongguo jiating lunli pian*中国家庭伦理片), where not only the individual is in conflict with the family (the Confucian clan in this film), but the family (the clan) as a collectivity is in crisis (Berry 2008: 235). Niu Jieshi's conflicts with the clan stem from its desire to discipline him and his resistance to be disciplined. As an intruder to the village, his behaviours and people's reactions lead to the destruction of the village; as a redeemer, he chooses to die for his own redemption and that of the clan – it makes them see their own cruelty and shed tears for it. However, there are some 'variations' from a 'standard' Chinese family melodrama. Niu Jieshi is not a virtuous hero but a ruffian; he is the destroyer rather than the victim – in fact, the villagers are victims of his pranks before they collude to get rid of him. His self sacrifice is out of the duty for his unborn child to live rather than for the family (clan) to maintain its operation and values. I argue that precisely because of these variations, *Design of Death* strictly conforms to the discussion of '*jiating lunli*' (家庭伦理) (or rather '*jiazu lunli*' 家族伦理, the ethics of the clan) in this film – ethical expectations of behaviour in a confined establishment such as the clan; and the analogy between the clan and the medical establishment provides superb opportunities to guide medical students to discuss the 'shady' aspects of medicine.

Hierarchy and pressure to conform

The film is shot in a traditional village of the Qiang 羌 ethnic minority in Sichuan Province (Chen 2012: 144). The village is enclosed by mountains and is a perfect symbol of a confined establishment. The physical size of the village is small, but with its layered architectures and complicated connecting alleyways, it radiates an air of mystery and depressiveness. The predominant colours in the village are grey and black. One standing on the upper-level dwellings can see the lower levels directly – 'the special "nesting" of hierarchised surveillance' (Foucault 1977: 171) is a display of the power structure in the village. It is a citadel in itself, with its strict rules and forms and rituals. The villagers live by 'The Seventy-two Rules of the Ancestors'. They are disciplined by these rules in everything they do in their life – when to get up, when to wash for the night, what to eat and not to eat, what to say to each other, how to be deferential to the elders and the authorities, how to behave on different occasions such as funerals and weddings. . . . These rules become sacred to the villagers, like the laws to the Israelites in the Old Testament. Then there is this Niu Jieshi – son of a petty passing tradesman who has forced his stay in the village, takes up the clan name 'Niu' of the village and afterwards dies of cancer – with his almost childish mischief, wreaks havoc on these sacred rules. But these rules are not to be messed with, for the penalty of 'sins' against them is death. Rebels must be punished and the sanctity of the rules maintained.

But Niu Jieshi is a free soul, reveling in life and is not hesitant to die. Even though he's been living in the village, among the villagers all his life – maybe because he grows up an orphan, he is not 'disciplined' enough. Compared with the villagers, he is free and full of vitality. Rules are nothing to him, he enjoys life to its fullest, laughing wherever he goes, satisfied with his pranks. He attracts the children. They are his faithful followers. This immediately bring to mind the image of the Monkey King (Sun Wukong 孙悟空) in the Chinese folklore story *Journey to the West* (*Xiyouji* 西游记). The Monkey King, an intruder and outsider, a mortal in the heavenly space, rebels against all rules set up by the Jade Emperor, the highest monarch in Heaven. But unlike the Monkey King who is buried under the mountains for 500 years, just waiting for the opportunity to serve the orthodoxy as his redemption, Jieshi chooses to redeem his 'sins' by sacrificing his life in order to save the life of his son, who is expected to be the new generation rebel. The other difference between Jieshi and the Monkey King lies in their deportment of the body. As depicted in various opera films and cartoons, the Monkey King is a martial arts hero with superb control of his body and can transform into 72 forms. On the contrary, Niu Jieshi apparently has no intention to control his body. His bodily movements lack coordination and he seems to be invulnerable to pain.

True to the concerns of the sixth-generation directors such as Guan Hu, hierarchy, resentment to conform, and an individual's rebellion against the establishment are central themes in the film. Niu Jieshi's chaotic freedom from the socialised body is the tool for rebellion. This film offers a great starting point to discuss these issues with medical students. They have to understand that their profession is a hierarchical field – after all, a senior surgeon has lamented to me openly that

'The nurses of the Peking University hospitals strut around like queens, whereas in hospitals with better traditions, like the PUMC hospital, nurses sidle along the walls'. Hierarchy exists not only between doctors and nurses, but between doctors and other healthcare professionals, between doctors of different ranks and specialties, with neurosurgeons perched at the top of the specialty pyramid. This strict hierarchical structure in the healthcare system is perhaps second only to the military. Research shows that in the process of their training, 'not all transformations medical students go through are positive. They move from being open-minded to close-minded; from being intellectually curious to narrowly focusing on facts; from empathy to emotional detachment; from idealism to cynicism' (Manhood 2011: 983). In the process of this transformation, they are constantly under 'hierarchical observation', therefore gradually take hierarchy for granted, and may at the same time be encouraged to climb the hierarchical ladder and guard the system. In fact, hierarchy and the pressure to conform to the 'norm' in the hospital is so intense that Japan, Taiwan, and South Korea have all made their own versions of the popular medical TV dramas entitled 'The Gigantic White Tower' (*baise juta* 白色巨塔) to explore these issues, amongst other themes. When we think of the emphasis on conformity, collectivism, and respect for authority and seniority in East Asian culture, we may understand why these TV dramas are so popular and why the producers in these three countries/regions are fond of the same title. In discussion with students, we have to make them aware that the medical establishment will discipline both the caregivers and those seeking care. They are expected to behave according to certain patterns – doctors should be authoritative, caring yet paternalistic, showing only 'detached concern' (Halpern 2001). Patients definitely have to be deferential, asking little but obeying all orders. . . . Medical students may feel that they are powerless in front of such cultural and institutional forces and that they cannot change anything but have to conform to survive. However, this doesn't mean they should conform blindly. In the now increasingly popular narrative medicine movement (even in China), medical students and healthcare providers are encouraged to write reflexively about their practices, their interactions with patients, colleagues, and society. They are also learning to listen attentively to the patients' stories to show true concern and bear witness to patients' suffering (Charon 2006: 177–202). With the 'aesthetic' analysis of the film, and the tools of narrative medicine, the power dynamics in the hospital can be altered and affiliation with patients and colleagues can be forged.

The pursuit of longevity and avoidance of death

'The Village of Longevity' has, since the Qing Dynasty (1644–1911), produced 18 people who have lived for more than 110 years, and there are numerous people aged 90 years old and above. Given this proud phenomenon, longevity has become the obsession of the villagers. Great grandfather is 119 years and three days old, bedridden and sustained by intravenous drips. He has a hobby of modest drinking since his youth days but the village head reproaches him when he 'catches' him drinking secretly: 'Stop drinking, Fourth Uncle. According to the rules of the ancestors, a man must not drink when he turns seventy-six. Don't you break that rule'. Great-grandfather is forced to live. The village head urges him to discipline himself for the reputation of the village in the form of personal achievement: 'If you can live a few more days, you'll break the record of longevity in this village'. But Niu Jieshi gives him alcohol from a venous dropper when he is alone with great grandfather. 'Turtles live a long life, but they spend their entire life in the shell. What's the meaning of such a life! Drink as you wish!' Great grandfather drinks from the dropper, smiling and nodding contentedly.

The Qing Dynasty had an elaborate system to celebrate longevity. The emperor would order that an honorific arch be built to honour a man who lived to be 100 years or older. Silk and silver were given as gifts from the emperor. For those (only men) who lived to be 120 years, the largess would double (Wang 2006: 38–48). Even though these material gains were not attainable in the Republican era, the pursuit of longevity with all means is retained to this day.

With the development of biomedicine, the relentless pursuit of longevity, or rather, the delay or avoidance of death by all means, has become the goal of medicine worldwide. Henry James writes, 'We are never old, that is, we never cease easily to be young . . . the whole battalion of our faculties and our freshness . . . on a considerably reluctant march into the enemy's country, the country of the general lost freshness' (James and Dupee 1983: 547). But this loss of freshness is unacceptable to the contemporary Chinese, who increasingly worship youthfulness and resent the process of aging. Even though this theme in the film is not the director's major concern, for medical students it provides a golden opportunity to discuss life, aging, death, and prolonged dying. This is especially necessary and relevant for Chinese medical students. Death is a taboo in Chinese culture, people don't talk about it and cannot bear to hear the word 'death'. It is usually replaced by many euphemisms when people have to talk about it. This is common in Confucian culture – for Confucius has famously said 'If life is not understood, how could death be fathomed?' By this, he exhorts people to concentrate only on life, and THIS life at that. He also teaches that, 'if one respects the spirits of the dead and the gods while keeping them at a distance, one can be called wise'. Furthermore, the Chinese believe that 'a bad life is better than a good death', which encourages people to cling onto life even if they are dying. Therefore, 'death' – a fact of life – is swept under the carpet, people simply pretend that this is something they don't have to face in their life. Those who are dying die in loneliness. Most families don't talk about death with their dying family members, assuming this avoidance will do them good – if death is undesirable and life is so good, then telling someone s/he's dying is cruel. One study shows that 57.7% of the families with cancer patients that took part in the research did not inform the sufferer that they had cancer, because the immediate association with a diagnosis of cancer is imminent death (Sun *et al.* 2007: 556–9). Another study shows 70.0% of patients with cancer that took part wished that healthcare professionals and their families 'do everything possible to save the lives of cancer patients even though they're suffering from severe pain'. However, 76.5% of these patients themselves did not mind discussing death (Zeng *et al.* 2008: 71–3). These studies indicate the disparities between dying persons' expectations to talk about death and the families' reluctance to discuss these issues; between the dying persons' acceptance of death and their desire to cling onto life. This is a rare occasion that the Chinese tradition and Confucian thoughts coincide with the precepts of biomedicine. The medical students are young and healthy, but will be attending to the weak and the dying, wielding their weapons of modern medicine and medical technology. It would be a shame if the message they get from the second study is that they should do everything technically possible to save the terminal patients' lives. A lot has been written about the harm of such 'heroic medicine'. At this stage, prolonging life (or rather, the process of dying) with all kinds of technology is prolonging suffering and squandering precious medical resources. 'To die with dignity' is a concept which is gaining increasing popularity in China today. 'Beijing Living Will Promotion Association' and their website 'Choice and Dignity' are being endorsed by more and more healthcare professionals. They advocate a natural process of dying without resuscitation and life-sustaining facilities at the end of life. In order for their will to be carried out at the end of life when people are unable to make decisions and express their desires, people are encouraged to write their 'living will' so that grieving family members will not ask physicians 'to do everything possible to save their lives' (Choice and Dignity 2017). Students must be aware that aging is not a disease, it's the natural passage of time. They should not be afraid to discuss death with dying patients and their families. When the restoration of health is not possible, he/she should help patients in their 'pursuit of personal goals with a minimum of pain, discomfort, or disability' (Pellegrino 2008: 165).

The doctor image

When watching this film, medical students at Peking University Health Science Center were acutely aware of the images of the two doctors. As a matter of fact, one student in the Q&A session after the screening of the film on campus asked Guan Hu why he made the doctor of Chinese medicine the 'good doctor' and the doctor of western medicine the 'bad doctor'. Students were obviously not convinced when Guan Hu said he didn't realise this until they asked.

The good doctor is sent to the Village of Longevity to investigate a rumoured 'plague outbreak'. He finds the almost dead Niu Jieshi on the cliffs and set out to probe the reasons of his death. As a matter of fact, the story is narrated mostly from his perspective – we can reasonably assume that this outside doctor is the embodiment of the director himself. The doctor puts forward hypotheses, searches evidence, 'interviews' witnesses and participants of events, and even dissects the 'dead' Niu Jieshi. He leads the audience in patching together evidence and reaches conclusions through logical reasoning. Is he the compassionate doctor – 'the good doctor' – from the beginning as students have assumed? Hardly. We see that this doctor is only doing his job dispassionately, with 'detached concern', like many doctors today. Students might be fooled by his fixed smile throughout the film and regard him as a benevolent doctor simply because of that. However, the smile, as well as the doctor himself, goes through a transition throughout the film. As he is 'researching his project', he is more and more fascinated by Niu Jieshi, and attempts to understand him as a person. He becomes identified with Jieshi, sympathetic to his attitude toward life, and is appreciative of his values. When he finally meets with the village head, he tries to recount to him the whole event from Jieshi's perspective – in this version of the story, life in the village is less rigid; people have more freedom; the relationship among the villagers is characterised by warmth. At the very end, he smiles peacefully and contentedly when Widow Ma leaves the village with the baby in glowing warm light.

Medical schools are now striving to foster empathy in their students. In the latest literature, empathy is defined as:

1 knowing another person's internal state;
2 matching the posture of the other;
3 coming to feel what the other feels;
4 projecting oneself into the other's situation;
5 imagining how another person is thinking and feeling;
6 imagining how one would think in the other's place;
7 feeling distress as witnessing the other's suffering;
8 feeling for another person who is suffering (Batson 2009: 3–15).

Measured against these features, we can see we have an example of a doctor who is becoming more and more empathic – he is going through a journey with Niu Jieshi. He not only adopts Niu Jieshi's perspective in the end, and feels for him; he even emulates in action in surveying the village on a bicycle in uncoordinated movements (no other person in the village has done so). Towards the end of the film, he even cuts his hair and adopts Jieshi's hairstyle. This is a journey the medical humanities educators intend to guide medical students to go through – from cool-headed scientific physicians to warm, empathic healers.

The bad doctor is the cold-blooded Dr Niu, the designer of death for Niu Jieshi. He agrees to come back 'to help' the village head to get rid of Jieshi out of personal vengeance. As a child the boy Jieshi used a hook to steal preserved meat from the ventilation holes of the house of Dr Niu's grandparents. The boy Dr Niu, to protect the family food, blocks up all ventilation holes as a precaution, causing his grandparents to die of carbon monoxide emitted from the stove. However, he firmly regards Jieshi, not himself, as the culprit of his grandparent's death. He is the only person in the village to speak in Mandarin, not in Sichuan dialect. Only on one occasion does he talk in the dialect – when the outside doctor finally finds out he is the chief instigator of the death plan, he says with a bitter smile (the only time he smiles at all): 'My grandparents shouldn't have died for nothing'. He insists on forcing Widow Ma to abort the fetus, 'to rid the weed with the roots', while the villagers are hesitant, believing that 'it's best to rid of the sore, not the skin'.

Contrary to the expectations of a doctor, Dr Niu is a killer and a liar. When the villagers ask him to think of a good way to 'get rid of Niu Jieshi', he asks 'do you all want to kill him?', shocking everyone with the word 'kill'. It's understandable that the medical students are concerned with the depiction of Dr Niu – who is a doctor of western medicine, the medicine THEY are learning. In recent media exposure of medical malpractice (some doctors of course are misrepresented) and conflicts between doctor and patients in China, the targets of blame are generally doctors of western medicine. This of course is related to the eminence of western medicine (or biomedicine) in the Chinese healthcare system, but the public belief is that Chinese medicine is more people-oriented and therefore more humane, while biomedicine is more technology-oriented and thus cold. This film provides a good introduction to doctor image in the new millennium – in the media, in films – and how that image affects high school graduates' decisions as to whether to take up medicine in college, as well as what can be done to improve the doctor image.

Decipher the metaphors and solve the riddle

'Metaphor is a matter of imaginative rationality' (Lakoff and Johnson 2003: 235). This sentence probably explains the extensive – some even say 'excessive' (Sun 2016: 35–6) – use of metaphors in this film. Rita Charon argues that close reading is an important means to train medical students in recognising metaphors in patients' illness narratives, which will help them better understand patients and make more accurate diagnosis, with the help of lab tests results and physical check-ups (Charon 2006: 107–30). The 'close reading' of this film is a challenging intellectual task, but as a group who are proud of their IQs, medical students at Peking University are delighted to take this challenge. Guan Hu uses a lot of flashbacks in the narration. Sometimes a short narrative from a particular character in the film is interposed to make a point – for example, when the important people in the village gather to discuss what to do with the maverick Niu Jieshi. For the audience, this nonlinear style of narrating is like guessing a riddle. In the popular Chinese film commentary website Douban, posts like '*Design of Death* kills a lot of brain cells' are common. For the medical students, it's like seeking evidence for the final diagnosis and they like this exercise of stretching their brains.

First of all, they have to understand the sequence of everything that happens, the cause and effect, to piece together the storyline. Second, the pervasive metaphors in the film increase the difficulty of that riddle. They have to identify these metaphors to better understand the plot and the director's intention in using these metaphors. For example, why is Widow Ma mute? Why is Jieshi's dwelling place in the village ancestral hall? Why does he always wear three keys on his neck? What do these keys symbolise, especially the fish-shaped one? Why are the children following him in smashing the ancestral hall when he learns the entire village are colluding to kill not only him but his unborn son? Why does he have to die in a blue coffin? What is the significance of the music box and the kite? Why does the music box only play 'Happy Birthday'? Why are the cast names at the end of the film shown against a cartoon background of the blue ocean and fish? Why does Dr Niu always wear his black leather gloves? (He does not wear them on one occasion, which excludes the possibility of scars or deformity of his hands.) Why is there a huge boulder propped up perilously at the highest point of the village?

Why is Niu Jieshi the only person in the film that has a name? (All other people are called by what they do, such as the midwife, the butcher, the blacksmith.) Why does the blacksmith always wear a fur collar on his bare chest? Why do the villagers wear black robes with black hoods at funerals (in contrast to the colour white which is worn in real Chinese funerals), howling toward the sky and beating their chests at the same time? Why are the predominant colours in the film black and grey, but toward the end, when Widow Ma escapes the village with the baby, there are suddenly warm colours surrounding her? Why is this film shot in such a cramped village? Some of these images are culturally specific – the mute Widow Ma represents the silenced women, especially widows, in traditional Chinese society; the ancestral hall symbolises tradition and rules that the villagers so revere. However, many of the metaphors have to be understood in the context of this film and the art of film making.

The ultimate question is: who has designed death for whom? Ostensibly, it's Dr Niu who has designed the death plan for Niu Jieshi, and all the villagers except the children participate. However, Dr Niu finally dies after eating the preserved meat 'with less cholesterol' – the poisoned piece the butcher offers Jieshi but Jieshi refuses to eat. The village head participates in the rain ceremony, a trick in the death plan – to make it more real to Jieshi; but as a result, he contracts a disease and subsequently dies of cancer, the disease which they try to convince Jieshi he has. The village head lives to be 99 years old, one year short of completing the designated age at which the Qing Dynasty would mandate that an honorific arch be established to commemorate a man's longevity. The villagers conspire together to 'get rid of Jieshi', but finally their howling at the funeral of the village head shakes the foundation of the boulder at the highest point of the village, and the ensuing earthquake destroys the whole village. Their intrigue to get rid of the maverick kills everyone. They have designed their own death.

Finally, students will see that there exist two versions of explanation as to what has happened: the villagers' perspective and the perspective of the outside doctor (hence that of Niu Jieshi). Charon argues that such process of 'close reading' (of the film) resembles the process of making diagnosis and adjusting treatment (Charon 2006: 111). Students learn to tolerate ambiguity, uncertainty, and confusion. They also learn to see things from different perspectives, perspectives other than their own, which is what empathy is all about. In this process, students learn to 'open [their] mind as widely as possible', so that 'signs and hints of almost imperceptible fineness . . . will bring [them] into the presence of a human being unlike any other' (Woolf as cited in Charon 2006: 109). They not only know the characters much better, appreciate the film more deeply, but also gain a lot of pleasure, even though the process is taxing on both the mind and the body.

The hidden curriculum

In the English-speaking world 'the hidden curriculum' is

> a set of influences that function at the level of organizational structure and culture . . . comprised of processes, pressures, and constraints which fall

outside the formal curriculum, and are often unarticulated or unexplored. In essence, the hidden curriculum represents what an institution teaches without intending or being aware it is taught.

(Stanek *et al*. 2015: 156)

In medical education, the hidden curriculum is usually enacted in such aspects as unspoken hierarchy, stratification, teaching by humiliation, unprofessionalism, patient dehumanization, and bad role modeling (Michalec and Hafferty 2013: 388–406; O'Callaghan 2013: 305–17; Martimianakis *et al*. 2015: s5–s13). However, in China 'hidden curriculum' (regardless of its Chinese translations) mostly refers to indirect, implicit ways to instigate desired values in students, such as responsibility, altruism, respect, caring, and beauty through extracurricular activities, rituals, and campus environment, like drama competition (Davy and Liu 2017: 309–21), speech contests, debates (Gan and Ou 2008: 92–3), white robe ceremony (Wang and Zeng 2016: 49–51), and sculptures and other art works that beautify campus (Liu 2015: 114). Films are excellent means by which the 'hidden curriculum' in the Chinese context can explore issues of the 'hidden curriculum' in the English-speaking world.

Bibliography

Batson, C.D. (2009) These Things Called Empathy: Eight Related but Distinct Phenomena, in J. Decety and W. Ickes (eds.) *The Social Neuroscience of Empathy*, Cambridge, MA: MIT Press, pp. 3–15.

Berry, C. (2008) Wedding Banquet: A Family (Melodrama) Affair, in C. Berry (ed.) *Chinese Films in Focus II*, New York: Palgrave Macmillan, pp. 235–42.

Charon, R. (2006) *Narrative Medicine: Honoring the Stories of Illness*, New York: Oxford University Press.

Chen Gang 陈刚 (2012) *Xinyou xiangsheng – Yu Song Xiaofei tan Shasheng de sheying chuanzuo* 心由像生 – 与宋晓飞谈《杀生》的摄影创作 (Emotions Arise from Image – Dialogue with Song Xiaofei on the Shooting of *Design of Death*), *Audio and Visual*, 4: 144–9.

Choice and Dignity (2017) Living Will, www.lwpa.org.cn/XZYZY/NewsIndex.aspx? accessed 27 August 2017.

Davy, J. and Liu, J. (2017) Using a Second-Language Drama Competition to Foster Medical Humanities Education, *Journal of Applied Arts in Health*, 8 (3): 309–21.

Foucault, M. (1977) *Discipline and Punishment*, London: Penguin Books.

Gan Qinghua 甘庆华 and Ou Shenghua 欧胜华 (2008) *Goujian kexue yinxing kecheng tigao rencai peiyang zhiliang* 构建科学隐性课程，提高人才培养质量.中国高等医学教育 (Constructing Scientific Hidden Curriculum and Improving the Quality of Students), *Chinese Higher Medical Education*, 1: 92–3.

Halpern, J. (2001) *From Detached Concern to Empathy: Humanizing Medical Education*, New York: Oxford University Press.

James, H. and Dupee, F.W. (1983) *Henry James: Autobiography*, Princeton, NJ: Princeton University Press.

Lakoff, G. and Johnson, M. (2003) *Metaphors We Live by*, Chicago: The University of Chicago Press.

Li Jiuru 李九如 (2012) *Duihua Guan Hu: douniu ruguoshi yige nanren, shasheng jiushi yige nüren* 对话管虎:《斗牛》如果是一个男人,《杀生》就是一个女人. (Dialogue with Guan Hu: If *Cow* Is a Man, *Design of Death* is a woman), *Film*, 4: 46–7.

Liu Xinxin 刘欣欣 (2015) *Yixueyuan yixue renwen kecheng tixi jiangou yanjiu* 医学院校医学人文课程体系构建研究 (Study on the construction of medical humanities courses in medical colleges), *Zhongguo xiaowai jiaoyu xunkan* (Extra-Curricula Education Research), 4:114.

Manhood, S.C. (2011) Medical Education: Beware the Hidden Curriculum, *Canadian Family Physician*, 57: 983–5.

Martimianakis, M.A., Michalec, B., Lam, J. *et al.* (2015) Humanism, the Hidden Curriculum, and Educational Reform: A Scoping Review and Thematic Analysis, *Academic Medicine*, 90(11): s5–s13.

Michalec, B. and Hafferty, F.W. (2013) Stunting Professionalism: The Potency and Durability of the Hidden Curriculum within Medical Education, *Social Theory and Health*, 11 (4): 388–406.

O'Callaghan, A. (2013) Emotional Congruence in Learning and Health Encounters in Medicine: Addressing an Aspect of the Hidden Curriculum, *Advances in Health Sciences Education*, 18: 305–17.

Pellegrino, E. (2008) *The Philosophy of Medicine Reborn: A Pellegrino Reader*, Notre Dame, IN: University of Notre Dame Press.

Stanek, A., Clarkin, C., Bould, M.D. *et al.* (2015) Life Imitating Art: Depictions of the Hidden Curriculum in Medical Television Programs, *BMC Medical Education*, 15: 156.

Sun Xiaoling 孙晓玲 (2016) *Yinyu de shenghua yu piancha – yi shasheng weili* 隐喻的升华与偏差 – 以《杀生》为例 (The sublimation and deflection of metaphor – taking Design of Death as an example), *Yalujiang Monthly*, 35–6.

Sun Yuqian 孙玉倩, Li Zheng 李峥, Sun Bingfu 孙秉赋 *et al.* (2007) *Aizhenghuanzhe jiashu dui gaozhi huanzhe zhenxiang de taidu ji yingxiang yinsu fenxi* 癌症患者家属对告知患者真相的态度及影响因素分析 (The attitude towards diagnostic disclosure of cancer patients' families and the analysis of influencing factors), *Chinese Journal of Nursing*, 42 (6): 556–9.

Wang Feiya 汪斐娅 and Zeng Ying 曾盈 (2016) *Yixue yuanxiao zai xinsheng jiaoyuzhou goujian renwen sushi jiaoyu yinxing kecheng de shijian* 医学院校在新生教育周构建人文素质教育隐性课程的实践 (The Practice of Constructing Medical Humanities Hidden Curriculum in the Freshmen Orientation Week in Medical Colleges), *Education and Teaching Forum*, 30: 49–51.

Wang Yanzhuo 王彦卓 (2006) *Qingdai zunlao youlao lizhi shulun* 清代尊老优老礼制述论 (The Rites of Honoring and Rewarding Longevity in the Qing Dynasty), *Historical Archives*, 4: 38–48.

Woolf, V. (1932) *The Second Common Reader*, New York: Harcourt Brace Jovanovich, as cited in Charon, R. (2006) *Narrative Medicine: Honoring the Stories of Illness*, New York: Oxford University Press, p. 109.

Zeng Tieying 曾铁英, Chen Fengju 陈凤菊, Yang Xiaomei 杨笑梅 *et al.* (2008) *Aizheng huanzhe dui zhongmoqi zhiliao he siwang de taidu diaocha* 癌症患者对终末期治疗和死亡的态度调查 (Investigation on attitudes of patients with cancer towards treatment of advanced cancer and death), *Journal of Nursing Science*, 23(7): 71–3.

9   *Blind Massage*
Sense and sensuality

Chris Berry

How can we analyse the depiction of blindness in the 2014 film, *Blind Massage* (*Tuina* 推拿)? This chapter approaches the task from various angles, to demonstrate how the film understands blindness through the lenses of sense and sensuality. First, the chapter focuses on representation to examine how the film depicts the social conditions of blind people in China. In the context of ongoing global debates about whether and how to integrate people with disabilities into mainstream society, this analysis shows that prevalent cultural understandings of blindness in China lead to social segregation, even in efforts to support the blind through education and employment possibilities. Second, it adopts an auteurist approach to account for both the narrative emphasis on the sexual desires and entanglements that result from the social segregation of the blind as depicted in the film, and for the use of camerawork, lighting, and more to communicate the atmosphere and character subjectivity associated with these feverish passions. It argues these characteristics are part of a pattern in the work of Lou Ye 娄烨, forming a focus on obsession that is also his own obsession and his signature. Finally, however, a crucial feature of the film is its effort to make the audience feel what the film believes it is like to be blind. Here, the chapter draws on the phenomenological turn in cinema studies to argue that the film attempts to give the audience an embodied experience. However, it achieves this embodied experience in a complex and anti-mimetic manner, and not simply by obscuring vision or making the screen black. In this way, *Blind Massage* becomes an investigation of cinema and the senses at the same time as it communicates an understanding of what the experience of blindness is.

Representing the blind

As Gayatri Spivak once famously pointed out, representation has two meanings: to depict and to act as an agent (Spivak 1988: 275–9). In her article, Spivak works hard to hold the two meanings apart. However, when someone depicts or 'represents' someone else, they are also in some sense acting as their agent, taking some control over the way in which someone different from them is shown and known to others. Lou Ye is not blind, and so this is his position as the director of *Blind Massage*. I am not blind or Chinese, so I cannot judge whether his effort to depict the experience of blind people in China accords with their own experiences. (And, of course, we must recognise that different blind people have different experiences.) However, we can note the other sense of representation and examine how the film depicts blindness as a social condition.

Blind Massage begins with the adolescent Xiao Ma 小马, who has been visually impaired since a car accident that also killed his mother. When Xiao Ma learns he has been deceived and will not recover his eyesight, he smashes a bowl and slashes the artery in his neck in a suicide attempt. After he recovers, we see him in a school for the blind before he gets a job in a blind massage centre specialising in an ancient therapeutic form of massage known as *tuina* (Pritchard 2015: 3–5), which is also the Chinese title of the film. The film then becomes an ensemble piece, following the stories of different characters in the massage centre.

The opening sequence depicting how Xiao Ma's life leads him to the blind massage centre raises questions about the social conditions of blind people in China. First, Xiao Ma is depicted as being educated in a special school for the blind. This indicates that blindness is recognised by the state and that special provisions are in place to support the blind. The fate of the son of the former Chinese leader Deng Xiaoping 邓小平, Deng Pufang 邓朴方, who became a paraplegic a result of his encounter with the Red Guards during the Cultural Revolution (1966–1976), raised the profile of people with disabilities (Salisbury 1989). It also enabled Deng Pufang to work to amalgamate various welfare associations and establish the China Disabled Persons Federation, of which he became president, in 1988 (China Disabled Persons Federation 2016a; see also Kohrmann 2003). The current 2008 Law on the Protection of Persons with Disabilities covers areas including education and employment (China Disabled Persons Federation 2016b).

Blind Massage is set around the turn of the century, which, we are told in the film, was a golden age for blind massage centres. According to a 1988 report, only 6% of blind children in China were entering education (Deng *et al*. 2001: 294). This pattern of low enrolment was found across the special needs categories, but by 1996 the rate of participation in education had been increased to 60% for all categories (Deng *et al*. 2001: 291). It was addressed partly by a learning in regular classrooms movement (Deng *et al*. 2001: 291–2), and partly by rapid expansion of special schools, including special schools for the blind, from 292 in 1980 to 1,437 in 1998 (Deng *et al*. 2001: 294). This situation suggests a combination of strategies, some of which would enhance mainstreaming and others of which might lead to social segregation but provide more specialised support.

Xiao Ma is also depicted as receiving vocational training in the school. This is reported to be an important element of special needs education in China, motivating more parents to send children to school (Deng *et al*. 2001: 295). However, the range of vocational options is consistently reported as being limited to massage and, although less frequently mentioned, music (see for example Cheng and Zhou 2015). What these professions share is an emphasis on the senses other than sight – either touch or hearing, in these cases. This suggests a cultural belief in China – as in many other places – that loss of one sense can lead to enhancement of the other senses. This belief also informs the film, which, as explored further, places great emphasis on touch and hearing, as well as smell.

The combination of special schools and a very limited vocational range contributes to the social isolation we see in the film, where the blind masseurs live and work together in the blind massage centre. This isolation may be in a mutually reinforcing relationship with social prejudice (e.g. Palmer 2014). In the film, a recurring theme is prejudice against having blind people in your family, presumably for fear that the condition might be hereditary. One of the clinic directors, Sha Fuming 沙复明, is an outgoing man and a good dancer. But when his girlfriend's mother meets him, she refuses to allow her daughter to have further contact with him. This prejudice extends to a sort of hierarchy among the blind: we discover that partially sighted Xiao Kong 小孔 has run away with a fully blind character we only ever know as 'Dr Wang' 王大夫 and they have come to the massage centre together, partly because her parents oppose their relationship.

An obsession with obsession

Beginning *Blind Massage* with Xiao Ma's childhood is a part of a restructuring of the narrative of the original novel, which was written by Bi Feiyu 毕飞宇 (Bi Feiyu 2008, 2016) and won the prestigious Mao Dun literary prize in China in 2011, along with other literary awards (Mao Dun Prize no date). The novel opens with Dr Wang and Xiao Kong in Shenzhen, a location which we barely see in the film, and it ends with a chapter about Dr Wang and then an epilogue in a restaurant. Not only does Lou Ye begin his film with Xiao Ma, but he also adds a final scene with Xiao Ma, who has unexpectedly recovered some of his sight after being hit on the head in a fight. Xiao Ma has left the segregated space of the massage centre and set up his own massage service elsewhere with the local sex worker, called Man 蛮 ('Mann' in the English subtitles), who he fell in love with while at the massage centre. By beginning with Xiao Ma, the film moves us into the confined space of the main setting – the massage centre – more quickly. It also raises issues of broader social engagement with the blind through the depiction of Xiao Ma's education and employment training, which we might not get by starting with Dr Wang.

Despite the social issues raised in this beginning, the fictional narrative of the film is less focused on its characters' engagement with such problems than it is with their sexual attractions. The focus on Xiao Ma is also part of this effect, emphasising his coming of age and various attractions over Dr Wang's attraction to Xiao Kong, which is more stable and less disruptive than Xiao Ma's passions. The social isolation of the blind masseurs is compounded by the fact that they not only work but also live together in the massage centre. When Xiao Ma arrives at the clinic, we are introduced to Sha Fuming, and Dr Wang and Xiao Kong turn up soon after. Xiao Kong immediately becomes the focus of male attention in the hothouse atmosphere of the massage centre, not only from Xiao Ma but also from Xu Taihe 徐泰和, who is already involved with another masseuse, Jin Yan 金嫣. Meanwhile, when Sha Fuming overhears his patients extolling the beauty of a third masseuse, Du Hong 都红, he starts to become obsessed with her. Quickly, passion overcomes reason and Taihe drops Jin Yan. By the time Xiao Kong starts to get more interested in Xiao Ma, he has discovered the nearby brothel masquerading as a hair salon and transferred his affections to Mann.

The theme of disruptive desire is also present in the novel, but other elements in the book, such as the details of running the business, are far less prominent in the film. This emphasis on the overwhelming quality of desire can be understood not so much as a characterisation of blind people, but more as a manifestation of director Lou Ye's auteur signature. Auteurism is the theory that takes the romantic understanding of the artist as a unique individual with a distinct signature and applies it to the cinema, arguing that the director is the artist among the various individuals involved in making a film. There have been numerous objections to this approach since it was introduced in the 1950s (Buscombe 1981). But it has persisted, especially where a director's work does manifest consistent features.

Indeed, Lou Ye is widely recognised to fit this pattern: in her *Variety* review of *Blind Massage*, Maggie Lee opens by referring to him as 'Chinese auteur Lou Ye' (Lee 2014). He is a regular on the film festival circuit, where his films have won many awards (www.chineseshadows.com/lou-ye). And a consistent signature appears across all eight of his feature films to date. That signature includes the theme of *amour fou* and sometimes illicit sexual passion. The title of his first film, *Weekend Lover* (*Zhoumo qingren* 周末情人 filmed in 1993, released in 1996), is clear enough. As Jerome Silbergeld has argued, *Suzhou River* (*Suzhou he* 苏州 河 2000) can be seen as reworking the core plot in Hitchcock's *Vertigo* (1958), where a man becomes obsessed with a woman who resembles another woman whose death he holds himself responsible for (Silbergeld 2004). Mistaken identity is also a feature of *Purple Butterfly* (*Zi hudie* 紫蝴蝶 2003), where two pairs of lovers mix sexual and political intrigue during the Japanese invasion of China. Sexual passion amongst students plays out against the backdrop of the 1989 student movement in Beijing in *Summer Palace* (*Yiheyuan* 颐和园 2006), while in *Spring Fever* (*Chunfeng chensui de yewan* 春风沉醉的夜晚 2009) a wife is furious when she discovers her husband cannot control his desire for another man. Sadomasochism features in *Love and Bruises* (2011). In *Mystery* (*Fucheng mishi* 浮城谜事 2012), Lou's last film before *Blind Massage*, he returns to adultery. This time the relationship is heterosexual, but the wife is no less furious and vengeful.

Lou Ye has acknowledged this consistent interest in sexual desire in his films, and commented:

> Sex is an indispensable part of a natural human being. Starting from sex, each individual human being can learn how to frankly face himself and the freedom he has, and learn how to listen to and follow himself instead of others.
>
> (Lim 2010)

Lou Ye's rhetoric here echoes the romantic individualist understanding of the artist as someone with a unique personality that must be expressed. In Lou Ye's description, sexual desire is the truth of the individual and its expression therefore has an absolute priority.

Lou Ye's own obsession with sexual obsession is not only thematic, but also shapes how his films use camerawork, lighting, and mise-en-scène to communicate the feelings of their characters and the atmosphere of their scenes. For example, as Andrew Chan says in his *Film Comment* review of *Spring Fever*, 'there's jittery handheld cinematography and dreamlike editing that emphasises the myriad sensations of the body' (Chan 2010). Indeed, the entire film was shot with a handheld digital camera in natural light to get around a five-year ban that Lou received for screening *Summer Palace* at Cannes without Chinese government approval. Stephen Holden, writing in the *New York Times*, acknowledges this history but expresses frustration that '[t]he indoor scenes are so dark that you can barely make out the outlines of the bodies' (Holden 2010). However, this characteristic could also be said to communicate the surreptitious urgency of the situation, as it pushes us to stare anxiously as we try to identify who is who and what they are doing. Andrew Hageman also notes how Lou's signature style communicates feelings and atmosphere in his essay on *Suzhou River*:

> Rather than representing social issues as something that can be conveyed through seemingly direct documentation, the combination of the hand-held aesthetic with erratic editing techniques such as rapid-succession jump cuts mixed with fast zooms and pans and non-linear narration in *Suzhou River* makes the spectator aware that the film is about more than just the plot line. It is also about how our minds and the world we inhabit are formal systems that are complex and inextricably coupled with each other.
>
> (Hageman 2009: 25–6)

Similar techniques can be found in *Blind Massage*. How do these techniques enable us to understand the specificity of blindness as a 'formal system' that links the mind and the world?

Seeing blindness, feeling blindness

At first, it seems *Blind Massage* is pursuing a realist or mimetic strategy in its efforts to communicate the experience of visual impairment. When the film opens with a sequence about Xiao Ma, the first shots are blurry, close-up and handheld images of a mechanism we later understand is a ticking clock that Xiao Ma carries around with him like a talisman. This seems like the subjective vision of someone with impaired sight. Techniques that appear to place the viewer right in a scene, reacting and following as though they were a character in the film, are common throughout the film.

One way of understanding this characteristic of *Blind Massage* is to turn to the phenomenological approach to cinema. If analysis of representation emphasises meaning and auteurism emphasises style as individual expression, then the phenomenological approach emphasises that the audience experiences a film with our bodies, and that our minds only make sense of what our bodies have already felt and perceived. One of the most famous essays that takes the phenomenological approach to film is Vivian Sobchack's on Jane Campion's film, *The Piano* (Sobchack 2004). In 'What My Fingers Knew: The Cinesthetic Subject, or Vision in the Flesh', Sobchack recounts her own experience of the first shot of the film, which, a bit like the blurry opening shots of *Blind Massage*, is an extreme close-up that is difficult to make out. In the case of *The Piano*, what we see turns out to be the flesh of the main character's hand, made translucent by sunlight. Sobchack remembers this as an intense moment of embodied response, when, as she puts it, '*my fingers knew what I was looking at* – and this *before* the objective reverse shot that followed' (Sobchack 2004: 63, italics in original). Perhaps we have a similar sense of embodiment in the opening seconds of *Blind Massage* before we retrospectively make sense of what we have seen and from whose perspective. Perhaps we have a physical knowledge of impaired vision before we name it as such.

In this way, how *Blind Massage* is filmed appears to be working to make us know in an embodied and experiential or quasi-experiential manner what it is like to be blind or visually impaired by making our experience of the film mimic the experience of the characters in a realist manner. In their discussion of medical humanities education for medical practitioners, Maura Spiegel and Danielle Spencer have noted that this kind of ability to inspire empathy is 'the most important if not only relevant feeling' (Charon *et al.* 2016: 41). However, although it is correct that the film is mobilising an embodied response to communicate some idea of what it might be like to be blind not only to medical professionals but to audiences more generally, in fact it is not following a mimetic approach to link our experience to that of the characters.

For the attentive audience member, this lack of mimetic correspondence between our experience and that of the characters is made clear by the opening lines of narration, read by a female narrator. She tells us of a blur of light followed by unconsciousness, and says:

> It was the last light Xiao Ma would ever see. From then on, it was as though he was in an endless night, surrounded by the scent of shadows. A car accident had taken his eyes and his mother, leaving him blind in a world filled with sound.

Immediately after this, we see Xiao Ma as a young man with the mechanism that we now recognise as a sort of clock. If the attentive audience member grasps that Xiao Ma is completely blind, at this point we understand the dark and blurry images are not attempting to replicate Xiao Ma's blindness in a mimetic manner, which would require sound but a black screen to be more accurate. However, it is still possible to understand this rendering as within a range of representations of blindness that could be considered realist, on the grounds that the film uses impaired vision to communicate something *similar* to Xiao Ma's experience, even if it is not exactly like it.

However, even that possibility is soon dispelled. First, after Xiao Ma has survived his suicide attempt and he has been compelled to understand that he has a lifetime of blindness ahead of him, the sequence cuts to the special school for the blind. At this moment, instead of blackness descending, paradoxically, the blurred vision disappears, and clear, focused cinematography follows. Furthermore, and again paradoxically, much later in the film, when Xiao Ma's sight is unexpectedly restored after he has been hit in a fight, the cinematography becomes blurry again.

Another example of this markedly anti-mimetic approach occurs when we get to the opening credits. The usual opening credits right at the beginning of the film are limited in the case of *Blind Massage* to a couple of slides announcing the production companies and producers, but not the director and so forth. Instead, approximately eleven and a half minutes into the film, after the Xiao Ma sequence, a scene of Dr Wang and Xiao Kong's call to Sha Fuming in search of work, and Sha Fuming's rejection by his girlfriend's mother, the female narrator reads out the credits over some shots of the lake near where Sha Fuming met his girlfriend's parents. She starts with, 'A Lou Ye film' and goes through the whole list including all the actors for the main roles. Of course, there are English subtitles, but there are no written titles in Chinese for the audience of the original film to read. This reading out loud takes approximately one minute, and so the audience cannot help but notice these unusual oral rather than written credits. Of course, this makes us think about what it means to be blind. Furthermore, the decision not only to read the opening credits out but also withhold the written form from the screen reproduces the frustration a blind person might feel when they are made aware that there is something visible but which is not being communicated to them. However, it achieves this without mimicking the blind person's experience. In this arrangement, we are seeing blindness, and our sight makes us feel blindness.

As well as seeing blindness, these markedly anti-mimetic moments draw attention to the cinema itself and make us grasp that the cinema itself is a specific arrangement of the senses. The cinema has sight and sound, but, except in some special effects exhibition venues, it does not have touch, taste or smell. In these circumstances, cinema forces us to use sight and sound to intuit the other senses, in a manner distinct from but analogous to how the blind are believed to use other senses to approximate or substitute for the sense they do not have – vision. In the opening moments of the film, discussed earlier, the narrator says, 'It was as though he was in an endless night, surrounded by the scent of shadows'. This connection of the senses, in the way cinema uses sight and sound to communicate other senses, or in the way shadows are said to have a scent by the narrator, is considered today to be synaesthetic.

As a condition, synaesthesia is described on the UK Synaesthesia Association's website as 'a joining of the senses. Sensations in one modality (e.g. hearing) produce sensations in another modality (e.g. colour) as well as its own'. (www.uksy naesthesia.com/2012synaesthesia.html). Seeing a colour while hearing music is one of the more common examples. When Vivian Sobchack *looks* at a close-up and *feels* something in her hands, she is experiencing a synaesthetic effect. To call this effect synaesthetic assumes a clear separation of the senses. Yet, this separation and classification may be a relatively recent cultural conception. Robert Jütte begins his book *A History of the Senses* with the following highly evocative quotation from Karl Marx's 1844 *Economic and Philosophical Manuscripts*: 'The forming of the five senses is a labour of the entire history of the world down to the present' (Jütte 2004: 8), and in their article on aphrodisiacs in ancient China, Greece, and Rome, Vivienne Lo and Eleanor Re'em note that in those times, 'the boundaries between what we now think of as the domains of individual senses were less distinct' (Lo and Re'em 2018: 326). Therefore, what we call 'synaesthesia' may also be understood as an unravelling of recent cultural constructions, and it may also open up further questions about the traces of ways of understanding our embodied relationship to the world around us. These might include an 'attention to the inner world' that Lo and Re'em call 'an early Chinese "sixth sense"' (Lo and Re'em 2018: 332). In the case of *Blind Massage*, we might understand Lou Ye's fascination with the sensual experiences of his characters as a particular kind of attention to this inner world.

As Sobchack and most theorists of the embodied experience of cinema point out, cinema depends upon this synaesthetic effect to produce embodied responses. Usually these responses are prompted by the cinematic techniques that produce identification and therefore projection. We watch a character cry, and tears well up for us, too. We watch as a car spins off a mountain road and hovers over a precipice, and we grip the armrest of our seats, moving forward, our stomachs in our mouths. However, Laura Marks famously writes about 'haptic cinema' as one that 'bypasses . . . identification and the distance from the image it requires' (Marks 2000: 171). She goes on to write of 'changes in focus, graininess . . . and effects of under- and overexposure' which 'discourage the viewer from distinguishing objects and encourage a relationship to the screen as a whole' (Marks 2000: 172). She claims that through such techniques, 'the eye is compelled to "touch" an object' (Marks 2000: 173). The opening shots of *Blind Massage* may be understood as haptic in this way, but when we see Xiao Ma looking at the clock mechanism a few shots later, the regime of identification is reinstated.

Indeed, we must be precise and acknowledge that in most cases what we experience in the cinema is not literal synaesthesia but a synaesthesia-like effect. When we see a rose on screen, it may make us feel that we can (almost) smell it. However, the website of the UK Synaesthesia Association specifies that some of the most common synaesthetic experiences for those with the condition are when symbols such as numbers are experienced in a synaesthetic way as a certain colour or sound. A true synaesthetic experience would be hearing a certain sound every time you saw a rose on screen, or having a certain bodily reaction. Cinema rarely if ever attempts to elicit such effects, because they are highly individualised and cannot be systematised. More commonly, it relies on mimesis and identification to prompt our synaesthetic projections of ourselves into a certain scene.

In this light, what is innovative about *Blind Massage* is its anti-mimetic strategy of organising the different arrangements of the senses between the cinematic experience, everyday experience and the experience of the blind to enable us to apprehend, not only rationally but also in an embodied way, something of what it might be like to be blind. Here, Lou Ye's signature interest in sexual desire serves as an excellent example of how this effect is achieved. Sexual desire is famously expressed in classical Hollywood cinema, and much other drama-based cinema, through a visual grammar that supposedly mimics the visual experience of people who desire each other: a shot that mimics one person's look at another person is followed by the reverse shot of the other person's vision as they meet the first person's look, and this exchange is repeated perhaps at ever-greater speed and with ever-closer shots to communicate building attraction followed by physical embrace. How does *Blind Massage* use the visual language of cinema to communicate the experience of desire amongst characters who cannot see each other?

A few examples can illustrate the deployment of the synaesthetic effect to make us see and feel the desire of blind people. First, smell. Once Dr Wang and Xiao Kong are settled in at the massage clinic, they are assigned separate beds in the men's and women's dormitories. Xiao Kong comes to visit her fiancé. His bed is above Xiao Ma's, so she sits next to Xiao Ma, while Dr Wang climbs down and sits on the other side of her. The camera frames Xiao Kong and Xiao Ma in the same shot, and we see Xiao Ma suddenly turn towards her and move closer as he catches her scent. The other characters cannot see what he is doing, but we can. So, our seeing makes us share his sense of smell. As the men in the room tease Xiao Kong, she demands Xiao Ma defend her, and then hits him when he fails to do so. However, in the tussle that follows, the camera cuts in close as Xiao Ma lies on top of Xiao Kong, burrowing his face into her body to get her full scent. Again, we move in as Xiao Ma does, and we see as he smells. We are encouraged to imagine ourselves smelling Xiao Kong, too, even as we sense her confusion.

Second, touch. Once Sha Fuming hears patients extol Du Hong's beauty, he is intrigued to the point of obsession and asks to talk to her. Suddenly, he starts running his hands across her face and says he wants to know how beauty *feels*. The camera cuts with his quick action and moves to a close-up of his hands and her distressed face. Again, the framing of the shot, which allows us to see the expression on her face and the movement to the close-up direct our vision so that we feel with her at least as much as with him – and with his hands – at this moment. The thematic idea of feeling as a possible way of seeing beauty further underlines the synaesthetic potential of the moment.

Sound is also important. In the scene where Xiao Ma smells Xiao Kong, the tone changes as the camera focuses on Dr Wang listening, and then, in a series of cuts, on each of the other men listening in silence. They have sensed that something is happening between Xiao Kong and Xiao Ma. As we look at them, our attention is directed to their effort to hear what we also cannot see any more. These patterns of intense focus with framing and close-up on moments of smell, touch, and sound are repeated throughout the film to signify to us not only the reliance of the blind on other senses but also to cue us to feel what it is like to rely on those other senses.

Conclusion

Blind Massage offers a certain representation of the world of the blind in China as one of social segregation, even as a result of the very institutions and mechanisms that are made available to support them and meet their needs. It uses intense sensual desire to communicate a hothouse atmosphere that results from a relatively small community working, living, and spending all their time together as a result of that segregation. But perhaps most powerful is the counterpoint the film builds between the senses of the viewing audience, the arrangement of senses available to the cinema itself, and the way in which the blind use the senses that are available to them. In the quotation about *Suzhou River* referenced earlier, Andrew Hageman writes about how 'our minds and the world we inhabit are formal systems that are complex and inextricably coupled with each other'. As we *look* at them *smelling* and *touching*, and strain even further because those senses are not available to us, we become aware – not just intellectually but also with our bodily senses – of the different 'formal systems' constituting blindness, the cinema, and sightedness.

Bibliography

Bi Feiyu 毕飞宇 (2008) *Tuina* 推拿 (*Massage*), Beijing: Renmin Wenxue Chubanshe.
―――― (2016) *Massage*, trans. H. Goldblatt and S.L Lin, Sydney: Penguin.
Buscombe, E. (1981) Ideas of Authorship, in J. Caughie (ed.) *Theories of Authorship*, London: Routledge & Kegan Paul, pp. 22–34.
Caughie, J. (ed.) (1981) *Theories of Authorship*, London: Routledge & Kegan Paul.
Chan, A. (2010) Review: Spring Fever, *Film Comment*, www.filmcomment.com/article/spring-fever-review/, accessed 14 August 2017.
Charon, R. *et al.* (2016) *The Principles and Practice of Narrative Medicine*, New York: Oxford University Press.
Cheng, L. and Zhou, J. (2015) China's Blind Cry Out for More Career Choices, *Shanghai Daily*, www.shanghaidaily.com/feature/news-feature/Chinas-blind-cry-out-for-more-career-choices/shdaily.shtml, accessed 15 August 2017.
China Disabled Person's Federation (2016a) The Historical Development of China Disabled Person's Federation, www.cdpf.org.cn/english/About/history_1798/, accessed 15 August 2017.
―――― (2016b) Law on the Protection of Persons with Disabilities, www.cdpf.org.cn/english/Resources/lawsregulations/201603/t20160303_542879.shtml, accessed 15 August 2017.
Deng, M., Poon-McBrayer, K.F. and Farnsworth, E.B. (2001) The Development of Special Education in China: A Sociocultural Review, *Remedial and Special Education*, 22 (5): 288–98.
Hageman, A. (2009) Floating Consciousness: The Cinematic Confluence of Ecological Aesthetics in *Suzhou River*, in S.H. Lu and J. Mi (eds.) *Chinese Ecocinema: In the Age of Environmental Challenge*, Hong Kong: Hong Kong University Press, pp. 73–91.
Holden, S. (2010) Revolving-Door Romances for Modern-Day Chinese, *New York Times*, www.nytimes.com/2010/08/06/movies/06spring.html, accessed 14 August 2017.
Kohrmann, M. (2003) Authorizing a Disability Agency in Post-Mao China: Deng Pufang's Story as Biomythography, *Cultural Anthropology*, 18 (1): 99–131.
Jütte, R. (2004) *A History of the Senses: From Antiquity to Cyberspace*, London: Polity.
Lee, M. (2014) Berlin Film Review: 'Blind Massage', *Variety*, http://variety.com/2014/film/asia/berlin-film-review-blind-massage-1201095936/, accessed 14 August 2017.
Lim, D. (2010) Parting Twin Curtains of Repression, *The New York Times*, www.nytimes.com/2010/08/01/movies/01spring.html?mcubz=1, accessed 18 August 2017.

Lloyd, G.E.R. and Zhao, J.J. (eds.) (2018) *Ancient Greece and China Compared*, Cambridge: Cambridge University Press.

Lo, V. and Re'em, E. (2018) Recipes for Love in the Ancient World, in G.E.R. Lloyd and J.J. Zhao (eds.) *Ancient Greece and China Compared*, Cambridge: Cambridge University Press, pp. 326–52.

Lu, S.H. and Mi, J. (eds.) (2009) *Chinese Ecocinema: In the Age of Environmental Challenge*, Hong Kong: Hong Kong University Press.

Mao Dun Prize (no date) "The 8th Mao Dun Literary Prize" (第八届茅盾文学奖), http://www.mdwenxue.com/8/, accessed 8 September 2019.

Marks, L.U. (2000) *The Skin of the Film: Intercultural Cinema, Embodiment, and the Senses*, Durham, NC: Duke University Press.

Nelson, C. and Grossberg, L. (eds.) (1988) *Marxism and the Interpretation of Culture*, Urbana: University of Illinois Press.

Palmer, J. (2014) Crippling Injustice, *Aeon*, https://aeon.co/essays/what-is-life-like-for-disabled-people-in-china, accessed 15 August 2017.

Pritchard, S. (2015) *Tui Na: A Manual of Chinese Massage Therapy*, London: Singing Dragon.

Salisbury, H. (1989) In China, 'A Little Blood', *New York Times*, www.nytimes.com/1989/06/13/opinion/in-china-a-little-blood.html, accessed 15 August 2017.

Silbergeld, J. (2004) *Hitchcock with a Chinese Face: Cinematic Doubles, Oedipal Triangles, and China's Moral Voice*, Seattle: University of Washington Press.

Sobchack, V. (2004) *Carnal Thoughts: Embodiment and Moving Image Culture*, Berkeley: University of California Press.

Spiegel, M. and Spencer, D. (2016) This Is What We Do, and These Things Happen: Literature, Experience, Emotion and Relationality in the Classroom, in R. Charon *et al.* (eds.) *The Principles and Practice of Narrative Medicine*, New York: Oxford University Press, pp. 37–60.

Spivak, G.C. (1988) Can the Subaltern Speak? in C. Nelson and L. Grossberg (eds.) *Marxism and the Interpretation of Culture*, Urbana: University of Illinois Press, pp. 271–313.

10 Cinemeducation and disability

An undergraduate special study module for medical students in China

Daniel Vuillermin

In the post-socialist era of the People's Republic of China the physically disabled subject in Chinese cinema is often portrayed as a figure of marginality and discrimination but also one that serves as a sociopolitical model of autonomy and self-improvement. This chapter seeks to examine representations of physical disability in Chinese cinema by drawing upon subjective viewer-response analyses by undergraduate medical students at one of China's leading medical schools, Peking University. The research base is a 4-week Special Study Module (SSM) that focused on cultural and social constructions of disability as portrayed in a selection of six films by fifth- and sixth-generation Chinese directors. Critical attention has been given to the historical and political contexts of the disabled subject in transnational Chinese cinema; however, there is, as Sarah Dauncey argues, a need to further 'understand how different disabilities are portrayed in the films and how they contribute to the formation and articulation of disabled identities in China' (Dauncey 2007: 498). For example, how do Chinese films represent aspects of disability such as (in)visibility, stigmatisation, and discrimination but also in what ways does the disabled subject serve as an exemplary model of independence, self-respect, and compassion? The SSM was designed to enable teachers and students to reflect on the role of cinemeducation – the use of film, television documentary or other audio-visual media to educate medical students about the cultural representations of illness and ethics of public healthcare – in a mainland Chinese context; an area of Chinese medical humanities that has not received research (Alexander *et al.* 2005: xiv). This introductory study seeks to identify a selection of responses from mainland Chinese students, which may serve to begin mapping Chinese cultural constructions of disability through the use of Chinese film.

This chapter surveys the emergence and challenges of cinemeducation at the School of Health Humanities (formerly the Institute for Medical Humanities) at Peking University. One such challenge is that Hollywood and European films dominate the curricula, which results in a paucity of research about the use of mainland Chinese films in Chinese medical pedagogy. A further challenge for the field of cinemeducation and Chinese films is that there is a need to balance 'in depth understandings of the Chinese social and cultural landscape with congruent understandings of disability and difference developed in the West' (Dauncey 2013: 75). In order to address this balance this study draws upon students' subjective viewer-responses in a student-centred teaching setting – students prepared for each of the classes by watching the films in advance and composed a set of discussion points and questions in order to engage in dialogues and debates in the classroom about two films that feature physical disability: *Ju Dou* (*Ju dou* 菊 豆 1990) and *The Common People* (*Guan yu ai de gushi* 关于爱的故事 1998). By drawing upon students' discussions of these two films this chapter will offer insights into the portrayal of disability in mainland Chinese film and consider the pedagogical usefulness of these films in analysing representations of disability in a Chinese context.

Cinemeducation and Chinese film

The past two decades have seen a vast expansion in the use of narrative cinema in medical education in the US, Europe, and more recently China. Medical educators have embraced film as a means of supplementing technologies such as PowerPoint presentations, apps, and other multimedia technologies to disseminate information and to facilitate discussion. Educating with films or Cinemeducation, the 'use of movies, television, YouTube, music videos or documentaries, either in their entirety or in short segments, to educate graduate and medical learners in the biopsychosocial-spiritual-ethical aspects of healthcare' is part of a set of ancillary medical humanities courses and research that may facilitate the development of communication skills and analytical thinking; expose students to a broad range of medical conditions in various historical and cultural contexts; enable examinations of the political, cultural, economic, and scientific aspects of healthcare; develop narratological skills in areas such as the doctor-patient relationship; and provide access to a broad range of conditions as well as processes of diagnosis and treatment (Alexander *et al.* 2005: 26). Although narrative cinema may not accurately represent clinical experiences of disease, medical educators can make use of film to uncover what Paul Longmore (2003: 146) describes as the 'unconscious attitudes and values embedded in media images'.

At the School of Health Humanities at Peking University several courses, including *Literature and Medicine*, *Medicine and Visual Culture*, and *Illness Narratives*, make use of films to engage students in visual and narrative analysis and to facilitate group discussion. For example, *Medicine and Visual Culture*, taught by myself and Vivienne Lo, Director of the China Centre for Health and Humanity at University College London (UCL), examines mise-en-scène of films such as *The Hours* (2002) to show how directors make use of light and shadow, interiors and exteriors, and non-diegetic sound to portray the main characters' psychological states. Other courses include an experimental 12-week 'engagement program' conducted in 2013–14 by a team of experienced teachers, Guo Liping, Wei Jihong, Li Yanfeng, and Li Han, that aimed to foster and improve empathy among postgraduate medical students by utilising three American films: *Scent of a Woman* (1992), *First Knight* (1995), and *The Emperor's Club* (2002) (Guo *et al.* 2016: 29–35). For the first stage of this empathic engagement program students discussed these films in class 'under the guidance of the teacher to extract the main themes of the films: empathy, love and integrity' (Guo *et al.* 2016: 32). Although this program did not result in a significant increase of empathy levels of the students in the pre-test and post-test surveys, it laid the foundation for the use of film in medical education at Peking University and signaled a shift towards the inclusion of multimedia in Chinese medical education.

Mainland Chinese films, however, remain on the periphery of medical humanities studies in the US, Europe, and, indeed, China. For example, the standard text *Cinemeducation: A Comprehensive Guide to Using Film in Medical Education* (2005) contains appendices that list films according to particular illnesses and conditions; a total of 16 mainland films were listed under the 'Cultural Diversity: Chinese American' film section. For the disabilities section of the appendix no mainland Chinese films were included. Moreover, the editors' 'Top Ten Cinemeducation Films' are exclusively Anglo-European. The exclusion of Chinese films not only reflects how medical humanities has been largely 'expressive' of Western cultural values but could also be ascribed to the political regulation of Chinese cinema since the founding of the People's Republic of China (Hooker and Noonan 2011: 79–84). As Sarah Dauncey (2007: 482) notes, 'With the establishment of the PRC in 1949 . . . the representation of impairment became exceedingly limited'. It was not until the late 1970s in the era of the Open and Reform Policies that mainland Chinese films would prominently feature disabled characters (Dauncey 2007: 481–506). Lastly, Chinese cinemeducation faces what Louise Younie (2014: 98) describes as the chicken and the egg problem of integration into medical curriculums in mainland China and internationally, that is, 'greater integration needs more research and more research is not possible without greater integration'. *Cinemeducation and Disability: A Special Study Module* is a small step towards integrating Chinese films into mainland Chinese medical curricula.

Cinemeducation and disability: a special study module

In March 2017, at the School of Health Humanities at Peking University, I conducted a four-week special study module (SSM) – *Cinemeducation and Disability: A Special Study Module* – for undergraduate medical students to examine mainland Chinese films that feature physically impaired characters and/or where physical disability is central to the narrative. Increasingly SSMs are being developed to augment medical curricula as part of a broader shift from the dominant biomedical model of medical education to a bio-psycho-social approach. As R.J. Macnaughton (1997: 49–51) writes, ancillary medical special study modules are suited to 'subjects which are not medical but which are directly relevant to the practice of medicine'. In the field of medical humanities SSMs can enable teachers to conduct experimental courses that examine representations of illness, disability, and mental health in cinema, life writing, literature, and the performing arts.

Related international SSMs have focused on the efficacy of film and related arts-based practices as a means of cultivating empathy, improving doctor-patient communication or making healthcare students become 'wiser, more observant, and more humane' (Fishbein: 646–651). Yet the results tend to be difficult to measure or show an array of inconsistencies. As Mark Perry *et al.* (2011: 141–8) demonstrate there is some evidence that art-based activities can improve diagnostic observation skills, yet due to a range of methodological issues the case that the visual arts, literature, and performance can positively change behaviour and attitudes is less convincing. With such inconsistencies in mind the *Cinemeducation and Disability* SSM was designed to use film as a means of facilitating class discussion for undergraduate medical students and to elicit responses from students to gain insights into mainland Chinese cinematic representations of disability.

Attendees

The *Cinemeducation and Disability* SSM attracted eight biomedical English majors and two clinical medicine majors. The biomedical English majors are highly engaged in social issues and cultural representations of illness in relation to health communication and public health. The two clinical medicine students each have a strong interest in the humanities, and one of them is undertaking a double major in clinical medicine and Chinese literature. The current generation of Chinese undergraduate medical students – commonly referred to as *Post 90s* – through their extensive use of the internet and smart phones as well as consumption of television shows and films are immersed in visual culture. Although the students are not formally trained in film analysis the students demonstrated sufficient visual literacy and narratological skills that enabled them to analyse and interpret the major themes, characters, and dialogue (Association of College and Research Libraries 2011). For this generation of learners cinema is an attractive form of communication and representation as they largely regard film as entertainment. For medical students in particular, cinema provides an alternative to rote learning and passive learning in the form of lectures and enables them to engage in analysing cultural discourses of illness.

Selection of films

For the *Cinemeducation and Disability* SSM students were required to watch two prescribed feature films per week over three weeks:

Class One: Physical Disability

Ju Dou (*Ju dou* 菊豆 1990)
The Common People (*Guan yu ai de gushi* 关于爱的故事 1998)

Class Two: Hearing Impairment

Silent River (*Wu sheng de he* 无声的河 2001)
Breaking the Silence (*Piao liang mama* 漂亮妈妈 2000)

Class Three: Visual Impairment

Life on a String (*Bian zou bian chang* 边走边唱 1991)
Blind Massage (*Tui na* 推拿 2014)

Due to time constraints clips were not used in class. The films were selected from a canon of Chinese films with medical humanities themes compiled by Vivienne Lo, Chris Berry, Michael Clark, and Patrizia Liberati as part of the China Centre for Health and Humanity's film studies program at University College London (UCL) (China Centre for Health and Humanity 2017). For the purposes of this chapter only two films will be discussed in detail: *Ju Dou* and *The Common People*. For all of the attendees this SSM was their first opportunity to focus exclusively on portrayals of disability in mainland Chinese cinema. Prior to the SSM the students had seen only one film – *Blind Massage* – as it was prescribed in the *Medicine and Visual Culture: The Body* course in 2016. This may be a surprise given that they are Chinese students studying medicine at an elite Chinese university; however, elective medical humanities courses at Peking University, as elsewhere, that make use of cinema as a pedagogical tool tend to focus on Hollywood and European films due to their popularity and artistic accessibility. For example, disabled characters are featured in Hollywood and European cinema in a wide range of genres from biopics, fantasy, crime, and action to horror, whereas in mainland China disabled characters are largely portrayed in the social-realist genre, the cornerstone of Chinese independent cinema. This is perhaps one factor as to why there is currently a lack of exposure to Chinese films that focus on disability and a paucity of analysis of representations of disability in Chinese medical education.

Facilitating discussion: student-centred teaching

Over the past two decades medical educators have been incorporating student-centred teaching to promote student engagement and facilitate independent learning. This is due, in part, to the emergence of information and communication technologies, which are profoundly reshaping traditional pedagogy at all levels of medical education. While many areas of medical education necessarily rely on teacher-centred learning, in the medical humanities there is a wider range of teaching modes – problem based learning, discovery learning, task-based learning, experiential and reflective learning, and project-based learning to name a few – available to teachers and students alike (Spencer and Jordan 1999: 1280–83). Student-centred teaching enables students to engage in active rather than passive learning, encourages individuals to participate in critical discussions and debates, decentres the teacher-student relationship, and provides a 'reflexive approach to the teaching and learning process on the part of both teacher and learner' (Lea *et al.* 2003: 321–34). For the SSM students did not choose which films they had to watch but they had control over 'how and why that topic might be an interesting one to study' (Harden and Crosby 2000: 334–47).

In order to prepare for the discussion students were required to watch the films before the class, prepare a list of questions and discussion topics, and select key scenes for close analysis. To begin the discussion I delivered a basic introduction to the film, which included a brief biography of the director, plot summary, descriptions of the main characters, and the major themes. The remainder of the class was led by students who engaged in open discussion; my role was to facilitate, to clarify, and to keep the discussion moving if necessary. One stereotype of Chinese students, domestically and internationally, is that they can be reticent in a classroom setting and enabling group discussion or eliciting opinions can be a challenge for instructors. In medical education this may be further pronounced as much of the learning that takes place in the classroom is necessarily teacher oriented. However, factors such as group size, familiarity with other students, the learning approach – role play, team-based learning, problem-based learning – each affect the dynamics of classroom discussion. Moreover, film, compared to texts, is popular among students as it has positive associations with entertainment, which allows students to engage in critical discussion as well as being able to express their personal feelings about the themes and issues presented (Dobson 2005: 166; Klemenc-Ketis and Kersnik 2011: 60). As Lisa Walker (2014: 44) claims, 'film allows students to develop more sensitive behaviours and attitudes because the medium is both familiar and nonthreatening, and the feelings movies evoke allow students to explore and analyse those feelings from a safe distance'. In the case of this SSM the small number of participants as well as their familiarity with myself and each other resulted in dynamic, robust, and candid discussion. One problem with this approach, however, is that it can be very difficult to predict the outcomes of the discussions. As will be seen in the following section the students in many instances opted not to focus on the core topic of disability but the related social issues presented in the films.

Student-led class discussions

Stepping back from my usual role as a teacher to that of a facilitator, the broad analytical framework of the SSM was to identify how a select group of medical students respond to representations of disability in Chinese film; how the portrayal of disability in Chinese cinema may diverge from Anglo-European cinema; whether the cinematic depiction of the disability/disabilities is clinically accurate; how disabled characters may be feared, stigmatised, stereotyped, or marginalised by non-disabled characters; and what positive images of disability are portrayed, for example, the disabled person who overcomes adversity. Although these major themes of disability are readily identifiable in numerous Anglo-European films that feature disabled characters, there are issues in transferring Anglo-European critical perspectives onto Chinese representations of disability. Thus, whilst this group cannot be considered representative, the discussion points raised may indicate some prevalent perceptions and attitudes towards disability in a Chinese context, in particular, post-90s university students. By drawing upon subjective reader response theory – how readers and viewers create meaning from their experience of a text or film – this pilot study is intended to be a step towards understanding how disability is portrayed in transnational Chinese cinema and how teachers may approach using films in medical education (Beach 1993: 1).

The first class – *Introduction* – was designed to provide an introduction to the SSM, cinemeducation in medical pedagogy, critical tools such as common Western representational stereotypes of disability (for example, the Disabled Monster, the Sweet Innocent, and the Prophet), a summary of the moral model, medical model, and social model of disability in Anglo-European contexts, an overview of film genres that feature disabled characters, and some examples of acclaimed films that feature physical disability, hearing impairment, and visual impairment. The remainder of the class provided students with a set of critical questions to assist with their analyses of the films. These sample questions were not prescriptive; rather they were intended to serve as a set of basic critical tools to enable film analysis. However, it was cautioned that this set of questions is rooted in Anglo-European cultural, social, and political perceptions of disability and that applying such theories may not be appropriate for the analysis of Chinese cinematic portrayals of disability. Students were, in turn, encouraged to identify what they might consider distinctly Chinese critical perceptions and disabled identities.

Class Two: Physical Disability

Ju Dou (*Ju dou* 菊豆), dir. Zhang Yimou, 1991.

'Filthy beast! You still want to hurt me? What's inside your pants? Nothing but shit! What's done is done. I want you to know you can do nothing about it'. Ju Dou in *Ju Dou*

Zhang Yimou's breakthrough film *Ju Dou* set in 'a small village somewhere in China in the 1920s' and focuses on the eponymous Ju Dou; a beautiful young woman who is sold into marriage to a dye-mill owner Yang Jinshan. Having killed two former wives for not producing a male heir, Yang Jinshan – seemingly in the pursuit of reproduction – soon begins to torment, beat, and humiliate Ju Dou through a series of sadistic acts. Yang Jinshan's adopted nephew Yang Tianqing, a worker at the mill, is enchanted by Ju Dou's beauty and soon they embark on an affair. Ju Dou produces a son, Tianbai, who Yang Jinshan assumes is his child. This unconventional and illicit romance soon takes a turn when Yang Jinshan suffers a stroke and is paralysed from the waist down and is forced to move about in a wooden bucket. Yang Jinshan's impairment renders him doubly incapable of reproduction – he is both infertile and unable to perform sexually. Moreover, Yang Jinshan's impairment empowers Ju Dou and Yang Tianqing who flaunt their affair and soon rumours of their affair spread throughout the village to the humiliation and anger of their son Tianbai. Tianbai, in acts that are anti-Confucian and Oedipal, kills both of his fathers. In the final scene Ju Dou, having lost her husband, lover, and her place in society, destroys the dye mill. Chinese and international critics have focused on aspects of gender and the sexuality of its main character, and its critique of feudal Confucian patriarchy and China's modern political system (Callahan 1993: 52–80; Cui 1997: 303–30; Zhang 2012: 57–74). The SSM participants similarly focused on the status of women in traditional and contemporary Chinese society; whether disability may be considered a form of punishment for Yang Jinshan; and whether the film is useful as a means of understanding disability in a Chinese context.

The students' first response to the film focused on its representation of the status and treatment of women in traditional Chinese society. This extended to Zhang Yimou's portrayal of feudal Chinese culture and whether his representation of the status of women could be considered accurate historically and in the present. One female biomedical English major, Li Xiuying (12 March 2017), found *Ju Dou*,

> very horrible because it shows the misery of Chinese women in our society. This is the situation politically right now and it's against our [women's] beliefs . . . I really wouldn't want to live in a society like that [the one presented in the film].

The students' adverse response to the treatment of Ju Dou was shared by all of the female students. In response Wang Wei (12 March 2017), a male student, argued that the 'film shows the way that Western people look at Chinese. Traditional Chinese society didn't really work like how it is shown in the film'. This perspective is akin to critics such as Zhang Yingjin (2012: 65) who have similarly argued that Zhang Yimou's early films 'resonate with a longstanding Orientalist view of a backward rural China'. Wang Wei further contended that the film was unrealistic as it did not resemble his own family history and continued to state that, 'In my family three or four generations ago they didn't buy wives. I don't think it is a realistic film'. However, following his description of his family background the female students strongly disagreed with his claim. Zhang Min, a female biomedical English major, drawing upon her experience of growing up in a village, maintained that historically and today that the main function of rural women in China is reproduction. Zhang Min (12 March 2017) described,

> Even nowadays in the countryside there is a prevalent notion that a woman's function is mostly about reproduction. Today the dominance of men is still upheld in the countryside and when a woman is married to such a man, the whole family will put great importance on her to give birth to a grandson. She is under such pressure that she can't help but to keep giving birth until a son is born. In my family I am the eldest and I have a sister and a brother. My brother is the youngest. You know why.

The students remained largely divided on the issue along gender lines. Critics to date have largely focused on Ju Dou and her 'individual struggle against her social placement as a woman in feudal China' as well as the film's possible allegorical critiques of the struggle against the ruling Communist Party of China (Callahan 1993: 53). But there has been little focus on Yang Jinshan, Ju Dou's sadistic husband who after having a stroke becomes a paraplegic. Although the students were significantly more engaged in issues of gender, sexuality, and paternalism in ancient and contemporary Chinese culture they offered some historical references in relation to Yang Jinshan's disability, an aspect of the film that has been largely overlooked by critics.

Following a stroke Yang Jinshan is paralysed from the waist down; however, he is able to communicate clearly and forcefully and is able to physically over-power Ju Dou. At the beginning of the discussion the students focused on whether Yang Jinshan's disability may be considered a punishment for his cruelty towards women. As Liu Yang (12 March 2017), a female biomedical English student, stated, 'I don't regard it as a punishment . . . I regard it just as an accident'. Wang Wei, however, argued that his disability was 'payback for his misdeeds'. Here the discussion stalled and the issue did not resonate among the students. As Liu Yang commented, 'In the West people will say that God will punish you with disability' but the students could not identify any religious or mythological examples of divine or supernatural forces that punish real or fictional wrongdoers with disabil-ity. The students, however, cited historical figures such as Sun Bin 孙膑 (d. 316 BCE), a military strategist who, accused of treason, had his kneecaps removed, and the historian and biographer Sima Qian 司马迁 (d. 86 BCE) who was cas-trated in lieu of a death sentence. It was subsequently debated whether castration could be considered a disability: the male students considered it a disability on account of the loss of the testicles – as Jeffrey Preston (2017: 34) notes disability is framed as a loss, therefore, 'to be disabled elicits the same fears and anxieties as being castrated' – yet the female students argued that although castration results in an inability to procreate it does not significantly impede sexual intercourse, thus, eunuchs cannot be considered disabled. Both the male and female students, how-ever, were incorrect about castration; in imperial China both the penis and testi-cles were removed (Chiang 2012: 30–31). The students' debate also demonstrates that their definitions of sex and gender conform to biomedical classifications of sex based on male and female reproductive systems and functionalities. The final part of the discussion tied together the two main areas of discussion: metaphors of Confucian patriarchy and how of each of the characters are ruined by cultural conventions and social order. As Li Xiuying stated, 'I don't consider this to be a movie about disability. I think it's about traditional society in China. It's not only a tragedy for Yang Jinshan but also for Ju Dou and Yang Tianqing. It's a tragedy for everyone'. In turn, Wang Wei agreed, 'Ju Dou and Tianqing's efforts to break tradition failed. This tradition must go on forever [laughs]'. The general response to this character from students was that they did not consider *Ju Dou* to be a useful film for studying disability in a Chinese context as it was not the primary focus of the film. Moreover, the students argued that Yang Jinshan's disability primarily serves as a narrative device and as a metaphor for repressive patriarchal Confu-cian values and, therefore, was of little use in understanding disability as a lived experience in historical or contemporary Chinese society.

The Common People (*Guan yu ai de gushi* 关于爱的故事), dir. Zhou Xiaowen, 1998.

'There are sixty million handicapped in our country. We have the same dignity and rights, the same ability to participate in life. I'll devote my whole life to this cause'. Ma Dali in *The Common People*

Zhou Xiaowen's docu-drama *The Common People* (1998) opens with a definition of cerebral palsy (CP) from an unspecified source:

脑性瘫痪 简称脑瘫
由于出生时窒息造成
主要特征：
1，思维很正常 2，行为受障碍
Cerebral palsy
A disease caused by suffocation at birth
Its main features:
1. Thinking normally 2. Having behavioural barrier

This definition differs from medical definitions, which emphasise how the neurological disorder affects muscle control, coordination, and fine motor skills (Mayo Clinic 2016). Although CP results from damage to the brain before or during childbirth such definitions do not first focus on the various cognitive abilities as the condition is unique to the individual. However, Zhou's definition differs from standard medical descriptions as it seeks to confront and dispel the common notion that people with CP are intellectually impaired (again this varies on an individual basis). The term 'normal' here carries significant weight in a Chinese context. While Anglo-European post-structuralist theorists and social justice activists deconstruct and rail against the multitude forms of normalisation – heteronormativity, white normativity, social normativity, among others – China, despite its many social and cultural changes over the past 30 years, remains a socially conservative society and many people aspire, especially those who have disabled children, to be accepted by the mainstream and its institutions. For example, having disabled children accepted into 'normal' schools is a major theme that runs through many Chinese films from the 1990s to the present including *Breaking the Silence* (*Piao liang mama* 漂亮妈妈 2000) and *Destiny* (*Xi he* 喜禾 2016). The second definition – Having behavioural barrier (*Xingwei shou zhangai* 行为受障碍) – which also translates as *impaired behaviour*, is in line with the standard medical definition that describes how the movements of the body are hindered or obstructed. The precedence of 'thinking normally' over the physiological aspects of CP demonstrates the director's aim to challenge the ways in which disability is framed and to create new perceptions of disability.

At the beginning of the group discussion students questioned the possible meanings of the English title 'The Common People'. Liu Yang stated that, 'one of the meanings is that disabled people can be functional like everyone else'. The theme of 'normality' was further discussed later in the class. In a further response to the translation of the title Zhang Min said,

> Another interpretation of the title is that disability is more common than people think. The film opens with a statement there are 60 million people with disabilities in China, I am not sure what the figure is today, but disability is more prevalent than people may think but we just don't notice it or it is hidden.

Deirdre Sabina Knight (2006: 99) speculates that the seemingly innocuous Chinese title – *Guan yu ai de gushi* 关于爱的故事 (*Stories of Love*) – was selected to avoid censorship issues but also to as a reflection of the film's 'presentation of alternative responses to severe disabilities'.

The film is divided into two parts–*First Story* and *Second Story*–and features two respective protagonists with cerebral palsy: Ma Dali, a young male who is acknowledged by the government as a 'model disabled person', with a small community of fellow disabled people, seeks to establish a small rehab centre; and Li Yun, a young woman who attempts to raise money to pay for the hospital bills of an injured acquaintance. Both characters are each in their own ways 'model citizens' who expose the ineffectual bureaucracies and economic inequities of medical services in China. Ma Dali, having visited a world-class and prohibitively expensive healthcare facility, organises a team of fellow disabled people to create their own Palace of the Disabled. As Knight (2006: 98) notes the Palace highlights the widening wealth gap in China but demonstrates how lack of access to facilities disables the impaired individual. In the *Second Story* Li Yun's attempts to pay for an increasingly complicated and therefore increasingly expensive medical procedure becomes farcical, if not tragicomic. Critics such as Knight (2006: 98–101) have examined how *The Common People* portrays 'the profoundly social nature of suffering' yet gives voice to the disabled. Each of the protagonists challenges discrimination by demonstrating 'uncommon courage and care for others' but also how inequity of healthcare services and the built environment as well as issues of funding further disable people with impairments.

For the class discussion the students focused on the *First Story*. From the discussion three major themes emerged: how the disabled *struggle* not so much with their impairment but with society, the notion of *normality*, and the *usefulness* of disabled people to improve the image of government officials and business people. Liu Yang opened the discussion by stating,

> After watching this movie I felt a little uncomfortable about the experiences of the main characters' in the two parts. It's like everything they experienced was a struggle. Everything in Dali's life doesn't change. The government or other people do not pay too much attention to him.

Unlike the 'triumph over adversity' narrative that is often featured in Hollywood cinema, Zhou's docu-drama utilises the suffering of disabled characters to highlight the disabling forces of society and the complex intersections between the worlds of the disabled and the non-disabled. This is evident in the portrayal of Dali's brief sexual and emotionally fraught relationship with a nurse, Liu Xiaorong. Whereas recent European and Hollywood cinema has embarked upon representing positive disability and sexuality narratives, for example, *The Sessions* (2012), Dali and Xiaorong's relationship abruptly, if not brutally, ends with Xiaorong choosing to have an abortion. *The Common People* is not a transformation narrative; rather it directly confronts the often unspoken social and sexual gaps between the disabled and the non-disabled. As Liu Yang commented,

> *The Common People* reflects a conflict about disabled people's lives, on the one hand they would like to be regarded as normal people but on the other hand they are still the Other.

The *First Story* further brings into question the public role of the disabled person, that is, that a disabled person should serve as a model citizen or inspirational figure. Liu Yang stated,

> When we see disabled people like Dali come to the stage and give a speech we assume he will talk about how to strive, how to fight against life . . . This is a stereotype; that disabled people are a special group that should inspire and motivate us.

The disabled person as an inspirational figure is prominent in both Anglo-European and Chinese cinema, media, and illness narratives. In China during the 1980s disabled people, in particular the writer Zhang Haidi, would become conduits to promote 'socialist spiritual civilisation' (*shehui zhuyi jingshen wenming* 社会主义精神文明), which Sarah Dauncey (2013: 182–205) describes as the 'Zhang Haidi Effect'. From propaganda posters to newspaper stories disabled people should embody one or more of the following attributes: self-respect (*zizun* 自尊), self-confidence (*zixin* 自信), self-improvement (*ziqiang* 自强), self-support (*zili* 自立), and serve as models for other citizens (Dauncey 2013: 191). The use of disabled people for political purposes was identified by the students. As Wang Wei said, the 'film is very "*hong* 红" (literally 'Red' but stands for communist), which was the atmosphere at that time'. This statement reveals the generation gap between young students today, who grew up during the relatively open Hu Jintao-Wen Jiabao era (2002–2012), and the socio-political climate of the period of the late 1990s in which the film is set. In one scene Ma Dali who is at a Party-sponsored banquet for other 'model handicapped comrades' states, 'We should love the Party and socialism. What does it mean to love the party and socialism? It means aspiration, self-respect, confidence and reliance'. Such speeches and political rhetoric were viewed skeptically by the majority of students. As Zhang Min stated,

> It was his own speech but they are clichés from the government. Disabled people are useful for propaganda but in reality they are marginalised and ignored. This is ironic. It gives the audience the illusion that disabled people are treated well but actually it's not the case. The ones that are rewarded are the lucky ones, they are a minority.

Although the students were cynical about how disabled figures can be utilised for propaganda purposes, in the engagements between disabled characters they identified genuine care. In the use of propaganda clichés they also recognised that the disabled characters expressed genuine care and solidarity. As Zhang Min commented,

> After the failure of his operation Dali said that I have to tell my experience to others who are considering going through this surgery, I have to let them know. Dali was not thinking just about himself but other people who may have the same experience as him. This shows he is not a selfish person but also helpful to others.

The explicit portrayal of disabled characters in *The Common People* stimulated more discussion about disability compared with *Ju Dou*. The students largely focused on the *First Story*, possibly because it is the more 'realistic' of the two stories. I attempted to steer discussion to the *Second Story* but the students appeared somewhat perplexed and were not interested in engaging in analysis. The students considered *The Common People* a useful and instructive film for analysing disability in a Chinese context but also noted that it is an 'old' film (the students were born in the mid 1990s) and therefore did not reflect contemporary notions of disability in China.

Limitations of cinemeducation and the special study module

To date Chinese films that feature disability have received very little attention by researchers and have yet to be integrated into medical curricula in China and internationally, making this study a small step forward in the field of cinemeducation. The *Cinemeducation and Disability* special study module had numerous limitations. As the SSM was a voluntary course – the students did not receive any formal credit – it was difficult to attract a large or diverse group of students. Medical students in China, as elsewhere, have very little time for extracurricular activities. I was fortunate to have a core group of highly motivated students who were willing to devote two hours on Sunday evenings (the only spare time many students have) over the course of four weeks to discuss and analyse the prescribed films. Although there is no specific number of classes for SSMs, *Cinemeducation and Disability* was limited to four weeks in response to the students' time constraints. Ideally an eight-week course would have allowed time for more in-depth discussions and variety of Chinese films. Another limitation was the range of perspectives. As this was not a controlled study the gender ratio of the students was imbalanced. On average eight females and two males attended the SSM over the four weeks. Based on my three years of experience teaching at Peking University, female students tend to be more active in class discussions; only one male student regularly offered his opinions during the four weeks, while the other male student mostly observed. A further imbalance was the range of medical majors. In my elective courses – *Illness Narratives* and *Medicine and Visual Culture* – I teach students from a range of majors including biomedical English, clinical medicine, dentistry, pharmacology, and nursing, among others, however, the SSM was dominated by biomedical English majors. This could be due to factors such as the students' confidence in their language abilities (the classes were mostly conducted in English) and as I have taught the biomedical English majors in several courses I have a strong rapport with this particular group. A further issue was how the discussions were guided. The open discussion was loosely framed in order to elicit responses from students and have them direct the conversation. I was cautious about imposing my own points of view, yet from time to time had to raise questions or issues so as to stimulate or redirect the conversation. One possible remedy is to make use of a video recorder and not be present in the class so as to allow students to openly discuss the films without interference from a teacher. Further SSMs will be conducted at the School of Health Humanities at Peking University to address these issues and further refine the process of eliciting more in-depth subjective viewer-responses from students.

Conclusion

Over the past 40 years mainland China has produced a remarkable body of national and transnational films that explore and critique a range of health issues, yet in China and internationally they are often overlooked in favour of Hollywood and European cinema. *Cinemeducation and Disability: A Special Study Module* is a small step towards addressing Louise Younie's 'chicken and the egg problem' of integrating Chinese films with a focus on disability into medical curricula and conducting related research. Cinemeducation offers educators and students alike an accessible and engaging means of analysing (trans) cultural representations of illness and stimulating discussion about a range of health issues. Although the students that participated in the SSM are not representative, they were strongly in favour of films that featured disabled protagonists and stories that focus exclusively on disability narratives, which are more conducive to in-depth analysis and discussion. A further factor to consider in the selection of films is the period of production. All films are products of their time but films such as *The Common People* represent a very different China than the one in which contemporary students came of age. While they may be fascinating from a historio-cultural perspective, students preferred contemporary films such as *Blind Massage* (*Tui na* 推拿 2014) and *Destiny* (*Xi he* 喜禾 2016) as they are more relevant to current social, cultural, and political environment. With further integration of mainland Chinese films into medical curricula new insights can be gained from into students' perceptions and responses, which may assist with identifying culturally specific representations of disability. Moreover, disabled people in China, as elsewhere, are largely 'invisible' and film can serve as a means of exposing students to the complex myriad of ethical, aesthetic, and political issues related to disability. For the international medical humanities community the ethical complexities and aesthetic richness of mainland Chinese films can serve to promote cross-cultural analysis of disability in cinemeducation.

Acknowledgements

I would like to thank all of the students for taking time from their busy schedules to watch the films and participate in the Special Study Module. All of the students' names have been changed to protect their privacy.

Filmography

Blind Massage (Tui na 推拿), dir. Lou Ye, 2014.
Breaking the Silence (Piao liang mama 漂亮妈妈), dir. Sun Zhou, 2000.
Destiny (Xi he 喜禾), dir. Zhang Wei, 2016.
First Knight, dir. Jerry Zucker, 1995.
Ju Dou (Ju dou 菊豆), dir. Zhang Yimou, 1991.
Life on a String (Bian zou bian chang 边走边唱), dir. Chen Kaige, 1991.
My Left Foot, dir. Jim Sheridan, 1989.
Scent of a Woman, dir. Martin Brest, 1992.
Silent River (Wu sheng de he 无声的河), dir. Ning Jingwu, 2001.
The Common People (Guan yu ai de gushi 关于爱的故事), dir. Zhou Xiaowen, 1998.
The Emperor's Club, dir. Michael Hoffman, 2002.
The Hours, dir. Stephen Daldry, 2002.
The Miracle Worker, dir. Arthur Penn, 1962.
The Sessions, dir. Ben Lewin, 2012.

Bibliography

Alexander, M., Lenahan, P., Pavlov, A., Bailey, S. and Scherger, J.E. (2005) *Cinemeducation: Using Film and Other Visual Media in Graduate and Medical Education*, Oxford: Radcliffe Publishing.

Association of College and Research Libraries (2011) *ACRL Visual Literacy Competency Standards for Higher Education*, www.ala.org/acrl/standards/visualliteracy, accessed 22 August 2018.

Beach, R. (1993) *A Teacher's Introduction to Reader-Response Theories*, Urbana, IL: National Council of Teachers of English.

Callahan, W.A. (1993) Gender, Ideology, Nation: *Ju Dou* in the Cultural Politics of China, *East-West Film Journal*, 7 (1): 52–80.

Chiang, H. (2012) How China Became a 'Castrated Civilization' and Eunuchs a 'Third Sex', in H. Chiang (ed.) *Transgender China*, Basingstoke: Palgrave Macmillan, pp. 23–66.

China Centre for Health and Humanities, University College London (2017) *HISTGC06: Chinese Film, Medicine and the Body, 2017–2018*, www.ucl.ac.uk/chinahealth/teaching/chinese_film_and_the_body, accessed 22 August 2018.

Cui, S. (1997) Gendered Perspective: The Construction and Representation of Subjectivity and Sexuality in Ju Dou in S.H. Lu (ed.) *Transnational Chinese Cinemas: Identity, Nationhood, Gender*, Honolulu: University of Hawaii Press, pp. 303–330.

Dauncey, S. (2007) Screening Disability in the PRC: The Politics of Looking Good, *China Information*, 12 (3): 481–506.

———. (2013) Breaking the Silence? Deafness, Education and Identity in Two Post-Cultural Revolution Chinese Films, in M.E. Mogk (ed.) *Different Bodies: Essays on Disability in Film and Television*, Jefferson, NC: McFarland & Company, Inc, pp. 75–88.

————. (2013) Whose Life Is It Anyway? Disabled Life Stories in Post-Reform China, in M. Dryburgh and S. Dauncey (eds.) *Writing Lives in China, 1600–2010: Histories of the Elusive Self*, Basingstoke: Palgrave Macmillan, pp. 182–205.

Dobson, R. (2005) Medical Students Should Watch Films that Inspire Compassion, *British Medical Journal*, 330 (7484): 166.

Fishbein, R.H. (1999) Scholarship, Humanism, and the Young Physician, *Academic Medicine*, 74 (6): 646–651.

Furmedge, D.S. (2008) Teaching Skills: A School-Based Special Study Module, *Medical Education*, 42 (11): 1140–1141.

Guner, G.A, Cavdar, Z., Yener, N., Kume, T., Egrilmez, M.Y. and Resmi, H. (2011) Special-Study Modules in a Problem-Based Learning Medical Curriculum: An Innovative Laboratory Research Practice Supporting Introduction to Research Methodology in the Undergraduate Curriculum, *Biochemistry and Molecular Biology Education*, 39 (1): 47–55.

Guo, L., Wei, L.H., Li, Y.F. and Li, H. (2016) Medical Humanities and Empathy: An Experimental Study, *Chinese Medical Humanities Review*, 1: 29–35.

Harden, R.M. and Crosby, J. (2000) AMEE Guide No 20: The Good Teacher Is More Than a Lecturer: The Twelve Roles of the Teacher, *Medical Teacher*, 22 (4): 334–347.

Hooker, C. and Noonan, E. (2011) Medical Humanities as Expressive of Western Culture, *Medical Humanities*, 37: 79–84.

Kennedy, K. and Wilkinson, A. (2018) A Student Selected Component (or Special Study Module) in Forensic and Legal Medicine: Design, Delivery, Assessment and Evaluation of an Optional Module as an Addition to the Medical Undergraduate Core Curriculum, *Journal of Forensic and Legal Medicine*, 53: 62–67.

Klemenc-Ketis, Z. and Kersnik, J. (2011) Using Movies to Teach Professionalism to Medical Students, *BMC Medical Education*, 11: 60.

Knight, D.S. (2006) Madness and Disability in Contemporary Chinese Film, *Journal of Medical Humanities*, 27: 93–103.

Lea, S.J., Stephenson, D. and Troy, J. (2003) Higher Education Students' Attitudes to Student Centred Learning: Beyond 'Educational Bulimia', *Studies in Higher Education*, 28 (3): 321–334.

Longmore, P. (2003) *Why I Burned My Book and Other Essays on Disability*, Philadelphia: Temple University Press.

Macnaughton, J. (1997) Special Study Modules: An Opportunity Not to be Missed, *Medical Education*, 31 (1): 49–51.

McCarthy, N., O'Flynn, D., Murphy, J., Barry, D. and Canals, M.L. (2013) Evaluation of the Educational Impact of a Special Study Module on Maritime Medicine for Medical Undergraduate Students, *International Maritime Health*, 64 (4): 195–201.

Mayo Clinic (2016) Cerebral Palsy, www.mayoclinic.org/diseases-conditions/cerebral-palsy/symptoms-causes/syc-20353999, accessed 22 August 2018.

O'Neill, B., Gill, E. and Brown, P. (2005) Deaf Awareness and Sign Language: An Innovative Special Study Module, *Medical Education*, 39 (5): 519–20.

Perry, M., Maffulli, N., Wilson, S. and Morrissey, D. (2011) The Effectiveness of Arts-Based Interventions in Medical Education: A Literature Review, *Medical Education*, 45 (2): 141–148.

Preston, J. (2017) *The Fantasy of Disability: Images of Loss in Popular Culture*, New York: Routledge.

Spencer, J.A. and Jordan, R.K. (1999) Learner Centred Approaches in Medical Education, *British Medical Journal*, 318 (7193): 1280–1283.

Walker, L. (2014) Teaching Compassion: Cinemeducation in Physician Assistant Programs, *The Journal of Physician Assistant Education*, 25 (2): 44–45.

Younie, L. (2014) Art in Medical Education, in V. Bates, A. Bleakley and S. Goodman (eds.) *Medicine, Health and the Arts: Approaches to the Medical Humanities*, Oxford: Routledge, pp. 85–104.

Zhang, Y. (2012) Directors, Aesthetics, Genres: Chinese Postsocialist Cinema, 1979–2010, in Y. Zhang (ed.) *A Companion to Chinese Cinema*, Oxford: Blackwell Publishing, pp. 57–74.

Part 4

Transforming self-health care in the digital age

11 Raising awareness about anti-microbial resistance

A nationwide video and arts competition for Chinese university students using social media

Therese Hesketh, Zhou Xudong and Wang Xiaomin

This chapter will describe a baseline investigation about antibiotic knowledge, attitudes, and use among Chinese university students, and the subsequent competition, which elicited submissions of artworks to raise awareness about anti-microbial resistance. The baseline investigation was carried out using the online Wen Juan Xing survey tool at six universities, representing all Chinese regions. A total of 11,915 respondents demonstrated widespread misuse of antibiotics, and an inverse correlation between knowledge and misuse. The findings led to a decision to launch a nationwide university competition for artworks, through social media networks and a dedicated website. Expressions of interest were received from 356 teams at 71 universities, across 29 provinces. This produced 142 submissions. A long list of 66 was reduced to 32 through a dual voting system: a panel of academics and student representatives from Zhejiang University, and a public vote via a WeChat public account. Around 50,000 people voted on the shortlist of 32. The shortlisted artworks were showcased and judged at 'The AMR Summit' at Zhejiang University in October 2016. Winners received monetary prizes and certificates, with dissemination of their work through social and mainstream media, and the World Health Organisation (WHO) website. The artworks not only demonstrate the talent and creativity of the students, but also the potential power of art forms and social media to deliver public health messages.

Background

Antimicrobial resistance (AMR) is one of the greatest threats to global population health this century, and a major contributor to rising healthcare costs worldwide (World Health Organisation 2012). The 2014 Review on Antimicrobial Resistance estimated that current annual mortality attributable to AMR is 700,000, and that this will rise to 10 million by 2050 if action is not taken to reduce our use of antibiotics. Predictions have been made of a 'post-antibiotic era', where people die from simple infections that have been treatable for decades, and where surgical procedures will be too dangerous to carry-out (World Health Organisation 2012). It is agreed that significant action is needed urgently.

Misuse of antibiotics, both in medicine and agriculture, is well-established as the major driver of AMR (The Review on Antimicrobial Resistance 2014). At a biological level, resistance results from mutations in bacteria and selection pressure from antibiotic use, in humans, agriculture, and aquaculture (Laxminarayan *et al.* 2013). This provides a competitive advantage for mutated strains. The most important causes of AMR are the routine inappropriate use of antibiotics as growth promoters in the livestock industry, their routine inappropriate misuse for self-limiting illnesses in medicine, as well as for prophylaxis (Ranji *et al.* 2008). In medicine, despite awareness by doctors that antibiotics should be used with care, defensive medicine and profit motives are driving the increase in antibiotic use in many countries (Laxminarayan *et al.* 2013).

In China overuse of antibiotics is highly pervasive (Li *et al.* 2012). This has led to very high and increasing rates of AMR in both hospital- and community-acquired infections (Reynolds and McKee 2009). This is exacerbated by poor practice of infection control measures in many hospitals. Spread of resistance, within and outside China, is facilitated by high population mobility, with massive rural-urban migration and increasing foreign travel (Sun *et al.* 2014).

The Chinese government is aware of the problem. In 2004 antibiotic sales without prescription in pharmacies were banned in China, yet the ease of access to antibiotics without a prescription has been well documented (Xiao and Li 2013).

In 2011, the Ministry of Health set up a special task force on antibiotic stewardship, resulting in strict rulings covering all aspects of antibiotic use in hospitals (Wei *et al.* 2017). As a result, the use of antibiotics in many hospitals, especially in tertiary settings, has reduced. However, overall use remains high. In hospitals in China, around two-thirds of in-patients and 60% of all out-patients are prescribed antibiotics (Chang *et al.* 2017). This high level of prescribing is largely blamed on the reliance on drug sales for health provider income, belief in the curative powers of antibiotics for many conditions (including self-limiting ones), which leads to patient demand, and simple habit on the part of doctors (Reynolds and McKee 2009). Misuse in China is high compared with most developed countries where regulatory frameworks control prescribing behaviours of doctors and pharmacists. But in many countries, especially low- and middle-income countries where such frameworks are absent or not enforced, doctors misuse antibiotics with impunity, and antibiotics can be easily purchased without prescription in retail pharmacies, shops, and markets (Review on Antimicrobial Resistance 2014).

The baseline research

Aims and methods

Against this background we started to observe what was clearly unnecessary consumption of antibiotics at our own university. Conversations with students and staff showed that unnecessary use was very common, with many individuals taking antibiotics as 'prophylaxis' for upper respiratory tract infections. This led to the plan to conduct a cross-sectional study in an attempt to quantify the use of antibiotics. The aim was to explore the knowledge, attitudes, and behaviours of university students at top Chinese universities. They represent the educational elite and future opinion leaders, and are also the next generation of parents of young children, who are known to be very high users of antibiotics (Wei *et al.* 2017). So the knowledge and behaviours of these young people are especially important to the future trajectory of antibiotic use in China. Specifically, we aimed to explore knowledge and healthcare seeking behaviours in relation to antibiotic use in university students from all six Chinese regions. The six participating universities were: Nankai, Zhejiang, Jilin, Lanzhou, Wuhan, and Guizhou. These represented the north, east, northeast, northwest, south, and southwest, respectively. The survey was conducted from November 2015 to February 2016. The chapter has been published (Wang, Peng, Wang *et al.* 2017) and we summarise it in the following.

The questionnaire comprised three sections: 1) socio-demographic information; 2) antibiotic knowledge, including indications for antibiotic use and awareness of dangers of overuse; and 3) health care-seeking behaviour focusing on self-limiting illness and the use of antibiotics.

To collect the data we used the electronic questionnaire tool, Wen Juan Xing (Chinese Survey Monkey). At the outset we set up a dedicated WeChat account for the research project. This facilitated all communication and allowed for rapid dissemination of ideas as the project evolved. At each university we identified two local researchers who would take the lead. This was crucial to the smooth running of the data collection. We aimed to achieve a sample size per university of around 1800 students across a range of disciplines, to include undergraduates and postgraduates. At each university students attending class on the main campus on the day of the survey were included. The investigator approached teachers, explained the aim of the survey and asked for permission to speak to students before the class began. No teacher refused. The investigator then explained the aim of the survey to the students, disseminated the printed QR code of the electronic questionnaires, and explained how to complete the electronic questionnaire. The first section of the questionnaire consisted of an information sheet and consent form which was signed-off by all participants. A gratuity of 3RMB (US$ 0.50) was paid automatically via WeChat to all students who completed the questionnaire.

Survey results

Completed questionnaires were obtained from 11,915 students. Their mean age was 20.8, and 44% were from rural areas. The overwhelming majority were aware that overuse of antibiotics was potentially dangerous. In contrast, knowledge of appropriate use was highly variable: in terms of knowledge of antibiotic use, 61% of the students thought that antibiotics are effective against viruses, 38% stated that antibiotics were effective for sore throat, 30% for the common cold, and 31% for diarrhoea, with 41% thinking that antibiotics can speed up recovery from flu.

In terms of behaviours in the past month 30% of the students reported experience of a self-limiting illness. Of these 68% had common cold, 36% sore throat,

19% diarrhoea, 18% fever, and 17% headache, with some obvious overlap between symptoms. Of these 27% went to see a doctor, and 66% were prescribed antibiotics, with 32% given by infusion; 23% said they specifically asked for antibiotics, because the doctor did not initially prescribe them, and in all cases the doctor did then prescribe antibiotics. Of those students who had an illness in the last month 51% treated themselves for their symptoms; of these 30% used antibiotics. In the past year 23% had taken antibiotics for prophylaxis and 56% had bought antibiotics from a pharmacy without a prescription. A stock of antibiotics was kept at home or in the dormitory by 63% of the students. Antibiotic use was higher in students from rural areas and was highest in Guizhou, the poorest province in our study. Students who scored higher on the knowledge questions were less likely to use antibiotics. While doctors are clearly inappropriately prescribing antibiotics, they are also responding specifically to patient demand for antibiotics, and students are clearly self-medicating through purchase of antibiotics at pharmacies, although as noted purchase of antibiotics without prescription has been illegal since 2004. Enforcement is virtually non-existent.

The aggregated results were sent via WeChat to all participants, with explanations of the correct answers, both to increase the understanding of those who got questions wrong, and to generally inform the students about AMR and rational use of antibiotics.

The competition

Process

The results showed very high levels of misuse of antibiotics among some of the best-educated individuals in the country. Consequently we started to consider ways, not only of increasing awareness of the dangers of overuse of antibiotics, but also of promoting the appropriate use of antibiotics in university students. We recognised that the key was to get students actively engaged and enthused about the topic, and hence encourage them to explore the topic for themselves. We finally came up with the idea of holding a competition, which would involve students developing works of art, which could deliver two key messages to a general audience: about the dangers of anti-microbial resistance, and about the appropriate use of antibiotics to a general audience.

Using the WeChat platform we had originally set up to support the research, and where we had reported the aggregated results of the research, we made an announcement of a nationwide competition open to all university students. The call was for artworks of any type, for example film, posters, fine art, cartoon/ animations, and logos. The remit was to communicate the message of anti-microbial resistance, its causes, its consequences, and its prevention to a wide, general audience. We explicitly encouraged students to work in multi-disciplinary teams, with a view to improving the quality and variety of the submissions, as well as increasing mutual learning and understanding between very different disciplines. For example, students from the arts and humanities, fine art, media studies or information technology would work with medical or biological sciences students, the latter providing the scientific knowledge and expertise, and the former the creative elements.

A dedicated website was set-up. Here we uploaded all the background information necessary to inform the accurate content of any submissions. This included: key academic papers on the importance of AMR from the human, animal, and environmental perspectives; the biological mechanisms of resistance; the epidemiology of AMR with a focus on China; the results of our university survey; selected recent global and national reports; and the official regulations about antibiotic use in China. We offered generous cash prizes to the six winners – one first prize, two second, and three third prizes.

In universities where we had specific existing links we identified so-called AMR champions, who actively disseminated information about the competition and who encouraged and advised potential applicants. By the end of June 2016 we had expressions of interest from 356 teams at 71 universities, in 29 provinces, including Tibet, and as well as Hong Kong. By the deadline at the end of August we had received 142 submissions.

The process of selecting the winners involved a number of steps. First, the team of four organisers viewed all submissions and developed a long list of 66. Overall criteria for selection were a clear message delivered in an accessible and entertaining way. Most of those who did not get through failed because of inaccurate messaging or a style which was too didactic.

This long list comprised: 31 short films, 14 posters, 10 logos, two powerpoint presentations, one fine art painting, two electronic magazines, a decorative drug box warning, plus a set of painted manhole covers on a university campus. They came from 35 universities, with three submissions representing collaboration between two universities. A large number of films made the long list. There were several entrants from a number of universities, for example, six from Peking University, Zhongshan University, and Shanxi Medical University respectively, and four from Fudan University. At these universities we had established 'AMR champions' who promoted the competition on campus.

We had planned to hold the finals of the competition to be called 'The AMR Summit' at Zhejiang University just after the G20 summit, which was to take place in Hangzhou. But restrictions on movement in Hangzhou around the time of the G20 made this impossible, so the so-called AMR summit was planned for the following month, on October 23. The timing around the G20 Summit was important because we knew that an announcement of a strategy to address AMR was to be made, demonstrating that the Chinese government was taking the issue seriously, and we wanted to capitalise on the interest which would be generated.

The long list of 66 needed to be reduced, to ensure the quality of the submissions which would be displayed at the AMR Summit. So we convened a panel of judges consisting of five academics from relevant disciplines at Zhejiang University, including medicine, microbiology, health promotion, and media, and five student representatives from these disciplines. The panel spent an afternoon evaluating and scoring the individual submissions, using an agreed protocol based on artistic merit, innovation, and strength and clarity of the health education message for a general population. A final total of 32 were selected for display at the Summit.

The final 32 included 14 videos, five cartoon-animations, three powerpoint presentations, nine posters, and the painted manhole covers. To select the winners we developed a dual voting process. This involved a public vote through the website and an expert vote which would take place at the AMR Summit.

So, first all 32 were uploaded to the dedicated website to allow the public to vote. The software was sophisticated enough to enable a fair system of voting. This allowed us to ensure that that individuals could only vote once, and that they could choose their three favourites, only after all the submissions had been viewed. This was designed to stop people just voting (frequently) for themselves or getting friends and family to vote (frequently) for them. A total of nearly 50,000 people voted and the system itself developed the ranking of all submissions. This process alone generated a lot of interest. Some of the contenders complained at the order of the submissions as they appeared on the website. Specifically, they felt that the submissions shown lower down the page would get fewer votes, so they asked for the order to be changed randomly on a daily basis. This proved harder than we expected, but we did manage to do change the order twice during the one month voting period. However, we have no evidence about whether it changed voting patterns.

The AMR Summit

The second element of the voting came at the AMR Summit on October 23, 2016 at Zhejiang University. A panel consisting of external experts in public health, health promotion, clinical medicine, and media studies judged all the entrants, by the same criteria used in the first phase of judging. All shortlisted candidates attended the Summit. A representative of each team personally presented their submission with some background explanation about how the ideas were developed and brought to fruition. The marks of the Summit judges and the public vote were combined on a 50:50 basis to select the winners.

The Summit itself was a memorable event. It was attended by about 350 people, including the general public.

We invited Jim O' Neill, the lead author of the highly influential 2014 review on AMR 'Antimicrobial resistance: tackling a crisis for the health and wealth of nations', and the China Director of WHO, Dr Bernhard Schwartlander, to provide short, supportive, and inspirational videos, which were shown at the start of the event. Local media were also present.

All winners, one first prize, two second prizes, and three third prizes, received monetary prizes and certificates. All other participants received certificates stating they were on the final short-list and that they had presented at the Summit.

The artworks

Before announcing the call we were genuinely concerned about the potential quantity and quality of the artworks. But we were very pleasantly surprised.

The 32 shortlisted artworks demonstrated great variety, imagination, and inno-vation, making the judging process a considerable challenge. Unfortunately, a very impressive and huge poster made from antibiotic packets, which would have come second, had to be withdrawn, having been found to be unoriginal. The films varied in length between 45 seconds and 12 minutes with most around 2–3 min-utes. The main focus of the submissions of all types can be divided into three areas: 1) the AMR apocalypse; 2) why overuse of antibiotics is harmful; and 3) the historical perspective – the discovery of penicillin through to the dangers of AMR in the future. Most focussed on human aspects of AMR, rather than animal or environmental, though a few touched on all three.

Very noticeably the videos used striking imagery (for example the world being taken over by superbugs), interesting voices (for example of young children), and the creation of compelling characters. In most, attention was paid to ensuring the back-ground music was particularly suitable and effective at strengthening the message.

The winning submission came from Fudan University. This was an impressive and highly original piece of filmmaking. Shot in black and white with captions in English and Chinese it was a hybrid of modern dance and silent cinema. It portrays a dream in which the protagonist takes over the world as the 'King' of the superbugs. It manages to combine simplicity – it was all filmed in a gymnasium, with students acting the roles of bacteria and antibiotics – with a highly imaginative use of music, dance, and symbolism. The credits included a choreographer and music director, demonstrating the very professional approach of the film. There was some critique from the judges: it was thought too long to be useful for education of the general public (it was over 12 minutes long, more than twice as long as any other film), it could have been easily edited in places (especially the dance sequences) without loss of impact, and the story, which was about acquiring resistance through expo-sure to antibiotics, could have been a bit simpler for a general audience. But this was overall a very impressive piece of cinematography (Figure 11.1).

Hand painting from Nanjing Medical University (Figure 11.2) is an anima-tion film, illustrating the story of bacteria and antibiotic resistance, distinguished not only by the vivid colours and expressiveness of the animations, but also by showing us the hand at work, so that we see the ingenuity of the hand painting technique.

Paperman History, also came from Kunming Medical University. It uses ani-mated paper figures and cut-outs to enliven a short lecture (Figure 11.3). The nar-rator's voice is gravelly and deadpan, which is an intriguing choice, and lends a unique quality to a film which delivers a very clear, but simple message about AMR.

One entrant was singled out for particular originality. This came from Shanxi Medical University where all the manhole covers on the campus were painted with messages about AMR, and successfully created a talking point for everyone working and living on the campus.

Reflections

The competition demonstrates the potential of the combination of a competitive element, social media, and creative artworks, to be successful at delivering public

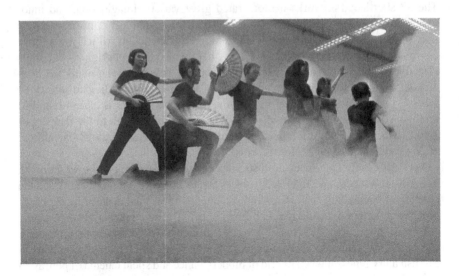

Figure 11.1 King Bac: Fudan University

King Bac is a winning hybrid of modern dance and silent cinema, with segments of dance alternating with intertitles and the whole held together by music. What is most striking is that the bacteria take human form and get 'larger', as the problem of antibiotic abuse worsens in China. Observers who do not speak modern standard Chinese easily engage with the human depictions of the bacteria and anti-biotics.

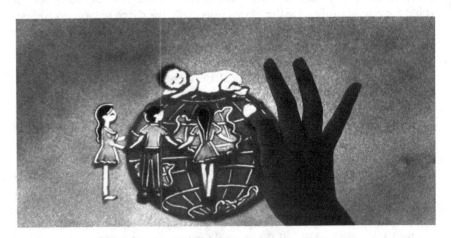

Figure 11.2 Hand Painting: Nanjing Medical University

This is a very elegant piece of animation which draws you in to understanding the issues despite the lack of words save some sparing use of subtitles. The animation illustrates the story of bacteria and antibiotic resistance and is distinguished not only by the vivid colours and expressiveness of the animations but also by showing us the hand at work, so that we see the ingenuity of the hand painting technique. The focus on the hand and its manipulations emphasises the central place of human action in dealing with the problem of antibiotic abuse.

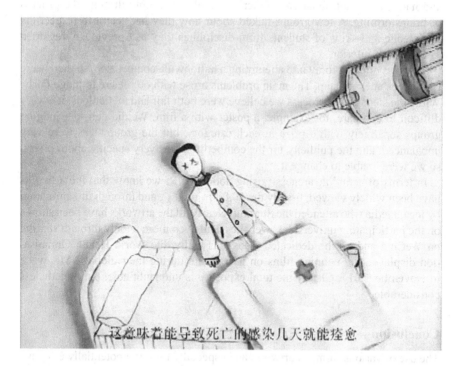

这意味着能导致死亡的感染几天就能痊愈

Figure 11.3 Paperman History: Kunming Medical University

Paperman History animates paper figures and cut-outs to enliven what is effectively a short lecture. The paper figure looks very fragile in the shadow of the giant doses of antibiotics. This entry is a more fact-laden animation than that in Figure 11.2, but nevertheless draws the viewer into the AMR message with its simplicity and charm.

health messages. The artworks were viewed by a large audience, which should of course increase awareness of AMR. The fact that 50,000 people voted is a success in itself, irrespective of the fact that many of them are simply family, friends, and classmates of the competitors.

From feedback we know that this was a very positive experience for the competitors. The majority were from medical and biological backgrounds, so nearly all had never taken part in an art competition. Nearly all worked in teams (with up to 10 members). Fifteen of the short-listed teams included students from both the sciences (mostly medicine) and the arts and humanities (mostly information technology and media studies). Many talked of the benefits of working in multidisciplinary teams. For example, one of the medical students said that she had learnt how to present messages about health education in an engaging and entertaining way, which she had never considered before. One group talked about how they had spent a lot of time brainstorming, both how to approach the topic, and how to explain the biological background to the general public in an understandable and accessible way. They had approached the challenge from different angles, and had learnt a lot about each other's disciplines, simply through the process of brainstorming. A few groups talked about how they had learnt to respect the knowledge and skills of students from disciplines they had previously regarded as somewhat inferior.

This was our first foray into attempting a nationwide competition, so there were challenges at every step. The main problems arose with our desire to judge fairly. While the steps of the process we believe were both fair and meticulous, it is very difficult to compare, for example, a poster with a film. We did consider judging groups separately with a prize in each category, but the group sizes were very unbalanced, and the publicity for the competition was very specific about prizes, so we were unable to change it.

In terms of actual awareness-raising about AMR, we know that the artworks have been widely viewed, first by the 50,000 'judges', and through dissemination by local media who attended the Summit. Nearly all the artworks have been shown on the participating universities' websites, and even more widely through sharing on WeChat and on the dedicated website. Finally, the World Health Organisation displayed the winning films on its website during their global AMR week in November 2017. Clearly the total exposure is unquantifiable, but nonetheless considerable.

Conclusion

The use of various forms of artwork, and especially film, is a potentially effective way of conveying the message of the dangers of AMR to the general public. The ubiquity of smartphones in China means that the films are easily downloadable and accessible to a potentially very wide population. But the most important question is whether increased awareness translates into behaviour change, that is, less misuse of antibiotics, and this is not clear. Two of the participating universities conducted small studies suggesting that knowledge of AMR had increased, and use of antibiotics decreased, compared with the original survey. But this is self-reported and actual use of antibiotics could not be measured. This approach, that is the encouraging of students to be creative and competitive, with the production of artworks of a very high standard, serves as one small contribution to the fight against antibiotic misuse and AMR.

Examples of seven of the shortlisted videos, including the winning film are available online as listed in the filmography.

Filmography

Antibiotics: things we should understand (*Kangshengsu: Kai liaojie de naxie shier* 抗生素：该了解的那些事儿), dir. Li Hongwei, Tianjin Medical University, 2016, https://mediacentral.ucl.ac.uk/Play/16566, accessed 18 March 2019.

Cartoon bugs, dir. Wang Feng, Tianjin Medical University, 2016, https://mediacentral.ucl.ac.uk/Play/16561, accessed 18 March 2019.

Chinese & English Graffiti style, dir. Li Jia *et al.*, Nanjing University of Chinese Medicine, 2016, https://mediacentral.ucl.ac.uk/Play/16558, accessed 18 March 2019.

Hand painting, dir. Chen Jie *et al.*, Nanjing Medical University, 2016, https://mediacentral. ucl.ac.uk/Play/16565, accessed 18 March 2019.

King Bac (Junwang 菌王*)*, dir. Yao Hao, Fudan University, 2016, https://mediacentral.ucl. ac.uk/Play/16570, accessed 18 March 2019.

Little Girl in Pharmacy, dir. Tang Wenlu *et al.*, Shanghai Medical College of Fudan University, 2016, https://mediacentral.ucl.ac.uk/Play/16555, accessed 18 March 2019.

Paperman History, Zhang Jingrong, Kunming Medical University, 2016, https://mediacen tral.ucl.ac.uk/Play/16563, accessed 18 March 2019.

Bibliography

Chang, J., Ye, D., Lv, B. *et al.* (2017) Sale of Antibiotics Without a Prescription at Community Pharmacies in Urban China: A Multicentre Cross-Sectional Survey, *Journal of Antimicrobial Chemotherapy*, 72: 1235–42.

Laxminarayan, R., Duse, A., Wattal, C., Zaidi, A.K., Wertheim, H.F., Sumpradit, N. *et al.* (2013) Antibiotic Resistance – the Need for Global Solutions, *The Lancet Infectious Diseases*, 13: 1057–98.

Li, Y., Xu, J., Wang, F., Wang, B., Liu, L., Hou, W. *et al.* (2012) Overprescribing in China, Driven by Financial Incentives, Results in Very High Use of Antibiotics, Injections, and Corticosteroids, *Health Affairs (Millwood)*, 31: 1075–82.

Ranji, S.R., Steinman, M.A., Shojania, K.G. and Gonzales, R. (2008) Interventions to Reduce Unnecessary Antibiotic Prescribing: A Systematic Review and Quantitative Analysis, *Medical Care*, 46: 847–62.

Review on Antimicrobial Resistance (2014) *Antimicrobial Resistance: Tackling a Crisis for the Health and Wealth of Nations*, London: Review on Antimicrobial Resistance.

Reynolds, L. and McKee, M. (2009) Factors Influencing Antibiotic Prescribing in China: An Exploratory Analysis, *Health Policy*, 90: 32–6.

Sun, Q., Tärnberg, M., Zhao, L., Lundborg, C.S., Song, Y., Grape, M. *et al.* (2014) Varying High Levels of Faecal Carriage of Extended-spectrum Beta-lactamase Producing Enterobacteriaceae in Rural Villages in Shandong, China: Implications for Global Health, *PLoS One*, 9: e113121.

Wang, X.M., Peng, D.D., Wang, W. *et al.* (2017) Massive Misuse of Antibiotics by University Students in All Regions of China: Implications for National Policy, *International Journal of Antimicrobial Agent*, 50: 441–6.

Wei, X., Zhang, Z., Walley, J.D. *et al.* (2017) Effect of a Training and Educational Intervention for Physicians and Caregivers on Antibiotic Prescribing for Upper Respiratory Tract Infections in Children at Primary Care Facilities in Rural China: A Cluster-Randomised Controlled Trial, *The Lancet Global Health*, 5: e1258–e67.

World Health Organisation (2012) *The Evolving Threat of Antimicrobial Resistance: Options for Action*, Geneva: WHO Library Cataloguing-in-Publication Data.

Xiao, Y.H. and Li, L.J. (2013) Legislation of Clinical Antibiotic Use in China, *Lancet Infectious Diseases*, 13: 189–91.

12 Queer comrades

Digital video documentary and LGBTQ health activism in China

Hongwei Bao

In July 2017, a gay man from Central China's Henan Province, identified by his surname as Yu, won an apology and compensation from a mental hospital which had administered so-called 'conversion therapy', a pseudo-scientific medical treatment designed to turn gay people straight, to him without his consent. He was admitted to the hospital by his wife and relatives in 2015 and was forced to take medicine and have injections over a period of 19 days. Although the court found that being forced into a mental institution infringed Yu's rights, insofar as he did not pose a danger to society, the ruling did not express an opinion on whether it was right for the hospital to practise gay conversion therapy (BBC News 2017). The success of the court case was celebrated by some as reaffirming the depathologisation of homosexuality since the removal of homosexuality from the third edition of the *Chinese Classification of Mental Disorders*, CCMD-3 (*Zhongguo jingshen jibing fenlei fang'an yu zhenduan biaozhun* 中国精神疾病分类方案与诊断标准, 第三版) in 2001. However, for others, it serves as yet another reminder of the ambiguous, and often problematic, status of homosexuality in China's public health discourse. The case also highlights some of the constraints and promises of health activism in contemporary China, whether practised by individuals such as Yu himself or through organised collective action, in this case represented by the 'rescue operation' carried out by the Guangzhou-based PFLAG (Parents and Friends of Lesbians and Gays) China and the legal support provided by the LGBTQ Rights Advocacy China. The collective action aimed at fighting for Lesbian, Gay, Bisexual, Transgender and Queer (LGBTQ) health rights, often carried out by Non-Governmental Organisations (NGOs), is the focus of this chapter.

In this chapter, I examine health activism in the People's Republic of China by focusing on China's LGBTQ community. Using *Queer Comrades* (*Tongzhi yi fanren* 同志亦凡人), a Beijing-based queer community video streaming website as a case study, I discuss some of the tactics that China's LGBTQ communities have adopted for health communication, including the strategic use of digital video (DV) documentaries by a community NGO and video streaming website, and examine how health activism effectively combined with media and community activism can help to build communities and promote LGBTQ rights while educating the public.[1]

Depathologising and repathologising homosexuality

Homosexuality is widely considered to have been depathologised in China since 2001. However, such 'depathologisation' is only partial. The CCMD-3 distinguishes between two types of homosexuality: ego syntonic homosexuality, i.e. those who feel comfortable with their sexual identity, and ego dystonic homosexuality, i.e. those who do not (Kang 2012). What constitutes 'feeling comfortable' or being 'in harmony with oneself' (*ziwo hexie*自我和谐), has only been vaguely defined and is thus open to interpretation. The CCMD-3 stipulates that ego-syntonic homosexuality is normal and requires no treatment. However, those who feel 'anxious, depressed, conflicted' about their sexual identity, and those who 'seek change of gender and sexual identity through treatment', are still seen as suffering from mental disorders (Zhou 2009: 125). This understanding of homosexuality is still prevalent in China today and it provides justification for medical and psychological interventions to 'treat' homosexuality.

A recommended text for mental health education, *Zixun xinlixue* 咨询心理学 (*Consulting Psychology*) (Qiu 2013) published by the Guangdong Higher Education Press, describes homosexuality as a 'disorder' (Norton 2016). The textbook recommends four ways of giving treatment: changing one's lifestyle and circle of friends so as to make a radical break with the past, forming a platonic relationship with a person of the opposite sex, using heterosexual images and audio recordings to 'transfer' one's sexual desire to the opposite sex, and finally, 'repulsion therapy', i.e. inducing nausea with forced vomiting or fear of electrocution when homoerotic thoughts emerge (BBC News 2017). The court case mentioned at the beginning of this chapter involves 'repulsion therapy', otherwise known as conversion therapy, aversion therapy, or reparative therapy. In this particular case, Yu was strapped to a hospital bed and force-fed drugs for 19 days (Beech 2016). The practice of using electroshock for conversion therapy on LGBTQ people in China is widely documented, including by a Chinese LGBTQ community webcast documentary *Cures That Kill* (*shenglai tongzhi* 生来同志) (dir. Wei Xiaogang 魏小刚, 2011), a UNDP and USAID report on LGBTQ issues in China (UNDP and USAID 2014), and a UK television documentary titled *China's Gay Shock Therapy* (Channel 4 2015).

In a book titled *Zhongguo tongxinglian yanjiu* 中国同性恋研究 (*Studies on Chinese Homosexuality*) published in 2005, one of the authors, Dr Lu, a neurologist from Nanjing Medical University, documented case studies of treating homosexuality by injecting 'gay patients' with apomorphine, a drug that induces nausea, and requiring them to keep a diary frequently checked by doctors (Liu and Lu 2005; Bao 2012). According to the book, Dr Liu gave advice to 2,534 gay 'patients' from 1987 to 1997. Among the 1,000 gay 'patients' whom he treated with his 'guided corrective psychotherapy', 79.8% came to him of their own accord, and 20.2% were referred by others, including family members and relatives. Among the 82 'patients' that he treated, a one-year follow-up study suggested that 13.5% had 'overall recovered'; 13.5% made 'considerable progress';

39% made 'some progress'; 34% 'showed no sign of change' (Liu and Lu 2005: 277). These statistics, problematic as they are, shed light on the precarious mental health of LGBTQ people in the 1980s and 1990s, as well as the pathologisation of homosexuality itself.

The medical, psychological, and psychiatric treatment of homosexuality in China stems from a deeply rooted belief that homosexuality is a disease and a form of mental disorder. This idea had its origins variously in the translation of Western theories of psychology and medical science into Chinese in the Republican era (Chiang 2010; Sang 2003; Kang 2009), in Maoist understanding of homosexuals as 'hooligans' (*liumang* 流氓) whose mentality and behaviour was incompatible with the socialist mindset required by the state, and in post-Mao Chinese intellectuals' obsession with a highly selective body of works in Western psychology, psychiatry, and medical science often equated with scientific objectivity and authority. The governance of non-heteronormative sexuality is not only a matter of public health, with its agenda of producing modern and healthy citizens, but also a concern for the state to establish a heteronormative, family-oriented and socially conservative moral and social order (Jeffreys 2006; Jeffreys and Yu 2015).

In this context, the high profile of mental health issues in China's LGBTQ community is hardly surprising. According to a national survey published by the United Nations Development Programme (UNDP) in 2016, only around 5% of LGBTQ people surveyed had chosen to 'come out', i.e. to disclose their sexual orientation and gender identity to family, friends, and the wider public. Gender and sexuality-based discrimination occurs most frequently in families (56.1%), followed by school (39.6%), and workplace (21%). Over 70% of LGBTQ people have been emotionally troubled by their sexual orientation and gender identity (UNDP 2016: 26–7). Some LGBTQ people have sought medical and psychological treatment; others have even attempted suicide. A survey of 1,000 gay men and lesbians in China by mental health experts found that 40% had attempted suicide, while a 2002 survey found that 33% of gays and lesbians had unsuccessfully attempted suicide. A mental health survey of 200 gay men, published in 2008, found that among them, 45% had anxiety symptoms and 57.5% had symptoms of depression (UNDP and USAID 2014: 40). There seems to be a strong correlation between the inability to reconcile with and articulate one's gender and sexual identity and LGBTQ mental ill-health.

As in many other countries, HIV/AIDS and other sexually transmitted infections (STIs) have posed serious threats to the lives and health of many LGBTQ people in China. The specificity of China lies in the simultaneity, or even overlap, of LGBTQ and HIV/AIDS issues, to such an extent that the gay identity, not long after it emerged in China's public discourse, became pathologised and stigmatised because of its close association with HIV/AIDS. This was hardly surprising because LGBTQ issues could only be legitimately talked about in relation to HIV/AIDS prevention in China's public discourse. It is worth noting that HIV/AIDS cases have spread rapidly since the identification of China's first reported case of HIV/AIDS in Beijing in 1985. Perceptions of HIV/AIDS have since evolved from a disease of 'the Other' – foreigners, minorities, and rural, peripheral, disadvantaged and vulnerable groups of people – to an epidemic that threatens the general populace (Yu 2012: 3). Despite this shift, gay people are still referred to as Men Who Have Sex with Men (MSMs) (*nan xingxingwei zhe* 男男性行为者) and are considered a high-risk group for HIV/AIDS infection in public health discourse. In 2006, the Ministry of Health pledged to send AIDS prevention volunteers to LGBTQ groups and also included MSMs in its Five-Year Plan. By 2008, the Chinese government had launched the first national programme devoted to the prevention of HIV/AIDS among MSMs (Hildebrandt 2012: 852). China's Health and Family Planning Commission (2015) officially estimates the prevalence of HIV/AIDS among MSMs to be 7.7% in 2015.[2] MSMs are estimated to represent over a quarter of new reported infections each year (UNAID 2013). The association of HIV with homosexuality has seriously stigmatised LGBTQ people, but it has also produced some unintended consequences of encouraging LGBTQ community building and promoting health activism.

LGBTQ health activism

Health activism is usually understood as 'action that involves a challenge to the existing order whenever it is perceived to influence people's health negatively or has led to an injustice or an inequality' (Laverack 2013: 137). Health activism has had a very significant influence on the Chinese healthcare system and national policy on health and well-being. In the past under China's socialist system, public health issues were taken care of by the Chinese state, and citizens were officially entitled to equal health rights. With the gradual deregulation and privatisation of the public health sector, together with an increasing awareness of health rights and citizen power, more and more ordinary citizens have taken action to fight for their health rights and to seek to change flawed public health policies. During the SARS (Severe Acute Respiratory Syndrome) epidemic in 2013, many Chinese citizens organised themselves in order to compel disclosure of government-censored information about the epidemic, pressure national and local governments to take quick actions against the spread of the epidemic, and help local communities to survive the epidemic (Yu 2009). In 2007, some citizens in Xiamen held a demonstration to protest against the construction of a chemical factory because they believed that the chemical PX (short for para-xylene) would be harmful to their health. This organised action, known as the 'PX-Incident' in China, successfully halted the project and served as yet another of the increasing number of successful instances of health activism in China today (Tang 2008).

To date, LGBTQ health in China has been primarily discussed in relation to HIV/AIDS. Perhaps not surprisingly, LGBTQ health activism in China has mostly been seen as HIV/AIDS prevention and treatment, and in relation to the state's control of civil society (Hildebrandt 2012, 2013; Jones 1999, 2007; Wei 2015). In an era when HIV/AIDS posed a tremendous danger to the LGBTQ community, and when LGBTQ identity was reduced to a pathologised and stigmatised MSM identity, the scholarly attention paid to HIV/AIDS was fully justified.

However, given that necessary international, national, and community resources have been pooled into HIV/AIDS prevention and treatment, and that China is no longer one of the high-risk countries, with a low national prevalence at 0.037% in 2015 (China Health and Family Planning Commission 2015), it is high time to pay attention to other health issues troubling the LGBTQ community, including sexual and reproductive health, as well as mental and psychological health.

Despite their ambiguous legal status and the difficulty of getting official registration as legitimate organisations in China, in addition to the Chinese government's tightened control over international support for China's civil societies through the Foreign NGO Law passed in 2016, NGOs play a vital role in health activism in China, especially in relation to HIV/AIDS (Hildebrandt 2013). China's HIV/AIDS crisis provided political as well as economic opportunities for many LGBTQ NGOs in China. As international HIV/AIDS funding began to enter China in the early 2000s, LGBTQ NGOs started to mushroom throughout the country. By 2012 more than 100 LGBTQ organisations had been established in various parts of mainland China (Hou 2014). It was estimated in 2014 that there was some semblance of an organised LGBTQ group in every major Chinese city (UNDP and USAID 2014). Because of the specific way in which HIV/AIDS funds are distributed (international funds have to be channelled through the Chinese government, primarily the National Centre for Disease Control (CDC), and then trickled down to local governments and NGOs), the HIV/AIDS NGOs in China have become increasingly dependent, financially and politically, on different levels of the Chinese government. Over time, different arrangements with the Chinese government have helped to shape NGOs in diverse ways. Some become partners of the state and shun gay rights advocacy, eventually getting 'de-pinked' HIV/AIDS NGOs; some act in partnership with the state but maintain a focus on gay rights advocacy; some focus on gay rights advocacy and neither partner with nor challenge the state. Very few NGOs challenge the state and focus solely on gay rights advocacy (Chua and Hildebrandt 2013: 1597–9). These different configurations of power relations shape the agenda and scope of health activism for China's LGBTQ NGOs.

Beginning in 2012, many international HIV/AIDS–related donors, including the Global Fund and the Gates Foundation, began to withdraw from China, partly because of China's established status as an 'upper middle-income country' (UNDP and USAID 2014: 51), partly as a result of the contained situation of the HIV/AIDS epidemic in China, and more importantly, because of increasing controls over the activities of international NGOs by the Chinese government. This has proven to be both a challenge and an opportunity for China's LGBTQ community. As many HIV/AIDS–focused NGOs disintegrate or change direction, an increasing number of LGBTQ NGOs have begun to devote their attention to identity building, community service, and public education. An example in case is the Shenyang Consultation Centre for AIDS and Health Services (*Shenyang aizhi yuanzhu jiankang zixun fuwu zhongxin* 沈阳爱之援助健康咨询服务中心, which is concerned both with LGBTQ health and LGBTQ community building. Since 2011, in collaboration with 16 LGBTQ grassroots organisations in Northeast China, the Centre has organised annual Northeast Gay Culture Festivals (*Dongbei tongxinglian wenhuajie* 东北同性恋文化节) and various other activities locally, regionally, and nationally. Some of the activities include Dalian Gay Pride Hiking (*Dalian caihong tubu* 大连彩虹徒步), a cross-dressing beauty contest, the Northeast Gay Relatives Talkfest (*Dongbei tongxinglian qinyou kentanhui* 东北同性恋亲友恳谈会), lesbians' rainbow weddings, a rainbow flag relay race across Northeast China, and gay rainbow cycling (UNDP and USAID 2014: 48).

LGBTQ health activism has thus shifted from a sole focus on HIV/AIDS prevention and support to community building and public education. In the process, there has been a reconfigured relationship between international funding support, the Chinese government, and LGBTQ NGOs. There has also been a deepened understanding of the diversity of the LGBTQ community and the disparate health needs of the community. Many NGOs have concluded that LGBTQ health issues are deeply connected to broad social and cultural issues; an improvement of LGBTQ physical and psychological health not only requires identity and community building but rights advocacy and public education as well. In the next section, I focus on Queer Comrades, a Beijing-based LGBTQ community video streaming website, and the ways in which it engages in health activism.

DV documentary and LGBTQ health activism

Founded in 2007, Queer Comrades (*tongzhi yi fanren* 同志亦凡人), originally named 'Queer as Folk Beijing' in English, is an independent LGBTQ video streaming website that aims to document queer culture and raise LGBTQ awareness in China.[3] It is one of the longest running and most popular community video streaming websites for China's LGBTQ community, with more than 20 million hits for its videos hosted on mainstream websites and an average of 15,000 hits on its own website every day (Deklerck and Wei 2015: 24). It regularly updates community news in text and three-to-five-minute short videos. It also hosts talk show programmes and makes community documentaries. Its programmes are mostly disseminated via its own website and on some major streaming websites in China and abroad including Sina, Tudou, and YouTube, often subject to frequent Internet censorship. Some programmes have been made into DVDs and sold at various screenings and fund-raising events.

Queer Comrades is a project administered by the Beijing Gender Health Education Institute (BGHEI) (*Beijing jiande jiankang jiaoyu zhongxin* 北京纪安德健康教育中心), a Beijing-based LGBTQ community NGO.[4] Wei Xiaogang 魏小刚 (aka Wei Jiangang 魏建刚) is the director of the BGHEI and many Queer Comrades programmes, and Stijn Deklerck, a Belgian national, is the producer of Queer Comrades.[5] Queer Comrades videos were predominantly made by Xiaogang, Deklerck, and a couple of regular film crew members, helped by community volunteers. Queer Comrades is mostly self-funded or supported by international foundations and organisations such as the Dutch Embassy in China, the Ford Foundation, and the European Union (Tan 2016: 45).

Queer Comrades is not the first, or the only, LGBTQ media platform in China to use digital media to engage in health activism. It is, however, one of the most successful organisations that consciously and effectively uses DV documentaries for health education, community building, rights advocacy and public education. It draws on, and forms part of, China's ongoing digital video revolution and the New Documentary Movement.

China's New Documentary Movement, which started in the early 1990s, witnessed a group of filmmakers including Wu Wenguang 吴文光 who departed from the highly orchestrated realism associated with state film and television studios and experimented with low-budget, experimental, and spontaneous filmmaking characterised by 'on-the-spot realism' (Berry and Rofel 2010: 5). These filmmakers also shifted the subject matter of their films from state sanctioned topics to the lives of people at the margins of society. The movement received a significant boost when the mini DV camera entered China in about 1997 (p. 8). The relative affordability and 'lightness' (Voci 2010), both in terms of weight and of technical and aesthetic qualities, of DV cameras have encouraged professional and amateur filmmakers alike to pick up their own cameras and document the lives they are most familiar with or concerned about, while the fast expansion of personal computers and the Internet in Chinese households has made it possible for these films to reach a wider audience. A variety of film festivals in China, including the Beijing Independent Film Festival, the Nanjing Independent Film Festival, the Yunfest, the Beijing Queer Film Festival, as well as numerous international film festivals, have promoted the production and dissemination of DV films (Berry and Robinson 2017). DV documentaries, made by professionals and amateurs alike and disseminated through various channels, have mushroomed in China and dramatically changed China's media landscape.

The development of DV culture coincides and intersects with the development of LGBTQ activism in China. In a country where public assemblies, demonstrations, and protests are considered politically sensitive and therefore shunned, LGBTQ activism mostly takes place in private homes, commercial venues, education spaces, and in the forms of dinners, karaoke parties, sporting events, film screenings, academic lectures etc. A historical coincidence has also shaped the trajectory of LGBTQ activism in China. Many of the early LGBTQ activists were Beijing-based filmmakers, writers, performers, and artists, and they all saw the potential of DV films and participated in filmmaking and film festival organisation.[6] There is no better media form than films for safely conveying 'public secrets' to the public in public spaces (Donald 2000); and there is nothing like a film festival or screening event for bringing people together in a seemingly less political and non-confrontational manner to share their feelings and experiences, thus effectively constructing identities, communities, and politics. Beginning in 2001, the Beijing Queer Film Festival (BJQFF) has become one of the most symbolically significant expressions of LGBTQ activism in contemporary China (Bao 2017). The Queer Comrades team is among the organisers and active participants of the BJQFF and the China Queer Film Festival Tour. Working closely together, China's LGBTQ Movement and the New

Documentary Movement have had a significant impact on the politics and aesthetics of Queer Comrades and on the health activism in which it engages.

The politics of representation

The popularity of the Queer Comrades webcast site owes as much to what it excludes as to what it includes. It excludes stigmatised, negative, and 'othered' representations of homosexuality and celebrates positive and diverse self-representations of LGBTQ people in China, and this has to do with the politics of representation: that is, with who represents whom and in what ways. Chao Shi-Yan (2010) and Luke Robinson (2012, 2015) have identified a key shift in the representation of homosexuality in DV documentaries. As more and more LGBTQ people take up DV cameras to make their own films, the film aesthetics and the queer subjectivity they construct have also undergone significant changes; 'the result is the emergence of a queer subject whose sexuality is less performed and documented than incorporated and networked' (Robinson 2015: 294). Most of Queer Comrades' production crew are self-identified LGBTQ people deeply committed to the LGBTQ community. They speak for, to, and as members of the LGBTQ community, rather than trying to cater to the voyeuristic gaze of the public. This is bound to have a tremendous impact on how LGBTQ identity and community is represented.

Producer Deklerck and Director Wei stated the mission of Queer Comrades in the following way:

> With our webcast, we show empowering LGBT images: our audience sees people who are not ashamed of their sexual orientation, people who are proud of who they are, people who talk openly about issues that our audience members might be struggling with themselves. We create a forum beyond taboos, a forum where people can gain positive insights into LGBT culture.
>
> (Deklerck and Wei 2015: 19)

Indeed, most of the Queer Comrades videos present positive images of the LGBTQ community. Take the first season for example: eleven talk shows, from April to June 2007, interviewed a number of LGBTQ celebrities, Chinese and international, and covered a wide range of topics, including so-called 'fag hags', 'gaydar', LGBTQ magazines, queer racism, drag culture, queer film, gay websites, gay athletes, lesbian sex, gay Shanghai, and the pink economy. The hosts and guests appeared confident, happy, and LGBTQ identified; the queer life the shows portrayed was diverse, colourful, and dynamic (Figure 12.1). If we consider how homosexuality was stereotypically and negatively portrayed in mainstream media and perceived by the wider society at a time overshadowed by HIV/AIDS, such positive representations were revolutionary. The Chinese title of the show, *tongzhi yi fanren* 同志亦凡人 (literally Queers as Ordinary People) and the English title at the time, 'Queer as Folk Beijing' vividly capture the longing for the 'ordinariness' of queer life without stereotyping and spectacularising it.

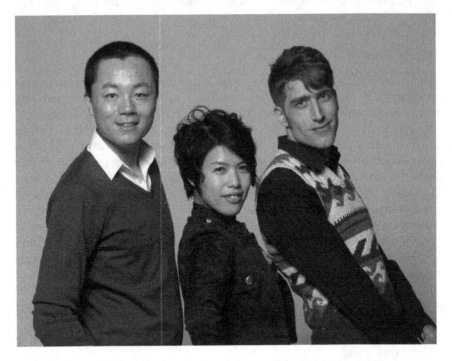

Figure 12.1 Queer Comrades talk show hosts, Xiaogang, Eva and Stijn, 2009

Source: Photo credit: Wei Xiaogang

Perhaps the queer life the shows represent is not so 'ordinary' after all. At a time when most LGBTQ people in China stay closeted and remain stigmatised, and many lead a precarious life affected by the stigma of being members of sexual minorities and by China's endorsement of neoliberal capitalism, such representations can only reflect a minority of queer lives, mostly those who are young, good-looking, urban, confident and middle-class, well-educated and widely travelled, multilingual, and cosmopolitan, partly because they were the ones who dared to 'come out' at the time. This is also evidenced by a large percentage of the production crew and interviewees being international expats or diaspora Chinese living in Chinese cities. In a city such as Beijing with a fast-developing pink economy, this is a niche market not to be missed and Queer Comrades has made a timely pitch for this market. As a result, some of the screening events and parties took place in relatively expensive bars and clubs in Chaoyang District, where many foreign embassies and international businesses are located. But the cost of consumption and the language barriers (English was the main working language) effectively prevented some local LGBTQ people from attending these events. Nevertheless, most LGBTQ people in China who access the video through online streaming can reasonably imagine an urban and cosmopolitan queer culture for themselves through the video viewing and sharing experience.

There has been criticism about the 'mainstreaming' of the programme, in that the show resembles a homonormative, middle-class, consumer culture in the West (Deklerck 2017; Robinson 2015). Addressing the use of traditional broadcasting techniques (the TV talk show format in this case) in some LGBTQ documentaries, Robinson (2015: 293) points out the complexity and ambiguity of the term 'mainstream' in the Chinese context. Queer Comrades, a video streaming website independent of the state, addresses politically sensitive issues; besides, the show is primarily funded by its producers and by NGOs, and made available online to the community for free. Seen in this light, Queer Comrades is far from being part of the 'mainstream'. Deklerck (2017) identifies some 'queer moments' in Queer Comrades, and comments on the specificity of queer politics in China, which cannot be reduced to the binary of gay identity politics (which advocates a 'coming out' strategy based on an essentialised notion of gay identity) and queer politics (which advocates a coalition politics for all gender and sexual minorities outside of mainstream gender and sexual norms), and which can best be described as 'nomadic activism', in the words of Lisa Rofel (2013). Both Robinson and Deklerck raise valid points, but they also risk romanticising LGBTQ activism in China as markedly Chinese and intrinsically subversive. I recognise the urban, middle-class and even consumerist and lifestyle bias of some Queer Comrades programmes, especially in the first season. However, starting from the second season, Queer Comrades has begun to pay more attention to the diversity of LGBTQ lives and experiences, including those from rural, working-class, and ethnic minority backgrounds.

It is useful to situate Queer Comrades in the context of a neoliberal 'desiring China' (Rofel 2007), which produces legitimate desires and desiring subjects demanded by the market economy promoted by the Chinese state. In legitimising some specific modes of queer desires, Queer Comrades excludes others. This is a type of 'homonormativity', understood as the gentrification of queer desires and the alignment of queer desires with the needs of the state and the market (Duggan 2004). In challenging heteronormativity, Queer Comrades also participates in, and contributes to, a transnational neoliberal hegemonic formation in which China takes part.

Having said this, the 'utopian' nature of Queer Comrades should not be overlooked. Even if these shows only represent a small LGBTQ minority in China, most of whom live sheltered lives largely free from real social problems, and thus seem utopian to many, they still break the monotony of the present and conjure up aspirational imaginations for many. As José Muñoz comments on the importance of imagination for a queer future, 'queerness is a structuring and educated mode of desiring that allows us to see and feel beyond the quagmire of the present'; it is 'essentially about the rejection of a here and now and an insistence on potentiality or concrete possibility for another world' (Munoz 2009: 1). Writing about lesbian activism in China, Anna Huang (2017: 226) also argues against 'pragmatic reformist politics' and for 'a queer politics of imagination'. Seen in this light, the representation of queer lifestyles in Queer Comrades can also be read as a strategy of activism that gives LGBTQ people in China hope and imagination, although such optimism can be 'cruel': insofar as it inspires aspirations for a good life, it also defines and sometimes confines such aspirations (Berlant 2011).

The 'technical quality' of Queer Comrades is worth noting. On the one hand, the format and aesthetics of Queer Comrades resemble the news, talk shows, and documentaries on mainstream television in China. For example, its talk show programmes 'blend elements of the chat show – studio shoots, the use of the host, and informal discussion with guests – with more classic *vérité* sequences and even elements of the music video' (Robinson 2015: 297). Its news programme uses voiceover which tries to imitate a state television newscaster but has traces of amateurism which can be easily discerned by the audience. LGBTQ identified journalists and newscasters report in the studio or on the street. Ordinary people are interviewed spontaneously and often without preparation. These programmes are reminiscent of the TV journalism influenced by China's New Documentary Movement (Berry *et al.* 2010) and its associated on-the-spot realist aesthetics of *xianchang* 现场 (Robinson 2012). The 'mainstreaming' of Queer Comrades in terms of programme format and aesthetics can be interpreted as reflecting LGBTQ people's wish to become normalised and accepted by mainstream Chinese society. But 'mainstreaming' can also be read as a subversive strategy. If we recall how LGBTQ people are usually portrayed as deviant, abnormal, and anonymous in mainstream Chinese television, Queer Comrades certainly turns against such representations: LGBTQ people's faces are not covered by mosaic; their voices are not disguised; their names are not hidden. They are mostly healthy, happy, articulate, and confident in front of the camera. They are, as the Chinese title of the video streaming website suggests, 'ordinary people'. In this sense, the use of 'mainstream' formats and aesthetics serves to 'queer' the mainstream.

In a parody of a news programme entitled *Breaking News from a Homosexual China*, Queer Comrades reports the discovery of a 'disease' called 'heterosexuality' in a hypothetically queer world. 'Ordinary citizens' interviewed expressed their lack of understanding of and even voiced their disgust against the 'abnormality' of heterosexuality. A 'medical expert' named Sun Haiyin 孙嗨淫 (a spoof of the name of the homophobic media celebrity Sun Haiying 孙海英), performed by queer activist Fan Popo 范坡坡, explained ways to prevent and to cure the 'disease'. This video is obviously a spoof of a mainstream television report on homosexuality. By replacing 'homosexuality' with 'heterosexuality' in news reporting, the video reveals the unconscious bias of a heteronormative society under the assumed scientific and journalistic 'objectivity'.

To avoid censorship, Queer Comrades used to adopt a non-confrontational political strategy by avoiding politically sensitive issues such as LGBTQ political rights. But after experiencing the forced closure of several editions of the Beijing Queer Film Festivals and the ILGA–Asia conference in Surabaya, Queer Comrades has now become more daring in clearly articulating a human rights agenda. However, such a political stance is quite rare and often ambiguous because survival is paramount.

Community participation and social engagement

Health communication is most effective when community participation is involved (Dutta 2011). Strategies created by communities for themselves can best address community health needs by forming a support network among community members and devising community-based strategies to solve these problems. Through actively participating in the process of health communication and activism, community members are empowered as responsible citizens and active agents in social changes. In the words of Deklerck and Wei, 'Queer Comrades aims to empower people to stand up for themselves and actively find solutions to the issues and problems they are dealing with in their lives' (Deklerck and Wei 2015: 32).

Queer Comrades does not avoid issues such as HIV/AIDS. In contrast to mainstream media which often take a condemnatory and moralising tone when reporting HIV/AIDS in the LGBTQ community, or regard LGBTQ identity solely as a pathologised and stigmatised MSM identity, Queer Comrades reports HIV/AIDS news in a positive light by focusing on community strength, tenacity, and solidarity in combatting HIV/AIDS. In the first season, Queer Comrades invited Professor Zhang Beichuan 张北川, a LGBTQ-friendly medical expert from Qingdao Medical University, to give tips about HIV/AIDS prevention. It also invited Dawei 大伟 (pseudonym), a gay man living with HIV/AIDS, to talk about his experience of fighting against HIV/AIDS. These individuals were celebrated in the programme as 'community heroes'. By placing individuals at the centre of the picture, while celebrating community strength and solidarity, Queer Comrades successfully communicates HIV/AIDs–related knowledge to the queer community.

In 2011, Queer Comrades made a documentary entitled *Cures That Kill* (*Shenlai tongzhi* 生来同志), which deals with the issue of LGBTQ mental health and 'conversion therapy'. Recognising that the root of conversion therapy lies in people's misunderstanding of homosexuality, both in and out of the community, Queer Comrades invites community members and mental health professionals to talk about their changing understandings of homosexuality. In interviews, several mental health professionals confessed their lack of understanding of, or even bias against, LGBTQ people before they met anyone from the community. A counsellor specifically mentioned her changing attitude from 'being able to tolerate in order to help these people' to eventually realising her deeply rooted prejudice and assumed moral high ground, thus being able to treat LGBTQ people as friends and learn from them. Two gay men, one Chinese and the other Dutch, narrated their experiences of receiving conversion therapy. Their experiences reveal the violence of medical, psychiatric, and religious institutions in forcing LGBTQ people to undergo conversion therapy; they also reveal that LGBTQ mental health is associated with complex social and cultural issues, such as loneliness and lack of emotional support, school bullying, family pressure for gay people to enter into heterosexual marriages, lack of access to correct information about sexuality, and lack of tolerance in evangelical religious communities. Queer Comrades suggests that these are social problems that require institutional or societal efforts to tackle, rather than individual psychological or psychiatric problems. This documentary has not only been shown inside the LGBTQ community, but also to mental health professionals in various parts of China and used as a tool for professional development and public education (Deklerck and Wei 2015: 25).

Most documentaries produced by Queer Comrades use mainstream TV documentary conventions such as interviews and talking heads. This is represented by *The Cream of the Queer Crop* (dir. Wei Xiaogang 2010), *Strong* (dir. Wei Xiaogang 2012), and *Chinese Closet* (dir. Fan Popo 范坡坡 2009). The significance of these documentaries lies in their unambiguous presentation of queer bodies and voices. 'Our refusal to use masking tools stems from the fact that the Chinese mainstream media often utilise these tools when interviewing LGBT people', Deklerck and Wei explain, 'it is for this reason that Queer Comrades has always promoted a very "out" LGBT identity'. (Deklerck and Wei 2015: 30). This serves as a strategy for 'digitally coming out': some LGBTQ people may not have the courage to come out to their parents, but they can come out to the community through DV films. These films, archived online and in DVDs, form part of China's ongoing LGBTQ history. In this sense, Queer Comrades is more than a video streaming website; it enables China's LGBTQ community to take shape, to present itself, and to make its own history.

Apart from community building, Queer Comrades also has a positive impact on mainstream Chinese society. Since 2011, the Beijing Gender Health Education Institute, in collaboration with Queer Comrades and other LGBTQ organisations, has been holding the China Media Rainbow Award Ceremony every year. At the ceremony, awards are given to journalists and media organisations which have given positive representations to LGBTQ issues, as well as individuals who have made significant contributions to China's LGBTQ community. The 2016 winners included *Vista* (*Kan tianxia* 看天下), Netease News (*Wangyi xinwen* 网易新闻), Phoenix Television (*Fenghuang weishi* 凤凰卫视), and *Global Times* (*Huanqiu shibao* 环球时报). Qiu Qiming 邱启明, a China Central Television (CCTV) (*Zhongyang dianshi tai* 中央电视台) newsreader, was given a Special Contribution Award for publicly supporting LGBTQ issues. By acting as a media watchdog and by encouraging mainstream media to pay attention to LGBTQ issues, the China Rainbow Award has become an important way in which the LGBTQ community influences mainstream media production and Chinese society.

Conclusion

This chapter has examined how LGBTQ community media such as Queer Comrades use documentaries and digital media platforms to engage in health activism. By producing DV films, and by using the digital platform to engage the community and the public, Queer Comrades has gone beyond a community NGO and has started to have an impact on China's media ecology and society. Also, by focusing on social, cultural, and community issues, and by encouraging community participation and involvement, Queer Comrades successfully communicates health issues to the LGBTQ community. If anything can be learned from Queer Comrades, it is that health issues are not simply individual problems that can be solved by medical, psychological, and psychiatric interventions; they are political and social issues that involve citizenship rights and societal support. In the recent past, immediately after homosexuality had been depathologised as a mental disorder, it was repathologised as an HIV/AIDS–related MSM identity in China. The process of depathologisation is a long, ongoing process that requires concerted efforts from the government, the society, and the community. Media, in particular community media, are playing a significant role in facilitating this process. After all, representation, by whom and in what way, matters significantly when it comes to identity, community, and health rights.

Notes

1 The Queer Comrades video streaming website: www.queercomrades.com, accessed 1 August 2017. Although the webcast programme was founded in 2007, its official website went online only on 1 January 2010. Prior to the establishment of its official website, the webcast programmes were mostly made available on mainstream websites, LGBT websites and video streaming websites.
2 This figure has been contested. A 2015 study in 11 major Chinese cities of more than 8,900 men who have sex with men shows the average prevalence of HIV infection to be 9.9%, with average incidence of 5.5 per 100 people, higher than the official figure (Shang and Zhang 2015).
3 The Chinese title (*tongzhi yi fanren* 同志亦凡人, literally meaning 'comrades as ordinary people') of the programme remains unchanged. The English title changed from *Queer as Folk Beijing* to *Queer Comrades* from the beginning of the third season in April 2009. *Tongzhi* 同志 (comrade) a term widely used in China's LGBT community to refer to themselves. For a discussion of the cultural politics of translating *tongzhi* and *tongzhi yi fanren*, see Bao (2011). For a history of the Queer Comrades video streaming website, see Deklerck and Wei (2015).
4 The webcast operated on its own in its first season from April to June 2007. In its second season, running from March 2008 to February, 2008, and third season onward starting in April 2009, the webcast operates as a project under the Beijing Gender Health Education Institute (Deklerck and Wei 2015).
5 Wei Xiaogang is also known as Wei Jiangang. Wei uses the name Xiaogang in most of his Queer Comrades productions and Jiangang primarily as director of the Beijing Gender Health Education Institute.
6 The names I have in mind include Cui Zi'en, Fan Popo, He Xiaopei, Wei Xiaogang, Shitou, and Mingming. For a brief account of the queer filmmaking scenes in contemporary China, see Bao (2018).

Filmography

Breaking News from a Homosexual China (*Shendu baodao* 深度报道), dir. Queer Comrades 同志亦凡人, 2014.
Chinese Closet (*Guizu* 柜族), dir. Fan Popo 范坡坡, 2009.
Cures That Kill (*Shenglai tongzhi* 生来同志), dir. Wei Xiaogang 魏小刚, 2011.
The Cream of the Queer Crop (*Tongzhi tatata tatata* 同志他他他他她她她), dir. Wei Xiaogang 魏小刚, 2010.

In the Name of Life (*Yi shengming de mingyi* 以生命的名义), China Central Television, 2005.
Strong (*Ni ruci jianqiang* 你如此坚强), dir. Wei Xiaogang 魏小刚, 2012.

Bibliography

Altman, D. (1997) Global Gaze/Global Gays, *GLQ: A Journal of Lesbian and Gay Studies*, 3: 417–36.

Bao Hongwei (2011) Queer Comrades: Transnational Popular Culture, Queer Sociality and Socialist Legacy, *English Language Notes*, 49 (1): 131–7.

———— (2012) On Not to Be Gay: Aversion Therapy and Transformation of the Self in Postsocialist China, *Health, Culture and Society*, 3 (1): 133–49.

———— (2017) Queer as Catachresis: The Beijing Queer Film Festival in Cultural Translation, in C. Berry and L. Robinson (eds.) *Chinese Film Festivals: Sites of Translation*, London: Palgrave Macmillan, pp. 67–88.

———— (2018) From "Celluloid Comrades" to "Digital Video Activism": Queer Filmmaking in Postsocialist China, *JOMEC Journal: Journalism, Media and Cultural Studies*, 12: 82–100.

BBC News (4 July 2017) Gay Chinese Man Wins Legal Battle Over Forced Conversion Therapy, www.bbc.co.uk/news/world-asia-40490946, accessed 1 August 2017.

Beech, H. (2016) *This Man Was Sectioned in China for Being Gay: Now He's Fighting Back*, http://time.com/4367925/china-lgbt-gay-conversion-therapy-rights/, accessed 1 August 2017.

Berlant, L. (2011) *Cruel Optimism*, Durham, NC: Duke University Press.

Berry, C. and Robinson, L. (eds.) (2017) *Chinese Film Festivals: Sites of Translation*, London: Palgrave Macmillan.

Berry, C. and Rofel, L. (2010) Introduction, in C. Berry *et al.* (eds.) *The New Chinese Documentary Movement: For the Public Record*, Hong Kong: Hong Kong University Press, pp. 3–14.

Berry, C. et al (eds) (2010) *The New Chinese Documentary Movement: For the Public Record*, Hong Kong: Hong Kong University Press.

Channel 4 (2016) Unreported World: China's Gay Shock Therapy, www.channel4.com/programmes/unreported-world/on-demand/60446-009, accessed 1 August 2017.

Chao Shi-Yan (2010) Coming Out of *the Box*, Marching as Dykes, in C. Berry *et al.* (eds.) *The New Chinese Documentary Movement: For the Public Record*, Hong Kong: Hong Kong University Press, pp. 77–96.

Chiang, H. (2010) Epistemic Modernity and the Emergence of Homosexuality in China, *Gender and History*, 22 (3): 629–57.

China Health and Family Planning Commission (2015) *2015 China AIDS Response Progress Report*, Beijing: China Health and Family Planning Commission.

Chua, L.J. and Hildebrandt, T. (2013) From Health Crisis to Rights Advocacy? HIV/AIDS and Gay Activism in China and Singapore, *International Society for Third Sector Research*, 25: 1583–605.

Deklerck, S. (2014) *Queer Comrades: A Visual Ethnographic Study of Activism in China's Contemporary LGBT Movement*, unpublished PhD thesis, University of Leuven.

————. (2017) Bolstering Queer Desires, Reaching Activist Goals: Practicing Queer Activist Documentary Filmmaking in Mainland China, *Studies in Documentary Film*, 11 (3): 232–47.

Deklerck, S. and Wei Xiaogang (2015) Queer Online Media and the Building of China's LGBT Community, in E.L. Engebretsen, and W.F. Schroeder (eds.) *Queer/Tongzhi China: New Perspectives on Research, Activism and Media Cultures*, Copenhagen: NIAS Press, pp. 18–34.

Donald, S.H. (2000) *Public Secrets, Public Spaces: Cinema and Civility in China*, Lanham, MD: Rowman & Littlefield.

Duggan, L. (2004) *The Twilight of Equality? Neoliberalism, Cultural Politics, and the Attack on Democracy*, Boston, MA: Beacon Press.

Dutta, M.J. (2011) *Communicating Social Change: Structure, Culture, and Agency*, New York: Routledge.

Hildebrandt, T. (2012) Development and Division: The Effect of Transnational Linkages and Local Politics on LGBT Activism in China, *Journal of Contemporary China*, 21 (77): 845–62.

———. (2013) *Social Organisations and the Authoritarian State in China*, Cambridge: Cambridge University Press.

Hou, H.L. (2014) LGBT Activism in Mainland China, https://www.solidarity-us.org/ node/4289#N1, accessed 1 September 2017.

Huang, A. (2017) Precariousness and the Queer Politics of Imagination in China, *Culture, Theory and Critique*, 58 (2): 226–42.

Jeffreys, E. (ed.) (2006) *Sex and Sexuality in China*, Abingdon: Routledge.

Jeffreys, E. and Yu, H. (2015) *Sex in China*, Cambridge: Polity.

Jones, R.H. (1999) Mediated Action and Sexual Risk: Searching for 'Culture' in Discourses of Homosexuality and AIDS Prevention in China, *Culture, Health and Sexuality*, 1 (2): 161–80.

———. (2007) Imagined Comrades and Imaginary Protections, *Journal of Homosexuality*, 53 (3): 83–115.

Kang Wenqing (2009) *Obsession: Male Same-Sex Relations in China, 1900–1950*, Hong Kong: Hong Kong University Press.

Kang Wenqing (2012) The Decriminalisation and Depathologisation of Homosexuality in China, in T.B. Weston and L.M. Jensen (eds) *China in and Beyond the Headlines*. Lanham: Rowman and Littlefield Publishers, pp. 231–48.

Laverack, G. (2013) *Health Activism: Foundations and Strategies*, London: Sage.

Lewis, B. and Lewis, J. (2015) *Health Communication: A Media and Cultural Studies Approach*, London: Palgrave.

Liu Dalin 刘达临 and Lu Longguang 鲁龙光 (2005) *Zhongguo tongxinglian yanjiu* 中国同性恋研究 (*Studies on Chinese Homosexuality*), Beijing: Zhongguo shehui chubanshe.

Munoz, J.E. (2009) *Cruising Utopia: The Then and There of Queer Futurity*, New York: New York University Press.

Norton, S. (2016) Woman Sues Chinese Education Ministry Over 2013 Textbook Describing Homosexuality as a 'Disorder', www.sbs.com.au/topics/sexuality/agenda/ article/2016/06/17/woman-sues-chinese-education-ministry-over-2013-textbook-describing-homosexuality, accessed 1 August 2017.

Qiu Hongzhong 邱鸿钟 (2013) *Zixun xinlixue* 咨询心理学 (Consulting Psychology), Guangzhou: Guangdong daodeng jiaoyu chubanshe.

Robinson, L. (2012) *Independent Chinese Documentary: From the Studio to the Street*, London: Palgrave Macmillan.

———. (2015) To Whom Do Our Bodies Belong? Being Queer in Chinese DV Documentary, in Z. Zhang and A. Zito (eds.) *DV Made China: Digital Subjects and Social Transformations After Independent Film*, Honululu: University of Hawaii Press, pp. 289–315.

Rofel, L. (2007) *Desiring China: Experiments in Neoliberalism, Sexuality, and Public Culture*, Durham, NC: Duke University Press.

———. (2013) Grassroots Activism: Non-Normative Sexual Politics in Postsocialist China, in W. Sun and Y. Guo (eds.) *Unequal China: The Political Economy and Cultural Politics of Inequality*, Abingdon: Routledge, pp. 154–67.

Sang, T.D. (2003) *The Emerging Lesbian: Female Same-Sex Desire in Modern China*, Chicago: The University of Chicago Press.

Shang Hong and Zhang Linqi (2015) MSM and HIV Infection in China, *National Science Review*, 2 (4): 388–91.

Tan Jia (2016) Aesthetics of Queer becoming: Comrade Yue and Chinese Community-Based Documentaries Online, *Critical Studies in Media Communication*, 33 (1): 38–52.

Tang Hao (2008) Xiamen PX: A Turning Point? www.chinadialogue.net/article/1626-Xiamen-PX-a-turning-point, accessed 1 August 2017.

UNAIDS (2013) *HIV in Asia and the Pacific: UNAIDS Report 2013*, Geneva: Joint United Nations Programme on HIV/AIDS.

UNDP (2016) *Being LGBT in China: A National Survey on Social Attitudes Towards Sexual Orientation, Gender Identity and Gender Expression*, Beijing: United Nations Development Programme.

UNDP and USAID (2014) *Beijing LGBT in Asia: China Country Report*, Bangkok: United Nations Programme.

Voci, P. (2010) *China on Video: Small Screen Realities*, New York: Routledge.

Wei Wei (2015) Queer Organising and HIV/AIDS Activism: An Ethnographic Study of a Local *Tongzhi* Organisation in Chengdu, in E.L. Engebretsen and W.F. Schroeder (eds.) *Queer/Tongzhi China: New Perspectives on Research, Activism and Media Cultures*, Copenhagen: NIAS Press, pp. 192–216.

Wei Xiaogang 魏小刚 (dir) (2011) *Cures that Kill* 生来同志. Beijing: Queer Comrades.

Yu Haiqing (2009) *Media and Cultural Transformation in China*, Abingdon: Routledge.

——— (2012) Governing and Representing HIV in China: A Review and an Introduction, *IJAPS*, 8 (1): 1–13.

Zheng Tiantian (2015) *Tongzhi Living: Men Attracted to Men in Postsocialist China*, Minneapolis, MN: University of Minnesota Press.

Zhou Dan 周丹 (2009) *Aiyue yu guixun: zhongguo xiandaixing zhong tongxinglian yuwang de fali xiangxiang* 爱悦与规训：中国现代性中同性恋欲望的法理想象 (*Pleasure and Discipline: The Legal Imagination of Same-Sex Desires in Chinese Modernity*), Nanning: Guangxi shifan daxue chubanshe.

13 Recovering from mental illness and suicidal behaviour in a culturally diverse context

The use of digital storytelling in cross-cultural medical humanities and mental health

Erminia Colucci and Susan McDonough

When we share our own stories, it makes me feel better! I feel more power in telling my own story. It is not shameful.

– (Kim, storyteller)

People from immigrant or refugee background access mental health services at lower rates than the local population (Minas *et al.* 2013; Colucci *et al.* 2014); socio-cultural and economic factors appear to contribute to this underuse (Whitley *et al.* 2006; Colucci *et al.* 2017). Mental health providers are struggling to provide services that are appropriate and accessible to increasingly culturally and linguistically diverse populations (NMHC 2014; DelVecchio Good and Hannah 2015).

Despite this persistent gap, the voices of individuals and families with migration or refugee experiences, who identify with minority ethno-cultural or faith communities, or prefer to speak a language other than English, are rarely heard in local mental health service planning or represented in governmental system reform debates. Relatively few mental health consumer and carer advocates have personal or family experience of migration and are in a position to lead conversations about diversity and cultural safety.

These are the concerns that informed the development of the small-scale community engagement project described here, which was conducted as part of an Australian national mental health initiative. The project provided people, who identified with the groups that the national initiative was designed to 'represent', with an opportunity to explore their personal perspectives, create a lasting record and, if they so wished, share this with others. We theorised that people with lived experience of mental ill-health, suicidal behaviour or emotional issues could influence wider public discourses on diversity and service delivery, as well as community responses to mental health and well-being issues, by telling their own story on their own terms. These narratives would function like windows onto local worlds and invite others to explore the links between 'personal troubles' and 'public issues' (Mills 1959: 15). In consultations with mental health consumers and carers from migrant and refugee backgrounds for another project (Diocera, Colucci, Minas, submitted), visual tools such as digital storytelling were identified as an especially powerful and effective way to engage directly with wider community members who prefer to speak languages other than English. These considerations led the coordinators to explore the possibilities of digital storytelling (DST).

Ten people of immigrant and refugee background, with a lived experience of mental health or emotional issues, participated in a four-day digital storytelling workshop, to create a story that expressed something about their personal encounters with mental ill-health and recovery. As many other DST projects have done before, this project used the power of first-person narratives and provided an opportunity for 'unheard voices to be heard' (LaMarre and Rice 2016: 5). The storytellers were supported to create their own accounts, share their experiences (in mainstream media, in policy and service settings, and for practitioner education), grow in self-confidence, and develop other capabilities.

The project was conducted as part of Mental Health in Multicultural Australia (MHiMA 2014)[1] and was designed in consultation with members of national consumer and carer representative working groups. Individuals from diverse cultural and linguistic backgrounds were invited to participate and explore any aspect of living with mental ill-health and recovery of importance to them. Community mental health practitioners and researchers coordinated the initiative and supported the well-being of participants for the duration of the project. Filmmakers from the Australian Centre for the Moving Image (ACMI) in Melbourne facilitated the workshop that helped each participant make his or her story idea a reality.

Participants learnt the basics of DST and received a copy of their own story in digital format. In the months following the workshop, a compilation DVD, *Finding our way*, featuring all ten stories was released and launched at public events. A national television news programme featured the stories on the national day that Australia celebrates multiculturalism. Two storytellers were interviewed about the project and their personal experiences by print and broadcast media agencies (Abo 2014; Jovic 2014; Price 2014; Savino 2014). Within weeks of completing the project, nine storytellers chose to make their story available on websites (MHiMA 2017; VTMH 2017) and six uploaded their story to a YouTube channel. A year later, stories from *Finding our way* were screened at a multicultural film festival where two storytellers also featured in a panel discussion (Colourfest 2015). Since this time, project coordinators and storytellers have shared the stories at community development events, academic lectures and workshops, health professional and social and cultural mental health conferences. Some storytellers continue to show these stories as part of their mental health advocacy and community education work. The stories have also been integrated into mental health cultural responsiveness education resources (see VTMH 2018).

This chapter describes the DST process and discusses its impact from the perspective of the two project coordinators (EC and SMcD) in consultation with six participants, five as storytellers and one support person. It also provides the perspective of a Mandarin-speaking participant in depth. The digital stories can be freely viewed at www.vtmh.org.au.

Visual methodologies, digital storytelling, and mental health

Visual methodologies offer a way to engage marginalised individuals from rarely consulted language and cultural groups (Colucci and Bhui 2015). DST is one of a range of participant-generated visual methodologies used in community development, health research, and service evaluation where participants are actively engaged in producing and interpreting the visual material that they create (Guillemin and Drew 2010).

The coordinators of this community engagement project wanted to offer people with personal or family migration and refugee experiences whose lives had been affected by mental health issues and emotional issues an opportunity to represent their experiences visually. We sought a personally empowering process that supported participants to produce accounts that could be used to inform conversations between service users, practitioners, and the broader community about diversity, mental health, and ways to support personal recovery.

DST is a well-established approach that has been shown to be an effective way to help individuals with few opportunities to be heard to explore intensely personal experiences and make meaningful multimedia presentations in a relatively short period of time. The DST method requires little or no pre-workshop technical know-how on the part of participants. Storytellers control every aspect of the stories that they create within a supportive workshop 'community' of other storytellers and story receivers.

The Digital Storytelling Program at ACMI uses an approach similar to the one pioneered by Lambert and Atchley in California in the 1990s. The methodology has seven core elements: identifying the story a person wants to tell; finding the emotional resonance of the story; describing a moment or moments when something changed; bringing the story to life in a visual way; exploring how voice and sound will enhance the story; and assembling the story (Lambert 2010). An editing software is used by the participants to create a story structure in a form that the creator may choose to share.

The priority placed on the person controlling how they present themselves, by organising their own ideas and directing the way the story elements are combined, is a fundamental tenet of the DST approach. Visual methods may provide a more effective way to tap the emotional aspects of a topic than verbal approaches alone. Images, especially ones created by participants, can evoke emotions and potentially facilitate the expression of personal feelings or attitudes (Pain 2011).

Hull and Katz argue that presenting one's own 'identities, circumstances and futures' in a digital story 'fosters agency' (2006: 44). As a method offering opportunities for self-expression and self-representation, DST is an especially effective way to reach 'traditionally powerless groups' (Kindon 2003: 115) and accessible to people who struggle to read, write or communicate using a dominant language.

Guillemin and Drew (2010) describe 'participant-generated visual methodologies', including DST, in terms of three production stages: before, during, and after. Conversations between facilitators and participants about protecting personal privacy and who owns any digital stories made in the workshop begin before image production. During the production phase, spoken words, images, music, and sound are arranged and edited. Audiences are already exerting an influence during this phase; workshop facilitators, fellow attendees, and the audience members whom the storyteller anticipates and imagines, all help to shape how the story is constructed. Finally, once the story is produced, the meaning that resides in the specific images and sounds, the narrative as a whole, the storyteller's circumstances, and the context in which the story was created becomes available for analysis and interpretation. This process may include participant-generated explanations, the interpretations of those who encounter the stories, and critical exploration of the knowledge perspectives 'deployed' and 'excluded' (Guillemin and Drew: 181–3). This chapter explores the ethical and practical considerations relevant to each of these phases.

A recent scoping review of 15 publications by De Vecchi and colleagues (2016) identified four broad ways in which DST has been used in mental health settings: as a mental health literacy intervention, e.g. with school students; as a way to teach interpersonal or technical skills to people who have experienced mental health issues; as a safe and supportive way to share personal lived experiences; or as a means of informing 'others', e.g. medical practitioners, by exposing them to stories that present the 'lifeworld' of persons 'living with a diagnosis of mental illness' (De Vecchi *et al.* 2016: 188–9). The latter two of these four ways resonate with the objectives of *Finding our way*. Drawing on our insights as project coordinators and participants, in the following section we describe the various steps of the project as well as explore the links between personal self-empowerment and capacity to contribute in public forums of advocacy and activism. Further information and reflections can be found in McDonough and Colucci (2019).

The project

Designing and developing the project

The project was designed and promoted as a participatory community project. Representing MHiMA, the project coordinators commissioned ACMI's DST Program to conduct the workshop in collaboration with them. This programme had conducted numerous community projects over many years, had the necessary facilities and equipment and could provide experienced filmmakers to facilitate the workshop and help edit the stories.

The agencies discussed ways to craft a culturally and emotionally safe, supportive, friendly workshop environment for storytellers, their support persons, the filmmakers/facilitators, and project coordinators where individual participants would take the lead in identifying what memories and experiences they wanted to represent and how. The usual workshop schedule was modified to four shorter working days across two weeks, instead of three full days in one week. No fees were payable by individuals and support persons for participating in the workshop. Other costs, such as transport to the venue and meals, were met by the funding agency so that individuals who faced ongoing challenges with daily living e.g. using public transport, or were on low income would not be disadvantaged. A well-equipped studio space, with nearby group and quiet rooms, was identified.

Recruiting and preparing participants

The project coordinators wanted to reach individuals living and coping with long-term mental health issues and social exclusion, of migrant or refugee background, who wanted to document their stories. This could include people who prefer to communicate in a language other than English. We approached mental health advocates whom we thought might be comfortable with discussing their lived experience. We also used our connections with community mental health agencies, bilingual practitioners, and cultural portfolio holders based at mental health services, and asked them to approach clients or former clients who might be interested in taking part.

We began looking for participants three months prior to commencing the workshop. Confirmed participants and nominated support persons were asked to come along to a group briefing session or to have a conference phone call with project coordinators and workshop facilitators in the weeks just preceding the workshop. Expectations were discussed, examples of other digital stories were shared and individual supports, including interpreters, were arranged. Family and other support persons were welcome to attend for part or the entire workshop if that was what the participant preferred. Participants were encouraged to start preparing their story and consider the images and ideas they might choose to represent in their story. They were reassured that no pre-existing computer or filmmaking skills were required.

Coordinators accepted individuals onto the project who had direct personal experience of emotional or mental health issues; were born overseas or born in Australia to overseas-born parents; who expressed a strong interest in telling a personal story of recovery; had grasped what the DST workshop process would involve; could commit to the proposed workshop schedule; and indicated that they were likely to want to share the digital story they created.

Conducting the workshop and launching the stories

A small group of filmmakers facilitated the workshop, guiding participants through the story writing and technical process (ACMI 2010), while coordinators and other support persons helped out as needed.

The DST workshop approach seeks to create 'transformative opportunities' (Lambert 2010: 24) that encourage peer feedback and the 'collective co-creation of individual narratives' (Willox *et al.* 2013: 132). Each participant shares their initial ideas in a story circle, then continues to support and inspire the others as their stories develop. It is this cooperative approach that helps to unite the distinct stories created by individuals as part of a single workshop and allows 'a rich, detailed, and nuanced tapestry of voices' to emerge (Willox *et al.* 2013: 132).

During the first day, each participant developed a script of about 300 to 500 words that they later read aloud and recorded. Most wrote and spoke in English. Two individuals drafted their story in English and then translated their own words into their preferred language. One wrote her first draft in her first language with the help of a family member and an interpreter. Three storytellers also added subtitles; this required filmmakers and storytellers and, in one case, an interpreter, to work together to align voice and text.

Participants found old photos, brought in artwork and mementos, created new images and short video sequences, and wove their recollections and aspirations into their narratives. They searched sound files for special effects and created a soundtrack. Using editing software they assembled voice, image, and music files and added titles and other credits to make their own stories. During the fourth workshop day *Finding our way* was proposed and chosen by participants as a fitting title for the project and the DVD compilation. Each person screened their story on the final day of the workshop and compiled final instructions for the filmmakers, e.g. to insert missing credits or improve image or sound transitions.

Forms giving permission to include the stories on a compilation DVD and licence ACMI to distribute and sub-licence the stories were discussed and signed before the end of the workshop. The filmmakers worked on each file and final versions were available within a few weeks. The coordinators worked with one of the storytellers to choose imagery which would subsequently be used to create a promotional postcard and DVD disc image (Figure 13.1). Each participant received a copy of their own story and the DVD. Participants who were interested attended some free media training sessions and the first launch event for agency staff, key stakeholders, and storyteller friends and families was held one month after concluding the workshop.

The following is an overview of considerations that emerged when coordinators and participants reflected on the *Finding our way* project in small and large gatherings, via phone calls, email, and face-to-face meetings, between 2014 and early 2017, that may help others embarking on similar projects. It is followed by a discussion of some of the effects that the project had, both anticipated and unexpected.

Storytelling

Generating the story

The DST process was used to support individuals to tell the story that they most wanted to tell (Lambert 2010). Digital stories 'and the voices and lived experiences within, are an important, rich, and powerful source of [information] that have not been written, pre-structured, or altered' by anyone else, whether a film director, service provider or researcher (Willox *et al.* 2013: 142).

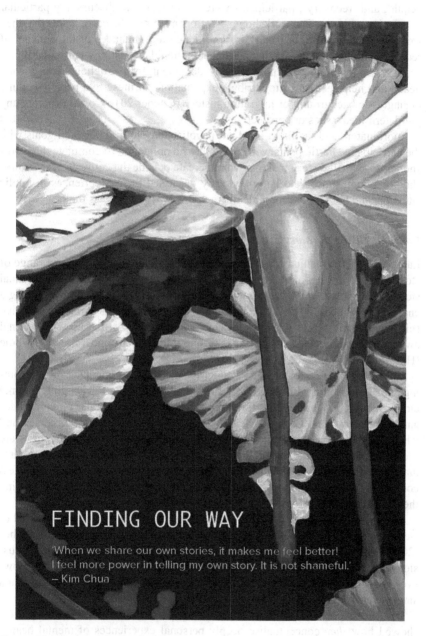

FINDING OUR WAY

'When we share our own stories, it makes me feel better!
I feel more power in telling my own story. It is not shameful.'
– Kim Chua

Figure 13.1 Postcard for the final DVD

While all group members all had some familiarity with 'migration', 'mental health', and 'recovery', participants were not expected to discuss any particular personal experience. The workshop facilitators informed the participants that they were interested to audio-visually explore the cultural nuances of the concept of recovery but did not suggest that participants should discuss any particular topics or themes. This project did not set out to document diverse beliefs about mental health and help seeking or to attribute explanations of these to a person's ethnic or linguistic background or migration history (Cooper 2016), or to promote any pre-determined issues or perspectives.

Coordinators and facilitators did not negotiate any formal personal goals with the participants. Participants were also under no obligation to complete the workshop or to share the story that they would create outside the confines of the workshop, although those who had previously discussed their experiences in public situations did help other group members to find ways to express theirs.

Conceptualising the story

Lambert's (2010) manual for DST encourages facilitators to consider a range of story types and notes that 'recovery stories' are among the kinds of 'personal stories' participants may want to tell. These include stories about 'overcoming a challenge' (Lambert 2010: 7) or, drawing on Bruner's theories about the narrative self, the 'turning points' or ways in which external events link up with internal awakenings and become tropes for how one thinks about one's life as a whole (Hull and Katz 2006).

The stories created as part of *Finding our way* contain elements of overcoming hardship, coping with illness experiences, and adjusting to changing external circumstances. Each story is informed by that person's particular circumstances and past experiences. Each storyteller chose how to represent him or herself and what experiences to share with others. Singly and as a collection, the stories are sad, hopeful, self-aware, and touching in their generosity and charm. The filmmakers and project coordinators took care to ensure that storytellers did not feel compelled to focus on any particular themes, yet some common and overlapping themes emerged.

As stories of recovery, however, *Finding our way* does not present the kind of 'recovery story' from 'descent, to crisis, to realization', that Lambert describes (2010: 7). Instead, they suggest possibilities for exploring contemporary discussions about mental health recovery that are beyond the scope of this chapter. However, we should state here that none of the ten *Finding our way* stories represent a single event, or experience that the storyteller had to 'overcome'.

DST, at its core, is a structured creative process. Participants in this project showed how *they* conceptualise deeply personal experiences of mental health, severe ill-health and emotional distress, and the growing sense of agency that recovery commonly involves (Drake and Whitely 2014). The storytellers chose to explore their own sources of suffering and fortitude. They explored challenges related to experiencing mental ill-health and loss of life opportunities and social roles, alongside personal accomplishments and ways to live meaningful lives. Knowing that about half of the group had had some previous mental health advocacy or public speaking experience, we as project coordinators were hopeful that some individuals would want to engage with broader conversations – within communities and among mental health practitioners and researchers – about what mental health recovery might mean within a socially and culturally diverse society such as Australia (see also Whitley and Drake 2010; Virdee *et al.* 2017).

Owning and sharing the story

The DST process also provides participants with experiences of ownership; participants own their stories and claim the persona of a storyteller. However, many thoughtful commentators on the use of visual methodologies also point out that once stories become public, they take on lives of their own and many other factors outside the images themselves will influence how they are interpreted by others (Guillemin and Drew 2010; Willox *et al.* 2013; Phelan and Kinsella 2013; Gilligan and Marley 2010). Writers also suggest that using visual modes inevitably leads a person to reveal information about themselves that they might not have disclosed if they had simply recounted their own story or had been interviewed (Brushwood Rose 2009; Phelan and Kinsella 2013).

Guillemin and Drew (2010) discuss the example of a young woman who experiences chronic physical ill-health and the publication of an image that she created as part of a photo-elicitation project. They explain that she felt '[so] strongly about wanting other people to know about her experiences that she declined the opportunity to choose a pseudonym and was adamant that her own name be used' (Guillemin and Drew 2010: 181). They describe the actions they took – encouraging consultation with other family members, exploring with the individual how she might feel in future if her image became more widely known to the public – before proceeding to publish. A similar experience occurred in *Finding our way*, as all the participants opted to use their real names and make their faces visible, and wanted their stories to be shared. Participants also chose to use their own names in the project follow-up publications.

Interpreting and analysing the stories

Researchers have applied various theoretical frameworks and analytical approaches to participant-generated photographic and video material (Mason 2005; Hull and Katz 2006; Pain 2011), choosing variously to emphasise the contexts in which they are produced and viewed, their internal narratives, the knowledge they produce, and their social effects. We adopted the approach, consistent with that of Willox and colleagues (2013: 142), that ultimately DST viewers-listeners have 'the responsibility and the privilege of listening deeply' to creator-tellers and 'bearing witness to the stories'.

Effects of participating in the DST process

One of the ethical demands on those responsible for facilitating or producing digital stories, especially with individuals from marginalised groups, is to understand the opportunities and risks for individual participants and beyond. These stories can be avenues for voicing rarely heard perspectives (Willox *et al.* 2013) and 'speaking back to dominant discourses' (LaMarre and Rice 2016), but they can also be used to perpetuate unhelpful stereotypes that can 'lend fuel to damaging representations' (Willox *et al.* 2013: 140).

The following discussion draws mainly on the reflections of five storytellers and one of the support persons who also attended, almost three years after concluding the project, about the effects of participating in the workshop and creating these stories.

We start this sub-chapter with a section specifically dedicated to the story of one of the storytellers, Kim (who gave permission to share her experience and use her real first name). Kim's and the other stories can be watched in the MHiMA (2017) and VTMH (2017) websites and we recommend readers to watch the videos before continuing to read this chapter (See Appendix A for Kim's story).

Kim's story

It has been more than 15 years since, while struggling with depression and personal troubles, a conversation with a Buddhist nun set Kim on a path that would see her re-build almost every aspect of her emotional and personal life. For Kim, this encounter marks the beginning of her 'second life', the moment she realised that a focus on acceptance and gratitude offered an alternative to self-blame. She still draws on these values in her everyday life and in her commitment to helping her local community.

Kim was born in Malaysia, a part of its Chinese cultural community, lived in Hong Kong, and then migrated to Australia. She worked extremely hard, holding down multiple jobs, running a family restaurant business, and raising her children. But her life 'fell apart' following a car crash; the business closed, her marriage ended and she lost her comfortable house and lifestyle. Shame, fear, and isolation led her to hide her experiences from her family and friends.

She came to realize first-hand the difficulties local Chinese-speaking communities in Australia have in addressing mental health issues. She began her long association with mental health services, a local community health centre, and a bilingual community-based counsellor and slowly set about piecing her life back together.

In *Spreading Joy*, Kim's digital story, she recounts how she lost 'everything'. She finds solace in making origami fish, varying their colour and size, yet repeating the creative act hundreds of times (Figure 13.2). She is working her way out of her distress, using pockets designed for gifting money to make fish, a sign of good fortune. Kim then uses these fish-gifts to re-connect with others in her local world.

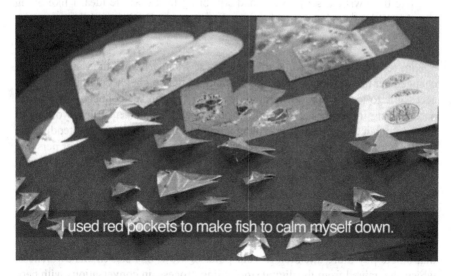

I used red pockets to make fish to calm myself down.

Figure 13.2 Kim's fish-gifts

Slowly regaining capacities that were lost to her, she also learns to become a 'laughter leader', rediscovering for herself how happiness feels and assisting others to laugh.

From there she also rediscovers her talent for cooking, starts a garden, and dedicates herself to community service. These interlinking tasks are ways to relate to others and express the gratitude that anchors her recovery and resonates with her Buddhist faith.

Her story ends with her own laughter, a key way to connect with feelings, spread joy, and care for herself.

Appendix A shows some extracts and interpretations of *Spreading Joy*.

Of *Spreading Joy*, Kim says, 'It's my story, so many people have been [like] me . . . people rescued my life, now it's my turn to rescue people. It's like karma, going in a circle. I don't want to waste the rest of my life. . . . The story is a record of my history, I love that'. Just recently, Kim was acknowledged in the state government volunteer awards for the way that she helps members of diverse communities to access and navigate health services.

By the time Kim learnt about the digital storytelling project and decided to participate, she was settled, had ongoing support in place, and was already well experienced in supporting others with personal struggles and advocating in her local community. She had become a 'laughter' exercise group leader, regularly prepared lunches at the temple, welcomes culturally diverse new arrivals to the housing estate where she lives, and tends her own vegetable plot.

Three years later, Kim describes the digital storytelling project as a 'once in a life-time' experience. At the time, she explains, it felt challenging.

I never thought I could make it, especially when we started writing our stories. I started with 500 words then reduced it down. I'd never written a story like that, write a script, short and still bring in the whole idea. I like doing that. I'd never done anything like that; write in English and then translate back to Chinese.

Kim recalls she did not initially plan to use Mandarin, her first language, but changed her mind when she realised the merit of making her account immediately accessible to local Chinese communities. Now she can see connections between participating in the digital storytelling project and her current roles, working at the local justice centre café and volunteering to support individuals attending the court. People tell her that they appreciate that she is willing to share her personal story with them and listen to theirs. Since the project, she explains, 'I can stand up, and tell people – you can stand up. I am the model that you can see. I can explain about myself, what happened to me, they say – 'nobody ever talks to me about this!''.

She also learnt that while it is hard to tell your own story in just a few minutes, succinctly communicating deeply personal and emotional experiences can mean that others pay more attention to your point of view. She shares this awareness, which she gained from the digital storytelling process, in conversations with people who are reluctant to accept the help of advocates in court.

Participation in the digital storytelling project has meant a great deal to Kim personally (Figure 13.3): 'I learnt that it's not only me, everyone [has] got their

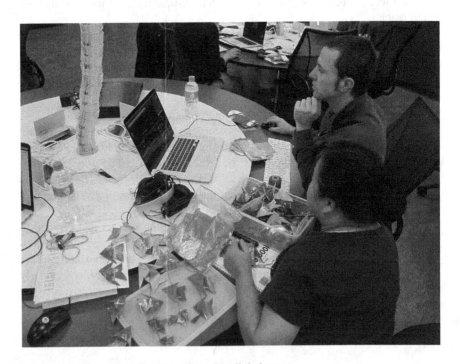

Figure 13.3 Filmmaker and Kim editing her digital story

stories'. When you have a mental illness, 'you are blaming yourself, why me, why me?'. 'When everyone [is sharing their story] I started to think, oh no, not only me'. She was not only reminded that she is not alone in living with the struggles of mental illness; she appreciated that her current situation, compared with many others, was now quite good.

Knowing Kim's long and deep commitment to learning to live well again and to help others, as project coordinators we were curious about these comments. Kim had been very involved in her local community and in self-help and advocacy projects for many years and yet she singled out the digital storytelling project. She explained:

> this one is my highlight, and also my changing point. . . . After this project, I was much stronger about myself. . . . Before I blamed myself. . . . But after [the project] my mental [health is] more stronger. . . . It's not only me . . . I am very strong. [After the project] I got this kind of feeling . . . I had done other [related courses and work] before . . . But I didn't have that strong feeling that I got after doing this project.

Personal growth

In their reflections on using visual methodologies, Guillemin and Drew (2010: 184) wonder 'about the consequences for participants [of] expressing what are clearly difficult or distressing experiences'. As project leaders, we were also very sensitive to the possibility of causing emotional harm. However, all the storyteller contributors to this reflective review have stressed that *Finding our way* was very helpful for them personally. Akeemi recalls thinking at the time that 'they' (the filmmakers) may not be used to 'us' (people who had experienced significant and lasting mental health problems). But the only way to make her digital story was to discuss her condition with the filmmakers, 'with people who weren't trained health professionals'. Akeemi recalled noticing 'I wasn't being judged, and it wasn't hard to say what I felt . . . that was the thing that made a lasting impression on me'.

Two years after the project, Monique, a support person for James who took part in the workshop, believes that the project shows the powerful ways in which art making and storytelling can work in people's lives. Storytellers offered these insights and self-assessments:

JAMES: I didn't know that I had a voice like that, that it would record as well as it did. 'A lot of people got really excited when they saw it'. Making the story 'gave me a kick along because I could show people what I'm on about'.

AKEEMI: 'Making the movie kind of empowered me, I'm still not open about [my mental health issues], but it empowered me to say something'. 'My story is a bit confronting, but I'm standing by it'. 'I feel like it is there in a nutshell – that's what I've been through – like I finally have something I can refer to'.

New and challenging experiences were also empowering:

> Kim explained that she enjoyed expressing herself in two languages, translating her own words from English to Chinese and learning to write a short, succinct script that told her 'whole story'.
>
> Monique noticed that James was particularly challenged by working on the DVD cover, but he got through it with the support of the group and is 'particularly happy with the way his work is presented there'. 'He grew from what became a productive experience, even though it was challenging for him at the time'.

Some storytellers have shown their stories to family and friends and some have not:

> Nevena explained that her children have shared the story with others through their online networks. She sees it as a lasting record that has 'captured' her family and cultural history.
>
> Akeemi has shared her story with her counsellors and presented her story at a public event but not with many family members. She explained, 'Maybe when I'm a bit braver, I'll share it with other people who are close to me'.

Hull and Katz (2006) ask a somewhat different question. They ask, what kinds of claims can we make about the development of agency and identity that participants experience through DST? Pain (2011) recounts a study that demonstrates the 'transformative potential' of using video with young people affected by asthma, where their quality of life and confidence in managing their symptoms improved significantly as a result. The authors 'concluded that the visual method itself acted as a 'therapeutic intervention'. Hull and Katz (2006) suggest that engaging in the DST process helps people believe in their own present capabilities and imaged futures and facilitates a sense of readiness for other opportunities. It would be extremely valuable to see future research explore the personal effects of DST on individuals and groups from diverse populations who have experienced mental health and emotional issues.

Public dialogues

Advocates have used the *Finding our way* stories to stimulate discussions with community members and policy leaders. Educators are using the stories as part of mental health practitioner training. Engaging in the project was a way to build personal readiness for sharing lived experience and assuming advocacy and consultation roles. As discussed above, the act of telling one's own story can itself be empowering. For example, Akeemi came along to the workshop motivated by a personal quest to create a story and learn visual editing skills. Initially she was frightened but later she shared her story at public events and has recently been involved in other diversity related mental health consultations.

Participatory projects provide opportunities for personal reflection, skill building and connection with others, for example, peers, health professionals, filmmakers, and others. In this instance, participants created a digital story that they could use when telling their own story in other contexts. Some individuals, including Maria and James, were already using their lived experience to inform their mental health advocacy and consultation roles. The workshop was an opportunity to revisit lived experiences, and to create a visual story that made their accounts even more compelling, and elicited strong responses from others.

In James' case, the digital story was a way to connect with others who also live with schizophrenia and to promote his own artistic work and the role of creative practice. James indicated that he sees his story as reaching out to other people with schizophrenia and to the general public who so often misunderstand the condition and the people who suffer with it: 'One of my things is to feel their pain, to feel the pain of the mentally ill and make an effort to understand'. James has also shown his story to mental health clinicians. His sister Monique explained that James uses it as 'a kind of calling card' to introduce himself at conferences and when introducing his work to new audiences (de Blas 2017).

Maria uses her digital story as an adjunct to telling her own story in community settings and, for example, shows her story as part of talks to school and community groups about living with mental illness. She says, 'It adds to the personal story I'm trying to tell'.

To summarise these possibilities, DST could be explored as a long-term strategy within the medical humanities and social sciences for developing existing and new advocates, for creating content that contributes to the plurality of voices that people can either listen to personally or privately on line, and for use in more formal education and discussions (for example, the education of health practitioners, or discussions with communities).

Conclusion

Mental health service users and carers from culturally and linguistically diverse backgrounds should have opportunities to tell their own stories in their own way. The participatory approach used in this workshop and the visual story telling method were integral to achieving empowerment. The approaches used in this project appeared to be effective ways to engage a vulnerable population to tell their stories. Similar findings were previously reported by Parr (2007), Pfeiffer (2013) and Wexlar *et al.* (2014). The story of a Mandarin-speaking participant illustrated the potential uses of DST in applied medical humanities.

Some of the key considerations emerging from *Finding our way* for developing similar projects are the importance of careful recruitment through established networks, the use of validated workshop processes with experienced personnel, thoughtful project planning, coordination, and evaluation, and adequate project resources.

Moreover, while stories have been shared and used on various platforms, similar projects in future should carefully prepare promotion and distribution plans, especially if aiming to reach culturally diverse and marginalised communities.

Supporting people to create the story they want to tell and ensuring that they maintain ownership of their story are critical elements of the DST method. Running DST projects in mental health contexts is suggesting ways to identify and develop mental health advocates. This should include the promotion of self-empowerment and coaching people in how to use and communicate their own lived experiences. Based on this reflection, we added a media training to this project. Agencies considering similar projects could consider linking to other real-world opportunities for learning and networking.

Acknowledgements

The contributions made to this project by each storyteller, their families and friends, and the filmmakers, practitioners, interpreters, and media advisers who provided assistance are gratefully acknowledged. Special thanks are due also to Kim who provided and approved her case study for this chapter.

This project was supported by Mental Health in Multicultural Australia (MHiMA), a project of the Department of Health of the Australian Government. We particularly acknowledge the support of Daryl Oehm (Victorian Transcultural Mental Health), Harry Minas (University of Melbourne) and other members of the MHiMA executive.

The Digital Storytelling Program of the Australian Centre for the Moving Image (ACMI) facilitated the workshop and produced the digital stories. SANE Australia helped both participants and project coordinators to prepare for media engagements.

Appendix A

Kim's story

Story: Spreading Joy - Kim Ling Chua

Spoken in Mandarin, with English subtitles, accompanied by ethereal music, of middle to high range, that includes some transitions and connotes 'SE Asian' sounds.

Voice	Visual	Codes*
00:00 [Opening credits. Title page]	Opening credits, 'Finding our way' Hand holding single gold fish on black background [Title] 'Spreading Joy'	
00:12 *After my mental breakdown, I found I was lost and couldn't concentrate on anything.*	Black screen Three red 'pockets' and a folded fish Two gold 'pockets' and a folded fish.	Feeling lost
00:22 *I started to make origami fish. I used red pockets to make fish to calm myself down. I started making fish whenever I could. I had made so many, maybe over three thousand of them.*	Two red pockets and two folded fish. Several images showing many pockets, silver, red, and green and folded fish made from each of these colours.	Finding a focus Making things to soothe self
00:38 *In the house there were fish everywhere, all over my table, chairs, and even the floor. Then I thought, where should they go?* [Pace of voice quickens a little]	Several fish, small and large. Image from past showing three people's hands, using scissors with materials spread over a tabletop. Stills in quick succession showing hands as they fold and cut the pocket fish.	Finding a destination, a purpose
00:53 *It was Christmas time, I took my fish and jumped on the city trams. I gave my fish to the tram drivers and passengers and said, "Merry Christmas".*	Continuing to show stills of hands cutting and folding a golden fish.	Connecting with others; giving as meaning-making

(Continued)

Voice	Visual	Codes*
01:06 *They were all surprised. Then I also began teaching my neighbours to make fish.*	Two images of mobiles of pocket fish hanging from a stairwell.	Teaching neighbours
01:09 *In 2003, I learned to be a laughter leader. At that time, I found out this is the only exercise I can do at anytime, anywhere.*	Two portrait photo images of Kim (made during workshop).	Learning to lead groups Finding and developing a skill
01:22 *Even in my situation, I could still laugh. Laughing makes me happy and it also brings happiness to others.* *Now I still go to different communities to bring my laughter to both old and young.*	Image of photo from local newspaper clip – about laughter group. The camera zooms in over part of image.	Laughing as coping mechanism Bringing joy to others Visiting community groups
01:40 *Once a month I cook a welcome lunch for the new residents moving into the housing estate. They are from many different backgrounds, Chinese, African, Aussie.*	Photo image showing people, from local community, sitting at a table, or standing nearby. A huge display of food, constructed to represent city buildings at an outdoor community event at a local park.	Cooking for others Welcoming new and diverse residents
1:50 *I also cook for different community events and at the Chinese Buddhist temple. People say my KLC (Kim Ling Chicken) is better than K.F.C. I love to cook. Every time I see people leaving an empty plate, it gives me great pleasure and a big reward.*	Another image of this event, showing hundreds of people in attendance, with some looking at the feast from a bridge. A third image showing more food. Final image showing empty plates where there was once a banquet.	Cooking and devotion Taking care of others Feeling gratitude
2:11 *Recently I started learning to grow seasonal vegetables.* *It makes me very happy to share food that I have grown and cooked myself.*	Several images showing a vegetable garden, garden beds and seedlings of green leafy vegetables.	Growing vegetables Sharing with others
2:21 HO! HO! HA! HA! HA!	Images of women at community event wearing aprons, smiling, clapping their hands.	Laughing, at a community event

Voice	Visual	Codes*
2:23 HO! HO! HA! HA! HA! HAHAHAHAHAHA	Complete image of news item about laughter group. Portrait image of smiling Kim.	Laughing, at a laughter group. Laughing for myself
2:30 – 2:47 [Closing]	"A digital story by Kim Ling Chua (Spoken in Mandarin)" Finding our way closing credit slides.	

* sets of codes relating to the combined effect of the narrative, visual imagery and sound of each segment.

Note

1 Between 2012 and 2015, Mental Health in Multicultural Australia (MHiMA) was funded by the Department of Health of the Australian Government, as part of the National Mental Health Strategy and operated as a consortium of four agencies – the Queensland Transcultural Mental Health Centre, the Centre for International Mental Health at the University of Melbourne, the School of Nursing and Midwifery at the University of South Australia and Victorian Transcultural Mental Health at St Vincent's Hospital Melbourne.

Bibliography

Abo, S. (2014) Films Unshackle Stigma of Mental Illness Faced by Migrants, *SBS World News*, 21 March 2014, www.sbs.com.au/news/article/2014/03/21/films-unshackle-stigma-mental-illness-faced-migrants, accessed 4 June 2017.

Australian Centre for the Moving Image (ACMI) (2010) *ACMI Digital Storytelling Program – Funded Workshops Information Sheet*, Melbourne: ACMI.

Brushwood Rose, C. (2009) The (Im)possibilities of Self-representation: Exploring the Limits of Storytelling in the Digital Stories of Women and Girls, *Changing English*, 16 (2): 211–20.

Colourfest (2015) Migrating Minds [Facebook event], Colourfest on Facebook event post, accessed 8 July 2017.

Colucci, E. and Bhui, K. (eds.) (2015) Special Issues: Arts, Media and Cultural Mental Health, *World Cultural Psychiatry Research Review*, 10 (3/4).

Colucci, E., Szwarc, J., Minas, H., Paxton, J. and Guerra, C. (2014) The Utilisation of Mental Health Services Among Children and Young People from a Refugee Background: A Systematic Literature Review, *International Journal of Culture and Mental Health*, 7 (1): 86–108.

Colucci, E., Valibhoy, M., Szwarc, J., Kaplan, I. and Minas, H. (2017) Improving Access to and Engagement with Mental Health Services Among Young People from Refugee Backgrounds: Service User and Provider Perspectives, *International Journal of Culture and Mental Health*, 10 (2): 185–96.

Cooper, S. (2016) Research on Help-seeking for Mental Illness in Africa: Dominant Approaches and Possible Alternative, *Transcultural Psychiatry*, 53 (6): 696–718.

de Blas, J. (2017) *The Divine Madman: The Psychiatric Superhero and the Quest for the Ultimate Medicine* [e-book], San Francisco: Blurb.

DelVecchio Good, M-J. and Hannah, S. (2015) 'Shattering Culture': Perspectives on Cultural Competence and Evidence-based Practice in Mental Health Services, *Transcultural Psychiatry*, 52 (2): 198–221.

De Vecchi, N., Kenny, A., Dickson-Swift, V. and Kidd, S. (2016) How Digital Storytelling Is Used in Mental Health: A Scoping Review, *International Journal of Mental Health Nursing*, 25: 183–93.

Diocera, D., Colucci, E. and Minas, H. (submitted) Undertaking Mental Health and Suicide Prevention Research with People from Immigrant and Refugee Backgrounds.

Drake, R. and Whitely, R. (2014) Recovery and Service Mental Illness: Description and Analysis, *Canadian Journal of Psychiatry*, 59 (5): 236–42.

Gilligan, C. and Marley, C. (2010) Migration and Divisions: Thoughts on (anti-) Narrativity in Visual Representations of Mobile People, *Forum: Qualitative Social Research*, 11 (2): Art. 32, www.qualitative-research.net/index.php/fqs/article/view/1476/3006, accessed 12 September 2017.

Guillemin, M. and Drew, S. (2010) Questions of Process in Participant-Generated Visual Methodologies, *Visual Studies*, 25 (2): 175–88.

Hull, G. and Katz, M-L. (2006) Crafting an Agentive Self: Case Studies of Digital Storytelling, *Research in the Teaching of English*, 41 (1): 43–81.

Jovic, M. (2014) Finding the Way, *Neos Kosmos*, 24 May 2014, http://neoskosmos.com/news/en/finding-the-way-maria-dimopoulos, accessed 4 June 2014.

Kindon, S. (2003) Participatory Video in Geographic Research: A Feminist Practice of Looking? *Area*, 35: 142–53.

LaMarre, A. and Rice, C. (2016) Embodying Critical and Corporeal Methodology: Digital Storytelling with Young Women in Eating Disorder Recovery, *Forum: Qualitative Social Research*, 17 (2): Art. 7, www.qualitative-research.net/index.php/fqs/article/view/2474, accessed 23 October 2017.

Lambert, J. (2010) *Digital Story Telling Cookbook*, Berkeley, CA: Digital Diner Press.

Lewin, T. (2011) Digital Storytelling, *Participatory Learning and Action*, 63: 54–62, http://pubs.iied.org/14606IIED.html, accessed 27 May 2017.

Mason, P. (2005) Visual Data in Applied Qualitative Research: Lessons from Experience, *Qualitative Research*, 5 (3): 325–46.

McDonough, S. and Colucci, E. (2019) People of immigrant and refugee background sharing experiences of mental health recovery: reflections and recommendations on using digital storytelling, *Visual Communication*, 18(4): 527–40.

Mental Health in Multicultural Australia (MHiMA) (2014) *Finding Our Way* [audiovisual], www.mhima.org.au , accessed 27 May 2017.

Mills, C.W. (1959) *The Sociological Imagination*, New York: Oxford University Press.

Minas, H., Kakuma, R., Too, L.S., Vayani, H., Orapeleng, S., Prasad-Ildes, R. and Oehm, D. (2013) Mental Health Research and Evaluation in Multicultural Australia: Developing a Culture of Inclusion, *International Journal of Mental Health Systems*, 7: 23.

National Mental Health Commission (NMHC) (2014) *Report of the National Review of Mental Health Programmes, Vol. 3: What People Told Us – Analysis of Submissions to the Review 30 November 2014*, Sydney: NMHC.

Pain, H. (2011) Visual Methods in Practice and Research: A Review of Empirical Support, *International Journal of Therapy and Rehabilitation*, 18 (6): 343–50.

Parr, H. (2007) Collaborative Film-Making as Process, Method and Text in Mental Health Research, *Cultural Geographies*, 14: 114–38.

Pfeiffer, C. (2013) Giving Adolescents a Voice? Using Videos to Represent Reproductive Health Realities of Adolescents in Tanzania, *Forum Qualitative Sozialforschung*,

14 (3): Art. 18, http://nbn-resolving.de/urn:nbn:de:0114-fqs1303189, accessed 13 September 2017.

Phelan, S.K. and Kinsella, E.A. (2013) Picture This . . . Safety, Dignity, and Voice – Ethical Research with Children: Practical Considerations for the Reflexive Researcher, *Qualitative Inquiry*, 19 (2): 81–90.

Price, N. (2014) Migrant Storytelling Project Inspires with Positive Tales Sharing Mental Health Strategies, *Melbourne Leader*, 23 May 2014, www.heraldsun.com.au/leader/central/migrant-storytelling-project-inspires-with-positive-tales-sharing-mental-health-strategies/story-fngnvlpt-1226928468352, accessed 4 June 2017.

Provencher, H., Gregg, R., Mead, S. and Mueser, K. (2002) The Role of Work in the Recovery of Persons with Psychiatric Disabilities, *Psychiatric Rehabilitation Journal*, 26 (2): 132–44.

Savino, N. (2014) Westmeadows Short Film Reveals Challenges of Life for Migrants with Mental Illness, *Hume Leader*, 10 April 2014, www.heraldsun.com.au/leader/north/westmeadows-short-film-reveals-challenges-of-life-for-migrants-with-mental-illness/news-story/eae500f5460291a871b8290bbfb19b72, accessed 26 April 2017.

Victorian Transcultural Mental Health (VTMH) (2017) *Finding Our Way* [audio-visual], www.vtmh.org.au, accessed 27 May 2017.

Victorian Transcultural Mental Health (VTMH) (2018) Free online learning resources, www.vtmh.org.au, accessed 4 Aug 2019.

Virdee, G., Frederick, T., Tarasoff, L., McKenzie, K., Davidson, L. and Kidd, S. (2017) Community Participation Within the Context of Recovery: Multiple Perspectives on South Asians with Schizophrenia, *International Journal of Culture and Mental Health*, 10 (2): 150–63.

Wexlar, L., Eglington, K. and Gubrium, A. (2014) Using Digital Stories to Understand the Lives of Alaska Native Young People, *Youth and Society*, 46 (4): 478–504.

Whitley, R. and Drake, R. (2010) Recovery: A Dimensional Approach, *Psychiatric Services*, 61: 1248–50.

Whitley, R., Kirmayer, L. and Groleau, D. (2006) Understanding Immigrants' Reluctance to Use Mental Health Services: A Qualitative Study from Montreal, *The Canadian Journal of Psychiatry*, 51 (4): 205–9.

Willox, A., Harper, S., Edge, V., 'My Word': Storytelling and Digital Media Lab, and Rigolet Inuit Community Government (2013) Storytelling in a Digital Age: Digital Storytelling as an Emerging Narrative Method for Preserving and Promoting Indigenous Oral Wisdom, *Qualitative Research*, 13 (2): 127–47.

14 Food-related *Yangsheng* short videos among the retired population in Shanghai

Xinyuan Wang and Vivienne Lo

Despite an emerging and significant impact upon daily life (Lomborg 2014), health and self-care in China, the popularity of smartphone-based short videos (*duan shipin* 短视频) has not yet drawn enough attention from either anthropological study or the Medical Humanities. The research of this chapter is part of an ongoing long-term (Feb 2018–June 2019) ethnographic research among the retired population in Shanghai, with a specific focus on the use of short videos and their influence and potential for influence upon everyday health and self-care.

Self-care in China has a unique history which is related to the practice of *yangsheng* 养生, literally translated as 'nourishing life', 'nurturing life', or 'cultivating life'. *Yangsheng* has more than 2000 years of history that refers to a broad range of ever-changing practices that have been taught and practised in domestic, religious, and educational contexts. The purpose of the practice is to promote well-being in individuals and communities, to generate strength and resilience, as well as an acuity of the sensory or spiritual faculties among the practitioners. Many activities are attributed *yangsheng* qualities: martial arts, sexual regimen, singing, calligraphy, and even the keeping of song birds or other pet animals (Dear 2012). This chapter looks at how *yangsheng* is achieved through the use of foodways, and the survival into our times of the close relationship between food and medicine.

In order to gain long-term participant-observation (Miller and Slater 2000; Pink 2001) among the ageing population, the ethnographer, Wang, moved into an ordinary residential compound called *ForeverGood*[1] in the city centre of Shanghai. Established in 1947, the gated *ForeverGood* compound consists of 23 residential buildings, housing more than 3000 residents and 941 households. The average age of the residents of *ForeverGood* village is around 60, with 32% over 60, 6% over 80, and two residents over 100. Besides in-depth interviews, field work has been conducted mainly along with/through various volunteer work and daily engagements in the residential compound – from helping the resident committee office (*juweihui* 居委会) to compiling the oral history of the community to giving free English lessons for the residents; from joining the local self-care group to making friends and keeping contact with individual neighbours offline and online (via social media). This chapter is based on ethnographical material gained among 35 retired participants through in-depth interviews and interactions on a daily basis over eight months from February 2018 to November 2018 (19 females, 16 males; average age 65).

After introducing the significance of short videos in the context of the transforming landscape of personal communication in the age of the smartphone, this chapter focuses on the everyday deployment of short videos (Mohammid 2017) in the discourse of health and *yangsheng*. Based on the observation of the general use of smartphone-based videos as well as historical inquiry into traditional beliefs in the close relationship between diet and the aims of *yangsheng*, the case studies lead to the discussion of the impact of the short videos upon Chinese traditional *yangsheng* practice.

Short videos in daily communication

One of the most common daily greetings in *ForeverGood*, shared with people all across China, is 'have you eaten?' (*chi guo le ma?* 吃过了吗?). The collective concern for regular feeding is a cultural idiosyncrasy which has been widely recorded and analysed in multiple academic researches and popular writings for how it reflects the significance of food in Chinese social life. Following closely behind this most commonplace greeting comes another opening line which triggers small talk among residents – a line which has been spotted only recently on a few occasions and seems to suggest the emerging importance of another popular daily activity – the sharing of short videos via smartphones.

'Have you checked the video I sent to you?', Ms Shi frequently opens her daily chit-chat with her neighbours when they meet at the after-dinner stroll in the neighbourhood. 'Yes, just watched, very useful! I have forwarded it to my family group. Have a look!' one neighbour, Ms Cai, replies, pulling out her smartphone. Ms Cai opens her WeChat[2] and quickly swipes down the screen, clicking on the video Ms Shi means, and passes the screen to other neighbours who are loitering in the vicinity. It is a one-minute video illustrating how to massage the acupuncture point *kunlun xue* (昆仑穴) near the ankle to treat sciatica and arthritis. Like many peers in their 60s and 70s, both Ms Shi and Ms Cai started to use the smartphone as well as social media around two to three years ago and soon became heavy users who would spend a self-estimated minimum of three hours per day on it.

The ownership of the smartphone among residents under 65 is more than 90%. Even though the majority (90%) over 80 do not use smartphones, there are a few who have taken it up with great passion. Experience and knowledge of smartphone use, they feel, is a sign that they are forever young. Activities facilitated by short videos account for a remarkable percentage of the usage time of smartphones. The length of the video on these platforms is one of key factors which defines its accessibility and popularity (also see Mohammid 2017), the majority being very short, from ten seconds to 2 minutes. For example, the logo of the short video platform *Miaopai* (秒拍) (lit. 'seconds shooting') is 'shoot a blockbuster in 10 seconds'. Being very short means that the video files (rather than web links) are small enough to be easily sent as messages.[3] In most cases, people received short videos from a variety of WeChat contacts.

The year 2017 witnessed a spurt in the availability of short video apps in mainland China. By the end of 2017, there were 334.1 million active users of short video apps in a month.[4] According to a recent report,[5] with 45 million downloads worldwide, *Douyin* (抖音), a newly launched Chinese short video app dominates the iPhone download. The popularity of short videos also emerges among the retired population who are generally regarded as the less digitally savvy population. Despite the fact that less than 10% of the participants had been to the cinema in the previous six months, all the participants watched short videos on smartphones; and more than 70% of them watched short videos on a daily basis. Almost one-third of them watch short videos for more than one hour per day.

In her early 60s Ms Jiang has become a big fan of short videos. In order to take her smartphone wherever she goes, Ms Jiang sewed a pocket into her apron. From time to time when she sits down for a short break in the middle of her housework, she pulls out the smartphone and clicks all the 'new-in' videos people have shared in four different WeChat groups (two alumni groups, one previous neighbours group, one family group) and those which were sent to her directly by a few of her good friends.

Like Ms Jiang, retirees are very keen on short videos and have accepted it as a form of daily communication as well as an important information resource (Okabe 2006). Mr Zhang in his 70s is also representative of this group. He explained why short videos have won his heart:

> They (videos) are much better than text, I need a magnifier to read small fonts on this small screen. But I can watch videos without any problem. Video has sound and moving pictures, very effective and engaging . . . nowadays the content of short videos is just so rich . . . I watch short videos everyday also to keep myself aware of the ever-changing world.

The majority of short videos Mr Zhang receives are less than one and a half minutes long, and some of them are just 15 seconds. In the previous week (16–22 April 2018) Mr Zhang had clicked through more than 100 short videos, ranging from funny cat videos to Traditional Chinese Medicine (TCM) *yangsheng* tips. From a cinematographic perspective, most short clips were made in a rather 'amateur' way. The majority of the video clips that circulated on smartphones were shot on ordinary smartphones without any choreographed camera direction or professional lighting. In many cases, the storytelling is as straightforward as one can imagine – either talking directly to the camera, or video/slides with background music plus voice-over. Also, in many cases, the videos are short cuts from a longer film or TV programme. The resolution of most short videos is therefore much below the quality needed for showing on the big screen. As Mr Zhang argues, the richness of short videos not only lies in their multimedia features, but also in the content. Common topics of the short videos shared among retired people include 1) funny or unusual videos of animals, people, and design; 2) entertaining performances such as singing, dancing, acrobatics, magic, etc.; 3) *yangsheng* tips; 4) news; and 5) lifestyle guidance and tips.

Among retired urban populations short videos about *yangsheng* are one of the most watched and shared in the genre. This fact leads us to explore further the daily practice of modern *yangsheng*, the classic TCM concept of self-care, as it is changing in the digital age. In order to do so it is first necessary to consider the historical relationship between *yangsheng* and food.

Yangsheng and food

Historically, food and drug culture in China was not limited to curing illness; the potential for herbal, mineral, and animal products to fortify and stimulate the body was well-known in ancient China. Food and drugs were an integral part of a regimen aimed at longevity, immortality, and even the preservation of the body beyond death. Recipe collections testifying to the antiquity of these traditions have been recovered from the tombs of Han China (Lo 2005). The early remedies often combined foodstuffs, common herbs, and household substances, with a view to healing specific illnesses, but also simply to promote health and well-being. Discovering the aphrodisiac qualities of food was a key context within which nutritional knowledge flourished at that time (Lo and Re'em 2018).

Over the following millennium each individual ingredient was systematically assigned medical efficacy according to classical Chinese scientific categories. The most fundamental of these categories were *yin* 阴 and *yang* 阳 which ordered the world in terms of complementary opposition. Something was not to be spoken of as *yin* or *yang* either absolutely or in isolation. In foodstuffs, the oppositions of heating and cooling or upward and downward (emetics and purgatives) are most often encountered.

Each substance not only had *yin* or *yang* qualities, but it also had a *wei* 味. Historians of Chinese medicine often translate wei as 'sapors' rather than 'flavor', the common translation, to distinguish medical rather than culinary virtues. *Wu wei* 五味, the five flavours, often cited in early Chinese literature, refer generally to the range of sensual pleasures that one might dream of consuming, but in a medical context, they were also specific flavours that could stimulate certain movements of qi 气, the essential 'stuff of life' that animated and invigorated the body, making a person astute, healthy, and effective (Unschuld 1986: 205–28).

By late medieval times there was an effective synthesis of all the observations and theories about the effects of food. Foods, like drugs, were classified according to their thermostatic qualities (hot, warm, neutral, cool, and cold), by flavor (pungent, sweet, salty, sour, and bitter), by the directions in which they induced movements within the body, by the organ system that they supported, as well as by the symptoms of illness that they could influence.

Sweet, for example, was thought slightly yang in nature and promoted an upward and outward movement. It entered the stomach and spleen channels. Mildly sweet foods, such as grains, nuts, fruits, and many vegetables, should form the main bulk of any diet. Stronger sweet flavours have a very warming and nourishing effect but should be avoided by people with signs of damp.

Saltiness moistened the body, while sour gathered and contracted, cleansing the body and moving the blood. Saltiness entered the kidneys and sour, the liver. Bitter was the most yin of flavours. It caused contraction and made qi descend and move inward reducing fever and calming agitation. It was also drying and therefore good for dampness. Bitter entered the heart clearing heat and calming the spirit (Lo 2005).

In general, medical priorities demanded restraint with a distinct moral overtone aimed at the leisure classes: too much strong meat, spice, oil, and fat would create excess heat, while raw vegetables and cold food and water were indigestible and harmed the stomach. Balance, harmony, and the careful intervention of the chef in cooking were keys to a healthy diet.

If we focus on the physiological effects of the foodstuffs and the mix of food and drugs in the pharmacological treatises, there is little to distinguish food from medicine. In practice, medical advice from the medieval period advised beginning with the gentler dietary therapy: Sun Simiao 孙思邈 (581?–682 CE) wrote:

> The nature of drugs is hard and violent, just like that of imperial soldiers. Since soldiers are so savage and impetuous, how could anybody dare to deploy them recklessly? If they are deployed inappropriately, harm and destruction will result everywhere. Similarly, excessive damage is the conse-quence if drugs are thrown at illnesses. A good doctor first makes a diagnosis, and having found out the cause of the disease, he tries to cure it first by food. When food fails, then he prescribes medicine.[6]

Thus, the best doctors diagnosed and treated the body with dietary advice before illness manifested. By attributing thermostatic and other physiological effects to every foodstuff, medical authors embraced nutrition within a larger framework of knowledge, thereby providing the rationale for what became an enormous and influential tradition of food combinations and prohibitions (Despeux 2007).

From the Han dynasty onwards we know that literate families shared recipes and recipe books as evidence of their participation in culturally elite patterns of consumption. By the Ming and Qing there were also formal *materia dietetica* modelled on the drug remedy books. By then much of this knowledge also formed part of the common knowledge of ordinary people. No doubt there were vibrant oral traditions at lower levels of literacy and between women. In the mid-twentieth century Chinese medicine was undergoing a revolution. Post-'liberation' 1950s China saw the creation of a new discipline of Chinese Medicine, which meant that the past was being used (and in many senses re-created and re-configured) to serve the present and the future. It was to become a medicine of the people (Taylor 2005), thoroughly modern and institutionalised. Whereas the norm elsewhere in constructing 'modern' scientific medical systems was to discard the 'pre-scientific' past, the new revolutionary government intended to incorporate and scientise Chi-nese medicine. Given that dietary medicine shared the same epistemological basis as Chinese pharmacology the standardised tenets of the new institutional Chinese medicine applied to nutrition, but the nutritional domain was always less profes-sional allowing lay authority to flourish.

Food-related *yangsheng* short videos in everyday life

The 30-member strong 'healthcare self-management' group of *ForeverGood* has started to self-teach itself the TCM acupuncture system of the channels (*jingluo* 经络). 92-year-old Ms Cai is a member of the group. In Ms Cai's flat, plastic bags filled to the brim with traditional medicines pile up on top of the closet. Like many older people, she has a very high opinion of the efficacy of traditional therapies. When she was suffering from a tumour in her lungs, one of her friends recommended traditional medicines, and now the nodule is much reduced. 'TCM is magical!' Ms Cai claimed. Ms Cai is not alone, the majority of older participants in Shanghai view TCM as one of the most obvious ways to maintain their health.

Mr Liang, a retired engineer in his 80s, had a heart operation last year, and since then he had to take three different kinds of 'western' medicines every day. *Yangsheng* is now what concerns Mr Liang, he said:

> *Yangsheng* is not about fixing the problem, it is very holistic, it is about keeping a well-balanced lifestyle. If you really follow the principles of *yangsheng*, then you won't even be vulnerable to getting ill and have to take western medicine. . . . Now I have to respond with western medicines to save my life, that is the cost I have paid for living unhealthily in the past decades, ignoring *yangsheng*.

As Mr Liang said, the concept of *yangsheng* is accepted and practiced as a healthy way of living. People also take western medicines when they are ill while still seeing TCM *yangsheng* as a long-term self-care practice engrained in everyday life. As mentioned in the last section, food has long been regarded as the most important part of *yangsheng*. It is very common to see the daily discussion and practice of *yangsheng* manifest itself in the extra attention paid to the medical function of food from a TCM perspective. Consequently, food-related *yangsheng* short videos, in particular, are popular among retired people.

Ms Mao, in her early 60s, prepares 'tonic' (*bu* 补) soup made from Chinese Angelica root (*danggui* 当归), ginger, and lamb for her good friend's husband who has lost his ability to take care of himself because of a stroke. Ms Mao learnt how to cook such tonic soup from her aunty, but recently she was delighted to find a short video which also teaches people how to prepare this soup (Figure 14.1). Besides watching how to cook healthy dishes, Ms Mao has also collected and stored more than 30 short videos on her smartphone about topics such as 'What kind of food should rheumatic patients take during the summer rain season (*meiyu* 梅雨)', 'During the hot summer, what kind of food will help rid the body of dampness (*shiqi* 湿气)', 'What kind of food people with liver problems should avoid', etc. Ms Mao explained:

> These short videos are straightforward, usually I can learn (a recipe) immediately when I watch it once. If you forget you can always go back

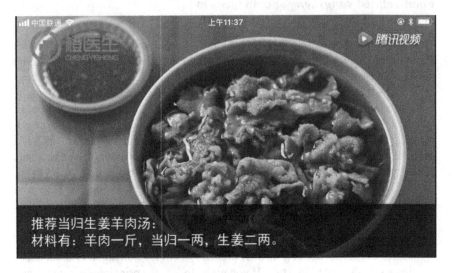

Figure 14.1 Screenshot of recipe for tonic soup

to check. It is also very convenient to share them with others who you care about, you simply click a few times. For example, I heard an old friend of mine was suffering from rheumatism, I sent him this video about the benefit of green bean soup . . . A previous middle school classmate of mine told me the other day that her daughter-in-law, 39, is pregnant again. I recalled a few days ago I watched a short video talking about food restrictions for older pregnant women, so I forwarded this video to her.

Another example comes from Ms Fan in her late 50s. Ms Fan is a retired middle school teacher, now regarded as a *yangsheng* expert among her friends. Knowing one of her neighbours, Ms Yu, suffers from mood swings and bad sleep, Ms Fan suggested:

I think you probably have liver Qi stagnation (*ganqi yujie* 肝气郁结). Try and have some *siwu* decoction (*siwutang* 四物汤). It is good for women, easy to prepare. I will send you the short video later when I am home.

'Liver Qi stagnation' is one of the most commonly experienced patterns identified in TCM, and it seems that all the participants above 50s have heard about such medical expressions, even if they have not entirely understood their meaning. As shown on the screenshots below, the two videos Ms Fan sent to Ms Yu via WeChat are both very short; the first one is about one minute, the second one two and half minutes. The first one is taken from a TV programme called *The path to health* (*Jiankang zhilu* 健康之路) on channel 10 of China Central Television (CCTV). In this TV program a TCM expert was invited to give a lecture on the benefits of the *siwu* decoction (Figure 14.2). This decoction is widely used to 1) tonify and invigorate the blood; and 2) regulate the liver, harmonise the menses, and alleviate pain. It is made from four herbs: processed Chinese foxglove root (*dihuang* 地黄), white peony root (*shaoyao* 芍药), Chinese Angelica root (*danggui* 当归), and Szechuan lovage root (*chuanxiong* 川芎). The second short video illustrates how to prepare the decoction with these four medical materials (Figure 14.3).

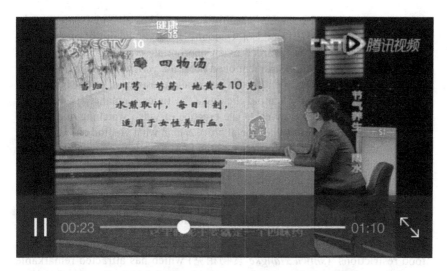

Figure 14.2 Screenshot of one-minute short video on the benefits of *siwu* decoction.

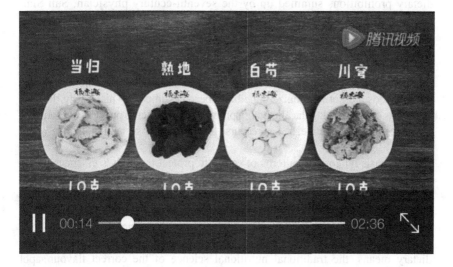

Figure 14.3 Screenshot of short video illustrating the preparation of *siwu* decoction

Ms Yu was pleased by the two short videos. Asked why she believes in the nutritional advice of these short videos, she replied,

> They are not random videos . . . they were sent by my old sister (*lao jiemei* 老姐妹), I know she has good knowledge of *yangsheng*. She is very kind and caring . . . so you can trust it. We were not well educated when we were young because we didn't have opportunities,[7] but we can still learn things from the internet and from each other.

To share a concern for another's health is perceived as an endorsement of the relationship (Chambers 2013). Also, to inquire about the health of others, especially the older people, is regarded as an appropriate way of showing respect as well as caring. In both cases mentioned here, the *yangsheng* short videos are not only regarded as convenient health information resources, but also the ideal media to express caring. By 'simply clicking a few times', social relationships are maintained at a relatively low cost. The practice of video watching and sharing has actually embedded in a wider social process than what we find online. People accessed online videos to get information and to build their knowledge, but the learning and dissemination of information is largely enacted in offline relationships that express caring and build solidarity among family members and friends.

Yangsheng short videos and food restrictions

Among the *Yangsheng* videos to do with food, there is one specific genre about 'food restrictions' (*shiwu xiangke* 食物相克) which has attracted remarkable attention among the ageing population. 'Taking the right food at the right time is very important, the failure to recognise food restrictions can cause a lot of problems'. Mr Zhu, a man in his late 60s, refers to an ancient tradition of dietary prohibitions summed up by the seventh-century physician, Sun Simiao. Sun emphasised the importance of dietary prohibitions in his chapter on dietetics:

> If the Qi of different foods are incompatible, the essence will be damaged. The body achieves completion from the flavors that nourish it. If the different flavours of foods are not harmonized, the body becomes impure. This is why the sage starts off by obeying the alimentary prohibitions in order to preserve his nature; if that proves ineffective, he has recourse to remedies for sustaining life.[8]

The emphasis on correct patterns of eating to protect the body's essences would mean that medical drugs were only appropriate when food combinations and prohibitions failed. There are multiple historical layers of food prohibition that underpin the restrictions recommended by residents of *ForeverGood*.

Traditionally food prohibitions embrace empirical knowledge about food hygiene and seasonal eating, Buddhist precepts that strive for purification through dietary means, the traditional nutritional science of the correct flavour/sapor combinations and their influence on inner organ function, not to speak of regional culinary wisdom about what combinations are unpalatable.

The way in which Mr Zhu and his wife regulate their daily food intake according to the principles of 'food restrictions' (*shiwu xiangke*) provides an illuminating example.

Mr Zhu has had high blood pressure for more than 8 years. His wife Ms Zhu takes close care of his daily food intake. 'Vegetable and fruits are the best for our health, meat does nothing good'. Ms Zhu would buy onions at least twice every week as onion is believed to be effective in lowering blood pressure as well as an anti-cancer agent. The couple also take honey with hot water in the morning, as it is said that honey every morning can help prevent constipation and can also battle chronic coughing. However, the couple believe that the two very healthy foods, onion and honey, are not supposed to be taken together. Ms Zhu said:

> Onion is good for everything, but you can't take onion and honey together as such a combination is not good for the eyes!

In order to drive home her point, Ms Zhu played a short video about food restrictions related to onions (Figure 14.4) which a good friend of hers had sent to her on WeChat a few weeks previously (Figure 14.5).

Besides making an effort to avoid harmful combinations of foods, the couple pay extra attention to what food they take during the period when they are taking TCM in order to maximise the effect of the medicines. They usually take some TCM medicine in the beginning of summer and winter to help the body to adjust to the changes of season smoothly – 'to tone your body' (*tiaoli shenti* 调理身体)

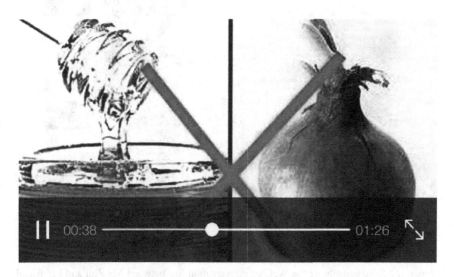

Figure 14.4 Screenshot of a one-and-half-minute long video clip about the prohibition against eating onion and honey

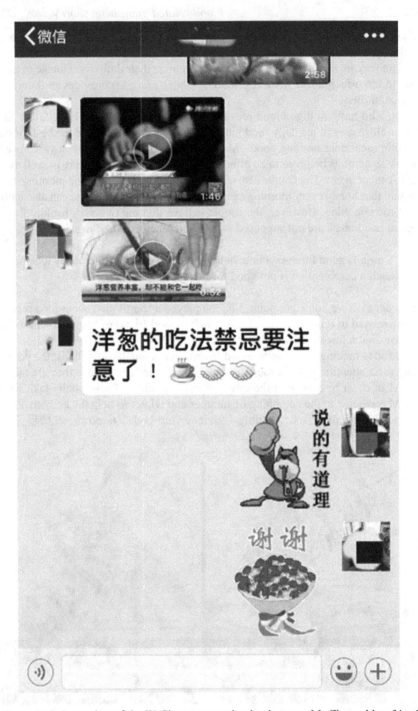

Figure 14.5 Screenshot of the WeChat conversation log between Ms Zhu and her friend who sent her the short videos of food prohibitions. The comment reads 'pay attention to the prohibitions of eating onion!', and Ms Zhu replies by two emoji: one says 'it makes a lot sense' with a cartoon character giving a thumbs-up gesture, the other says 'thank you' with a bunch of flowers.

as they said. Recently, they have been taking a TCM soup with ingredients like ginseng (*rensen* 人参), and atractylodes (*cangshu* 苍术) to strengthen *Qi* in summer, and they avoid taking turnips (*luobo* 萝卜). Mr Zhu explained:

> Ginseng is to strengthen the Qi while turnip's properties promote digestion and eliminate excessive Qi. So basically, these two are doing contradictory things to Qi. Therefore, we need to avoid turnips if we are taking ginseng.

Ms Zhu used to keep a long list of detrimental food combinations in a cutting from a local newspaper. She kept it sandwiched underneath the transparent mat on her dining table, 'I put that newspaper cutting on food restrictions just at the right corner of the table where I sit, so that from time to time when I was having meals I could look down and learn it by heart'. That yellowed paper cutting disappeared when they changed the dining table. However, Ms Zhu no longer needs that piece of paper as she can always check WeChat.

It is common to see retirees keeping the knowledge of 'food restrictions' in the form of newspaper clippings or handwritten notes. Ms Wang (71) still keeps a handwritten list of food restrictions underneath the transparent mat of her dining table (Figure 14.6).

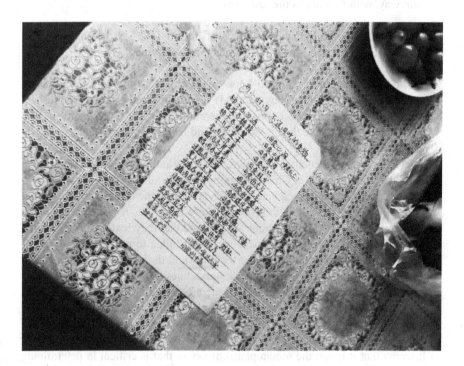

Figure 14.6 Handwritten list of food prohibitions by Ms Wang

CCTV, China's state television station, has taken a strong stance against the TCM concept of 'food restrictions' labelling such belief in the poisonous interactions of certain food combinations as spreading 'false rumors'. In 2018, the 'March 15th National Day for protecting consumer's rights' Gala, covered by CCTV-2 channel, included a programme segment in which food prohibitions such as shrimps and red dates, crab with tomatoes, durian fruit and milk, were debunked by laboratory testing.

Short videos showing CCTV debunking food restrictions are also available online, however they do not find an audience among retired people. When the ethnographer showed the retired engineer Mr Liang a video of CCTV debunking the food restrictions, Mr Liang commented:

> *Yangsheng* is Chinese wisdom of hundreds of years; it is beyond anything western science can test, don't you know? These tests are not long-term, I think it is short-sighted to value a thing only with reference to lab results. Many things cannot be lab tested.

Compared to him, Ms Yu seemed more convinced by the video, saying:

> Ah, good! It's good to know the consequences of eating the 'fatal combination' is not that deadly. But to be honest, I would never eat these two together anyway, with or without the restriction.

Meanwhile, the couple Mr and Ms Zhu, who follow food restrictions strictly in their daily life, expressed some reservations. Mr Zhu opined:

> When you get older, you will know that not everything can be explained properly and neatly. Our body system is very complicated. These food restrictions are the experience of many generations. For the sake of my health, I would rather believe than ignore them and feel regret later on.

This feedback is representative of general attitudes among the retired population towards the wider debate in China about the efficacy of TCM vis-à-vis a 'western' medicine based on lab science. The survey among the informants shows that when people really had a health problem, more than 75% received both 'western' treatment and TCM. Only about 5% claimed that they had never broken the rules of food restrictions as most of them (65%) failed to recall the long list of what exactly they should avoid taking together, and the majority of them (80%) think the rules of food restrictions work as guidelines for a healthy lifestyle rather than rules to be adhered to rigorously. Generally speaking, people regard TCM as associated with long-term *yangsheng* practice, whilst western medicine is for hospitals, operations, and short-term treatment – these two can therefore co-exist and work together harmoniously.

It seems that it is not the media platform *per se* that is critical in determining what it is that people choose to believe (Wang 2016; Miller *et al.* 2016): CCTV, the mainstream mass media platform, is no more convincing to the elderly than the short video. The ethnography also seems to show that even though there are contesting voices about the veracity of traditional food restrictions on short video platforms, audiences are not necessarily more highly exposed to different or challenging ideas than they were in the pre-digital age (Miller *et al.* 2016). Since the short videos are shared with regular contacts who, in many cases, share similar ideas, social media can easily perpetuate ingrained attitudes.

Conclusion

Being extremely short, accessible, and social, the video clips this chapter introduces are an unprecedented form of communication in this digital age. The short video as a genre cannot be said to enhance the status of film as a high art form. Quite the contrary, the short videos played on smartphones held in people's palms represent the most mundane form of film one can possibly imagine. However, exactly because of these mundane characteristics, it requires the lens of historical and ethnographic analysis (Banks and Morphy 1997) to make sense of how and why the short video has become an integral part of the daily life of the retired population in Shanghai.

How people gain *yangsheng* knowledge, as well as maintain social relationships by watching and sharing short videos, leads us to reflect on the relationships between short videos, health, and personal relationships in the age of smartphones. It is impossible to make any sense of short videos without taking into account the context in which they get circulated and consumed online and offline (Okabe 2006; Pink 2001; Miller *et al.* 2016).

Traditional TCM *yangsheng* practice has been transformed by the digital age. As a platform, the short video, shared on social media, is neither traditional nor modern, neither a product of the east nor the west – it simply provides a new and safe place where the debate about traditional knowledge can continue, and where local authority finds ways both to challenge and to integrate into top-down public health directives. It is evident that the short video facilitates the dissemination of *yangsheng* traditions among the retired population and, in doing so, makes a major contribution to the ways in which the elderly can express care for each other (Dijck 2008). As part of an amplified regime of *yangsheng* in China, the new visual cultures of self-care encourage the users to actively shape what they understand as China's ancient heritage to their own immediate needs, taking ownership of critical elements of their well-being – even as, within what otherwise might be enclaves of the isolated and elderly, they participate in the most cutting-edge and youthful technology.

Recent ethnographic research (Miller and Sinanne 2017) argues that the visual material on social media has introduced a 'new visibility' where the comparatively cost-free and effortless digital technology of smartphone and social media has enabled images to be produced, consumed, posted, and shared with unprecedented speed and coverage. Thanks to the availability of smartphones, faster mobile internet and a boom in short video apps, the exchange of short video clips has gained great popularity among the retired population.

Along with this development in digital technology, there is an ever-growing and ever-deepening visual language among the elderly in mainland China (Wang 2016). Given the challenges that China faces with its ageing population and the breakdown of the family as the unit of care, understanding what sorts of clips are more likely to be watched and understood and circulated, and why, becomes critical. How the combination of the topic, the view, and the properties of the clip itself interact requires greater investment from the field of health-related communication to understand the potential of short videos to transform healthcare in China.

Notes

1 According to ERC research ethics the names of the participants as well as the residential compound are anonymised.
2 WeChat is the dominant smartphone-based social media platform in mainland China.
3 Having said so, one of the main concerns about the short video among the retirees is that it can take up a lot of space on their smartphones.
4 Figures for monthly active users (MAU) measure the success rate of online social games, social networking services and, increasingly, mobile apps. Typically, metrics are measured by counting the number of unique users during a specific measurement period, such as within the previous 30 days.
5 Huang Zheping (2018) The world's most popular iPhone app isn't Facebook or WhatsApp, 8 May 2018, https://qz.com/1272285/bytedances-music-video-app-douyin-tik-tok-is-the-most-downloaded-iphone-app-in-2018s-first-quarter/, accessed 20 March 2019.
6 *Beiji qianjin yaofang*, j.26, p. 465.
7 By saying 'we didn't have the chance' Ms Yu indicates the fact that her generation went through the Cultural Revolution in China (1967–1977), during which period schools nationwide ceased normal teaching and a whole generation of the young people at that time lost the chance of receiving proper education.
8 *Beiji qianjin yaofang*, j. 26, p. 465.

Bibliography

Pre-modern sources

Beiji qianjin yaofang 備急千金要方 (Recipes for Emergency-Preparedness Worth a Thousand GoldCoins) 652, Sun Simiao 孫思邈 (1955), Beijing: Renmin weisheng chubanshe.

Modern sources

Banks, M. and Morphy, H. (eds.) (1997) *Rethinking Visual Anthropology*, New Haven, CT: Yale University Press.
Chambers, D. (2013) *Social Media and Personal Relationships: Online Intimacies and Networked Friendship*, Basingstoke: Palgrave Macmillan.
Dear, D. (2012) 'Chinese Yangsheng: Self-Help and Self-Image', *Asian Medicine*, 7 (1): 1–33.
Despeux, C. (2007) Food Prohibitions in China, trans. P. Barrett, *The Lantern: A Journal of Traditional Chinese Medicine*, 4 (1): 22–32.

Dijck, J.V. (2008) Digital Photography: Communication, Identity, Memory, *Visual Communication*, 7: 57–76.

Huang Zheping (2018) The World's Most Popular iPhone App Isn't Facebook or Whats App, *Quartz*, 8 May 2018, https://qz.com/1272285/bytedances-music-video-app-douyin-tik-tok-is-the-most-downloaded-iphone-app-in-2018s-first-quarter/, accessed 20 March 2019.

Lo, V. (2005) Pleasure, Prohibition and Pain: Food and Medicine in China, in Roel Sterckx (ed.) *Of Tripod and Palate*, London: Palgrave Macmillan, pp. 163–86.

Lo, V. and Re'em, E. (2018) Recipes for Love in the Ancient World, in G.E.R. Lloyd (ed.) *Comparing Ancient Greece and China: Interdisciplinary and Cross-Cultural Perspectives*, Cambridge: Cambridge University Press, pp. 326–52.

Lomborg, S. (2014) *Social Media, Social Genres: Making Sense of the Ordinary*, New York: Routledge.

Miller, D. and Slater, D. (2000) *The Internet: An Ethnographic Approach*, Oxford: Berg.

Miller, D. and Sinanne, J. (2017) *Visualising Facebook*, London: UCL Press.

Miller, D. *et al.* (2016) *How the World Changed Social Media*, London: UCL Press.

Mohammid, S. (2017) Digital Media, Learning and Social Confidence: An Ethnography of a Small Island, Knowledge Society, PhD thesis, RMIT University.

Okabe, D. (2006) Everyday Contexts of Camera Phone Use: Steps Toward Techno-social Ethnographic Frameworks, in J. Höflich and M. Hartmann (eds.) *Mobile Communications in Everyday Life: An Ethnographic View*, Berlin: Frank and Timme, pp. 79–102.

Pink, S. (2001) *Doing Ethnography: Images, Media and Representation in Research*, London: Sage.

Taylor, K. (2005) *Chinese Medicine in Early Communist China, 1945–63: A Medicine of Revolution*, London and New York: RoutledgeCurzon.

Unschuld, P. (1986) *Medicine in China: A History of Pharmaceutics*, Berkeley: University of California.

Wang, X. (2016) *Social Media in Industrial China*, London: UCL Press.

Glossary of Chinese Films

A jihua xuji　A計劃續集 (*Project A II*), dir. Jackie Chan, 1987.
Beixi moshou　悲兮魔兽 (*Behemoth*), dir. Zhao Liang, 2015.
Bian zou bian chang　边走边唱 (*Life on a String*), dir. Chen Kaige, 1991.
Chunmeng　春梦 (*Longing for the Rain*), dir. Yang Lina, 2013.
Chunmiao　春苗 (*Spring Shoots*), dir. Xie Jin 谢晋, 1975.
Di Renjie zhi tongtian diguo　狄仁傑之通天帝國 (*Detective Dee and the Mystery of the Phantom Flame*), dir. Tsui Hark (Xu Ke 徐克), 2010.
Di Renjie zhi shen dou longwang　狄仁傑之神都龍王 (*Young Detective Dee: Rise of the Sea Dragon*), dir. Tsui Hark, 2013.
Donggong xigong　东宫西宫 (*East Palace West Palace*), dir. Zhang Yuan, 1996.
Dubi dao　獨臂刀 (*One Armed Swordsman*), dir. Jimmy Wang Yu, 1967.
Gaobie Yuanmingyuan　告别圆明园 (*Farewell Yuanmingyuan*), dir. Zhao Liang, 1995.
Guan yu ai de gushi　关于爱的故事 (*The Common People*), dir. Zhou Xiaowen, 1998.
Guizu　柜族 (*Chinese Closet*), dir. Fan Popo 范坡坡, 2009.
Shendu baodao　深度报道 (*Breaking News from a Homosexual China*), dir. Queer Comrades 同志亦凡人, 2014.
Hong gaoliang　红高粱 (*Red Sorghum*), dir. Zhang Yimou, 1987.
Hongse niangzi jun　红色娘子军 (*Red Detachment of Women*), dir. Xie Jin, 1961.
Hongyu　红雨 (*Red Rain*), dir. Cui Wei, 1975.
Jiating luxiangdai　家庭录像带 (Home Video), dir. Yang Lina, 2001.
Judou　菊豆 (*Ju dou*), dir. Zhang Yimou, 1991.
Kongque　孔雀 (*Peacock*), dir. Gu Changwei, 2005.
Laotou　老头 (*Old Men*), dir. Yang Lina, 1999.
Lao An　老安 (*The Love of Mr. An*), dir. Yang Lina, 2008.
Lao tangtou　老唐头 (*Shattered*), dir. Xu Tong, 2011.
Lan Yu　蓝宇 (*Lan Yu*), dir. Stanley Kwan (Guan Jinpeng), 2001.
Li chun　立春 (*And the Spring Comes*), dir. Gu Changwei, 2007.
Longhu dou　龍虎斗 (*The Chinese Boxer*), dir. Jimmy Wang Yu, 1970.
Longxiong hudi　龍兄虎弟 (*Armour of God*), dir. Jackie Chan, 1986.
Maishou　麦收 (*Wheat Harvest*), dir. Xu Tong, 2008

Nannan nünü 男男女女 (*Men and Women*), dir. Liu Bingjian, 1999.

Ni ruci jianqiang 你如此坚强 (*Strong*), dir. Wei Xiaogang, 2012.

Niezi 孽子 (Crystal Boys), dir. Kan Ping Yu, 1986

Piao liang mama 漂亮妈妈 (*Breaking the Silence*), dir. Sun Zhou, 2000.

Qingchun 青春 (*Youth*), dir. Xie Jin, 1977.

Shasheng 杀生 (*Design of Death*), dir. Guan Hu, 2012.

Shang Fang 上访 (*Petition the Court of Complainants*) dir. Zhao Liang, 2009.

Shanghai zhi chun 上海之春 (*Shanghai Spring*), dir. Sang Hu, 1965.

Shentan Di Renjie 神探狄仁杰 (*Detective Di Renjie*) Series 1–6, dir. Fu Dalong, Wang Jing, Yang Mu, Wang Shulei, 2004, 2006, 2007, 2010, 2017, 2018.

Shenglai tongzhi 生来同志 (Cures That Kill), dir. Wei Xiaogang, 2011.

Suanming 算命 (*Fortune Teller*), dir. Xu Tong, 2009.

Tongzhi tatata tatata 同志他他他她她她 (*The Cream of the Queer Crop*), dir. Wei Xiaogang, 2010.

Tuina 推拿 (*Blind Massage*), dir. Lou Ye, 2014.

Weiai zhi jianru jia jing 微爱之渐入佳境 (*Love on the Cloud*), dir. Gu Changwei, 2014.

Wode linju shuo guizi 我的邻居说鬼子 (*My Neighbors and Their Japanese Ghosts*), dir.Yang Lina, 2008.

Wu qiong dong 无穷动 (*Perpetual Motion*), dir. Ning Ying, 2006.

Wu sheng de he 无声的河 (*Silent River*), dir. Ning Jingwu, 2001.

Wuxia 武侠 (*Dragon*), dir. Peter Chan, 2011.

Xi he 喜禾 (*Destiny*), dir. Zhang Wei, 2016.

Xi zao 洗澡 (*Shower*), dir. Zhang Yang, 1999.

Yanming hu pan 雁鸣湖畔 (*By the Yanming Lake*), dir. Gao *Tianhong*, 1976.

Yecao 野草 (*Wild Grass*), dir. Yang Lina, 2009.

Ye Men 葉問 (*Ip Man*), dir. Wilson Yip (Ye Weixin), 2008, and sequels 2010, 2016.

Yi shengming de mingyi 以生命的名义 (*In the Name of Life*), China Central Television,2005.

Yingxiong wulei 英雄無淚 (*Heroes Shed No Tears*), dir. John Woo, 1986.

Yingzhou de haizi 颖州的孩子 (*The Blood of Yingzhou District*), dir. Ruby Yang (Yang Zeye 楊紫燁), 2006.

Yiqi tiaowu 一起跳舞 (*Let's Dance Together*), dir. Yang Lina, 2007.

Zai jiang bian 在江边 (*Return to the Border*), dir. Zhao Liang, 2005.

Zai yiqi 在一起 (*Together*), dir. Zhao Liang, 2010.

Zhao le 找乐 (*For Fun*), dir. Ning Ying, 1993.

Zhi feiji 纸飞机 (*Paper Airplane*), dir. Zhao Liang, 2001.

Zhongguo hehuo ren 中國合伙人 (*American Dreams in China*), dir. Peter Chan (Chen Kexin陳可辛), 2013.

Zui ai 最爱 (*Love For Life*, also known as *Tale of Magic, Life Is a Miracle and Til Death Do Us Part*), dir. Gu Changwei, 2011.

Zui yu fa 罪与罚 (*Crime and Punishment*), dir. Zhao Liang, 2007.

Index

Note: Page numbers in *italics* indicate a figure on the corresponding page.

Printed in the United States
by Baker & Taylor Publisher Services